GERALD E. SWANSON M.D.
9601 UPTON ROAD
MINNEAPOLIS. MN 55431
TELE: 881-6869

 GERALD E. SWANSON, M.D.
9601 UPTON ROAD
MINNEAPOLIS, MN 55431
TELE: 881-6869

COLORECTAL DISEASE

Colorectal disease

edited by

James P. S. Thomson MS, FRCS
Consultant Surgeon and Dean of Postgraduate Studies, St. Mark's Hospital for Diseases of the Rectum and Colon. Consultant Surgeon, Hackney Hospital. Honorary Lecturer in Surgery, The Medical College of St. Bartholomew's Hospital, London.

R. J. Nicholls BA, MChir, FRCS
Consultant Surgeon, St. Mark's Hospital for Diseases of the Rectum and Colon. Senior Lecturer in Surgical Oncology, Imperial Cancer Research Fund Department of Medical Oncology, The Medical College of St. Bartholomew's Hospital, London.

and

Christopher B. Williams MA, BM, BCh, FRCP
Consultant Physician, St. Mark's Hospital for Diseases of the Rectum and Colon and St. Bartholomew's Hospital. Honorary Consultant Physician, Hospitals for Sick Children, Great Ormond Street and Queen Elizabeth's, Hackney, London.

with illustrations by

Geoffrey Lyth BA

Foreword contributed by

Malcolm C. Veidenheimer MD, FRCS(C), FACS
Head, Section of Colon and Rectal Surgery, Lahey Clinic Medical Center, Burlington, Massachusetts.

APPLETON-CENTURY-CROFTS/New York
A Division of Prentice-Hall, Inc.

First published 1981

Copyright © JPS Thomson, RJ Nicholls and CB Williams 1981

ISBN 0-8385-1178-3

Library of Congress Catalog Card Number: 81-71411

Printed and bound in Great Britain.

CONTENTS

CONTRIBUTORS

Suzanne L Alexander MB, BS
Honorary Consultant Dermatologist, St. Mark's Hospital for Diseases of the Rectum and Colon
Consultant Dermatologist, Ilford and District Hospital, St. Andrew's Hospital, Bow, and Queen Mary's Hospital, Stratford
Honorary Lecturer in Dermatology, Guy's Hospital Medical School, London

J Alexander-Williams MD, ChM, FRCS, FACS
Consultant Surgeon, The General Hospital, Birmingham

CI Bartram MB, BS, MRCP, FRCR
Consultant Radiologist, St. Mark's Hospital for Diseases of the Rectum and Colon and St. Bartholomew's Hospital, London

Donald V Bateman MA, MB, BChir, FFARCS
Consulting Anaesthetist, St. Mark's Hospital for Diseases of the Rectum and Colon, London
Consultant Anaesthetist, St. Margaret's Hospital, Epping, Essex

A Bennett PhD, DSc
Professor of Pharmacology, King's College Hospital Medical School, London

AJ Blackshaw MA, MB, BChir, MRCPath
Consultant Histopathologist, St. Bartholomew's Hospital and Hackney Hospital, London

SR Bloom MA, MD, FRCP
Reader in Medicine, Royal Postgraduate Medical School
Honorary Consultant Physician, Hammersmith Hospital, London

HJR Bussey OBE, BSc, PhD
Consulting Research Fellow, St. Mark's Hospital for Diseases of the Rectum and Colon, London

RD Catterall FRCPEd
Director and Consultant Physician, Department of Venereology, The Middlesex Hospital, London

AM Connell MD
Professor of Internal Medicine, University of Cincinnati Medical Center, Ohio

GC Cook MD, DSc, FRCP, FRACP
Professor of Medicine, The University of Papua New Guinea

W Duncan MB, ChB, FRCP Ed, FRCS Ed, FRCR
Professor of Radiotherapy, University of Edinburgh
Consultant Radiotherapist, Western General Hospital, Edinburgh

RH Grace MB, BS, FRCS
Consultant Surgeon, Royal Hospital and New Cross Hospital, Wolverhampton

PR Hawley MS, FRCS
Consultant Surgeon, St. Mark's Hospital for Diseases of the Rectum and Colon, London

RJ Heald MChir, FRCS
Consultant Surgeon, Basingstoke District Hospital, Hampshire

MM Henry MB, BS, FRCS
Senior Surgical Registrar, The Central Middlesex Hospital, London

MJ Hill PhD
Director, Bacterial Metabolism Research Laboratory, Colindale, London

KEF Hobbs ChM, FRCS
Professor of Surgery, The Royal Free Hospital School of Medicine, London

Sir Francis Avery Jones CBE, MD, FRCP, FRCS(Hon)
Consulting Gastroenterologist, St. Mark's Hospital for Diseases of the Rectum and Colon and to the Royal Navy
Honorary Consulting Physician, St. Bartholomew's Hospital and The Central Middlesex Hospital, London

RHS Lane MS, FRCS
Consultant Surgeon, Royal Hampshire County Hospital, Winchester

JON Lawson MB, BS, FRCS
Consultant Paediatric Surgeon, St. Thomas's Hospital, Westminster Children's Hospital and Queen Mary's Hospital, Roehampton, London

JE Lennard-Jones MD, FRCP
Professor of Gastroenterology, The London Hospital Medical College
Consultant Gastroenterologist, St. Mark's Hospital for Diseases of the Rectum and Colon, London

MR Lock MB, BS, FRCS
Senior Surgical Registrar, Westminster Hospital, London

Sir Hugh Lockhart-Mummery KCVO, MD, MChir, FRCS
Consulting Surgeon, St. Mark's Hospital for Diseases of the Rectum and Colon
Consultant Surgeon, St. Thomas's Hospital, London

CV Mann MA, MCh, FRCS
Consultant Surgeon, The London Hospital and St. Mark's Hospital for Diseases of the Rectum and Colon, London

CG Marks MChir, FRCS
Consultant Surgeon, The Royal Surrey County Hospital, Guildford

Adrian Marston MA, DM, MCh, FRCS
Consultant Surgeon, The Middlesex Hospital and Royal Northern Hospital
Senior Lecturer in Surgery, The Middlesex Hospital Medical School, London

DM Millar MB, BS, FRCS, FRCS Ed
Consultant Surgeon, Essex County Hospital, Colchester and Notley Hospital, Essex

JJ Misiewicz BSc, MB, FRCP
Consultant Physician, Department of Gastroenterology, The Central Middlesex Hospital
Honorary Consultant Physician, St. Mark's Hospital for Diseases of the Rectum and Colon, London
Member of External Scientific Staff, Medical Research Council

Betty Moore SRN
Clinical Teacher (Stomatherapy), St. Bartholomew's Hospital School of Nursing, London

Basil C Morson VRD, MA, DM, FRCP, FRCS, FRCPath
Consultant Pathologist, St. Mark's Hospital for Diseases of the Rectum and Colon, London and to the Royal Navy

RJ Nicholls BA, MChir, FRCS
Consultant Surgeon, St. Mark's Hospital for Diseases of the Rectum and Colon, London
Senior Lecturer in Surgical Oncology, Imperial Cancer Research Fund Department of Medical Oncology, The Medical College of St. Bartholomew's Hospital, London

NS Painter MS, FRCS, FACS
Senior Surgeon, The Manor House Hospital, London

Sir Alan Parks MA, MD, MCh, FRCP, PRCS
Consultant Surgeon, The London Hospital and St. Mark's Hospital for Diseases of the Rectum and Colon, London
President of The Royal College of Surgeons of England

TG Parks MCh, FRCS
Reader in Surgery, The Queen's University of Belfast, Northern Ireland

AV Pollock MB, ChB, FRCS
Consultant Surgeon, Scarborough Hospital, Yorkshire

Jeremy Powell-Tuck MB, ChB, MRCP
Senior Registrar in General Medicine and Gastroenterology, Charing Cross Hospital, London

AB Price BM, BCh, MRCPath
Consultant Histopathologist, Northwick Park Hospital, London

Jean K Ritchie MA, DM, MRCP, FRCR
Director of Research Records Department, St. Mark's Hospital for Diseases of the Rectum and Colon, London

KRP Rutter MA, MB, BChir, FRCS
Consultant Surgeon, Frimley Park Hospital, Surrey

WS Shand MD, FRCS, FRCS Ed
Consultant Surgeon, St. Bartholomew's Hospital and Hackney Hospital
Visiting Lecturer in Surgery, St. Mark's Hospital for Diseases of the Rectum and Colon, London
Penrose May Surgical Tutor at The Royal College of Surgeons of England

Maurice L Slevin MRCP
Senior Registrar, Department of Medical Oncology, St. Bartholomew's Hospital and Hackney Hospital, London

Soad Tabaqchali MB, ChB, MRCPath
Senior Lecturer, Department of Medical Microbiology, The Medical College of St. Bartholomew's Hospital, London

BM Thomas MB, BS, MRCP, FRCR
Consultant Radiologist, University College Hospital and St. Mark's Hospital for Diseases of the Rectum and Colon, London

James PS Thomson MS, FRCS
Consultant Surgeon and Dean of Postgraduate Studies, St. Mark's Hospital for Diseases of the Rectum and Colon
Consultant Surgeon Hackney Hospital
Honorary Lecturer in Surgery, The Medical College of St. Bartholomew's Hospital, London

Ian P Todd MS, MD, FRCS
Consultant Surgeon, St. Bartholomew's Hospital and St. Mark's Hospital for Diseases of the Rectum and Colon, London

Christopher B Williams MA, BM, BCh, FRCP
Consultant Physician, St. Mark's Hospital for Diseases of the Rectum and Colon, and St. Bartholomew's Hospital, London
Honorary Consultant Physician, Hospitals for Sick Children, Great Ormond Street and Queen Elizabeth's, Hackney, London

BA Wood PhD, MB, BS, BSc
Reader in Anatomy, The Middlesex Hospital Medical School, London

Peter FM Wrigley PhD, FRCP
Consultant Physician, Department of Medical Oncology, St. Bartholomew's Hospital and Hackney Hospital, London

Foreword

St. Mark's Hospital has been a vital part of the British surgical scene for nearly 150 years. Through much of this century members of St. Mark's Hospital have assumed a leadership role of an international nature in surgery, pathology, and gastroenterology. The influences of the Hospital have long ago passed the shores of England to play an important role in the care of patients with diseases of the large intestine in all parts of the world. Members of the staff of this fine institution have become important ambassadors of Great Britain as they have travelled to many lands speaking about St. Mark's Hospital's concepts regarding colorectal diseases. Their international reputations have, in turn, attracted many visitors from around the world to St. Mark's Hospital and other British institutions.

One of the attractive features of St. Mark's Hospital for many years has been the series of lectures members of the Hospital staff present to the young doctors who are preparing for the Fellowship Examination of the Royal College of Surgeons. The material contained in this book is an enlargement of these lectures presented by friends and associates of St. Mark's. It is a full and complete description of all facets of colorectal disease and is presented in a most practical manner by persons who have had great personal experience.

The compilation of these chapters into one publication serves as a ready reference for all who are interested in colorectal diseases. The book is useful to the practicing physician or surgeon and to those still in training. Those of us who cannot attend the St. Mark's Hospital Course will also be able to profit from the collected writings of these fine teachers.

Malcolm C. Veidenheimer

Section of Colon and Rectal Surgery
Lahey Clinic Medical Center
Burlington, Massachusetts

Preface

This book has been compiled by staff members, associates and friends of St. Mark's Hospital to provide the general surgeon or physician with an account of current colorectal practice. The title has been changed from that of its predecessor, Dr Basil Morson's *Diseases of the Colon, Rectum and Anus*, since the style and content have also been extensively changed. Certain chapters are unique, such as those explaining (particularly for physicians) the fundamentals of colorectal operations, (for surgeons) the basis of paediatric coloproctology, and (for anyone) the proctological implications of trauma and sexually transmitted disease. The style of all sections has been unified as far as possible in an attempt to produce a simple, balanced and orthodox view of the subject which we hope will be of interest to a wide readership. We have intentionally encouraged a rather didactic approach in the interests of clarity, with a few selected references or suggestions for further reading rather than detailed referencing of each statement.

We are grateful to our contributors, illustrator and publishers for their patience with us. It is a pleasure to acknowledge the secretarial skills of Mrs Mary Groves and the help given to us by Dr Sheila Ritchie with the references, Dr Donald V. Bateman in proof-reading and William Heinemann Medical Books in the design and production of the book.

James P. S. Thomson
R. J. Nicholls
Christopher B. Williams

St. Mark's Hospital
1981

1. Investigation

CLINICAL ASSESSMENT

In the majority of patients with symptoms referable to the large intestine the precise diagnosis may be made by a careful clinical assessment. This involves an adequate clinical history, examination of the abdomen and a complete rectal examination consisting of inspection, palpation, sigmoidoscopy and proctoscopy.

Further assessment may be needed by means of radiology, endoscopy and pathology. All these aspects of gaining information from the patient will be discussed, but a full clinical investigation is always the initial stage.

CLINICAL HISTORY

The main symptoms which lead to a diagnosis of large bowel disorders are abdominal and anorectal but it should not be forgotten that general symptoms such as breathlessness – the result of anaemia – may be the only pointer to the large bowel. Conversely, large bowel symptoms may be part of a general disorder, e.g. diarrhoea in thyrotoxicosis or colicky pain (irritable bowel syndrome) in psychological problems.

The abdominal symptoms include pain, which is often colicky, the presence of a mass, abdominal distension, borborygmi and altered bowel habit. Although pain may sometimes be localised to the area of large bowel producing it, it is more often central in distribution and may be referred to the back or upper thighs. Assessment of a patient's bowel habit may be difficult because the use of the term 'diarrhoea' and 'constipation' may not have the same meaning when used by different patients. It is, therefore, essential to determine not only the frequency of

defaecation, but also the colour and consistency of the stool –
formed, pelletty, loose or watery. The time spent at defaecation
will give some indication of any difficulty that may be present
and the degree of straining may be relevant to the assessment of
pelvic floor problems. Finally, the use of laxatives should be
noted, including dosage, as constipation may be masked taking
such medicines.

The anorectal symptoms include perianal irritation and soreness, pain, the presence of a lump, prolapse, incontinence and,
of course, bleeding. It is noteworthy that the patient may
describe all these symptoms as 'piles'.

Perianal irritation or itching is usually called pruritus ani and
its assessment and management are discussed in Chapter 11.

Anal pain usually stems from an organic problem e.g. fissure,
abscess and fistula, thrombosed haemorrhoids or perianal
haematoma. If a diagnosis is not readily made an examination
under anaesthesia is necessary to exclude, in particular, intra-anal
sepsis (e.g. intersphincteric abscess).

Anorectal prolapse describes the passage of a structure through
the anus from the colon, rectum, or anal canal. Examples
include complete rectal prolapse, large benign rectal tumours,
pedunculated colonic tumours, haemorrhoids, fibrous anal
polyps and condylomata acuminata. Prolapse may occur at
defaecation or at other times of straining (e.g. lifting heavy
objects) and may be reduced spontaneously or digitally by the
patient. The description of 'something coming down' is characteristic.

Anorectal bleeding is the most important symptom of all. One
in every eight patients who complain of bleeding has a serious
or potentially serious problem (Williams and Thomson, 1977);
the correct diagnosis will usually be made by simple means at
the initial visit (Fig. 1.1).

Some idea of the site and severity of the bleeding can be
obtained by whether it occurs when wiping after defaecation, or
into the lavatory pan. Bright bleeding usually comes from the
anal region and dark blood, perhaps with clots, or a history of
passing blood without stools, suggests a source of bleeding
higher in the bowel. Black melaena will suggest upper gastrointestinal bleeding. Bright red blood which coats the outside of
the stool or drips and spurts after defaecation is suggestive of
haemorrhoids. However, no feature is absolutely characteristic
and all these patients must have as a minimum a full clinical
assessment including sigmoidoscopy.

EXAMINATION

A routine *general examination* is always appropriate including,
for instance, an accurate measurement of the heart rate (relevant

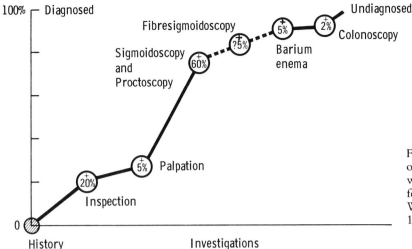

100% ⌐ Diagnosed

Undiagnosed

Fibresigmoidoscopy

Sigmoidoscopy
and
Proctoscopy

Barium
enema

Colonoscopy

Palpation

Inspection

0

History   Investigations

Fig. 1.1 The diagnostic yield of investigations in patients with anorectal bleeding as a feature of presentation (after Williams and Thomson, 1977).

to the diagnosis of thyroid dysfunction), inspection of the mouth and tongue and a search for enlarged lymph nodes, especially those of the left supraclavicular triangle, which may be the site of secondary carcinoma. Finger clubbing, skin or joint signs may be important in suspected inflammatory bowel disease.

Examination of the abdomen

Examination of the abdomen is essential. The caecum and left colon may be readily palpable as a soft swelling as a normal finding, especially in thin patients. The presence of a hard lump in the line of the colon may suggest either a tumour or constipation. The right upper abdomen should also be examined for abnormalities in the liver. Distension of the abdomen needs careful assessment as if it is not due to obesity it may be due to excess flatus, perhaps associated with visible peristalsis, ascitic fluid or faeces. In some patients with chronic long-standing constipation a large hard mass of faeces may be found arising from the pelvis. Finally the groins should be examined for enlarged lymph nodes which may be secondarily involved in some anal canal disorders.

Examination of the anorectum

In nearly all patients the anal canal and rectum can be readily examined following the sequence described below. Facilities should be such that this may be undertaken in the out-patient department or at the bedside. Examination under anaesthesia should only be needed if there is a painful lesion, if there is difficulty in the initial examination and perhaps in some children. In the United Kingdom it is usual to examine the patient

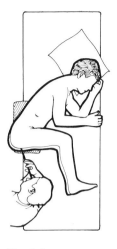

Fig. 1.2

in the left lateral position – Sims position – (Fig. 1.2) although some prefer the knee-elbow (Fig. 1.3) or jack-knife (Fig. 1.4) positions. If the left lateral position is used the patient must be made to lie *across* the couch with the buttocks protruding 15 cm over the edge, supported with a sandbag and the knees drawn well up; failure to position correctly will make inspection and

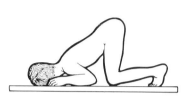

Fig. 1.3

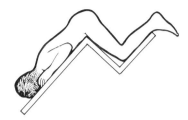

Fig. 1.4

especially the subsequent sigmoidoscopy difficult and possibly inaccurate. Good illumination of the perianal area is required. For the initial examination no special preparation is required.

Inspection

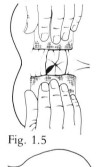

Fig. 1.5

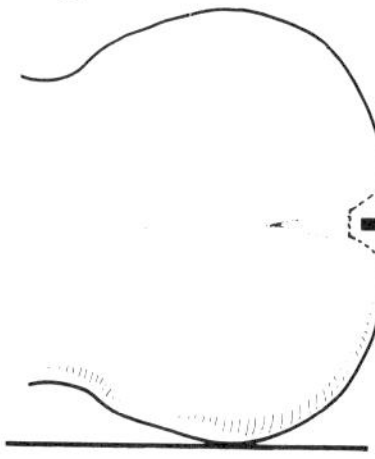

Fig. 1.6

Palpation

Careful inspection of the perianal area will reveal many different lesions. At this stage three additional manoeuvres are useful. By pulling the buttocks apart to open the lower anal canal most fissures become visible (Fig. 1.5). This is a very valuable part of the examination as it makes the diagnosis without causing the patient any increased discomfort. Laxity of the anal sphincters may also be seen. Next the patient should be asked to strain as at defaecation (Valsalva manoeuvre); this may reveal (Fig. 1.6) descent of the perineum (the result of prolonged straining at defaecation over the years with weakening of the pelvic floor muscles) or the type of anorectal prolapse. Finally, the patient may be asked to tighten the anal sphincter which gives some indication of the strength of the external sphincter and levator ani. In patients with pelvic floor problems a touch with a pin on the perianal skin may not produce contraction of the external sphincter (anal reflex).

The perianal area is first palpated with a well lubricated finger covered with a finger cot to detect induration which may be produced by sepsis or a tumour. The finger is then inserted into the anal canal and subsequently the rectum.

Within the anal canal such disorders as fistula, polyps and

tumours may be felt; haemorrhoids are not usually palpable. Useful information about the function of the anal sphincter may also be obtained: spasm is produced by a painful disorder, such as fissure or abscess; laxity is a sign of pelvic floor dysfunction. The ability of the anal sphincter to contract over the finger may be assessed during this part of the examination.

The faecal content of the rectum is assessed and then the wall palpated for polyps and tumours. Finally, structures outside may be examined, including the prostate, uterus and ovaries and finally the lymph nodes behind the rectum.

Sigmoidoscopy should be the next step in the examination. *Sigmoidoscopy* Palpation with the finger will have covered the lower third of the rectum and the remainder of the rectum and lower sigmoid colon are reached only by using the sigmoidoscope. The proctoscope is for examining the anal canal and the anorectal region.

Initially no bowel preparation is used so that the contents of the lumen may be assessed – the consistency and colour of the stool and whether or not blood, mucus or pus are present. If the rectum is very loaded the patient should be given a simple 100 ml phosphate enema (Fletcher's enema) and re-examined. The importance of correct positioning of the patient before sigmoidoscopy has already been stressed.

The instrument is lubricated and gently inserted into the anal canal, passing along the rectum and hopefully into the sigmoid colon under direct vision by inflating the bowel above the scope with the aid of the double bellows. The sigmoidoscope should at least be passed to 15 cm (the rectosigmoid junction) but may be passed to its full length. It is important not to force the rigid sigmoidoscope as this will cause the patient much discomfort, will not add much information and can even perforate the bowel, whereas the flexible fibresigmoidoscope will easily and safely cover this area.

The normal rectal mucosa appears pale pink in colour and the intramucosal blood vessels or vascular pattern are clearly seen. The abnormalities which may be detected by sigmoidoscopy are proctitis and the presence of polyps and tumours.

The first sign of proctitis is a loss of vascular pattern and generalised reddening of the mucosa. Granularity, contact bleeding and ulceration are the appearances which indicate increasing severity of the condition. Proctitis is a sigmoidoscopic appearance, not a pathological diagnosis and the conditions which may produce this change are shown in Fig. 7.1. The precise diagnosis may be difficult and a rectal mucosal biopsy for histological examination is essential.

The word 'polyp' is a clinical term to describe a tumour or

elevation which projects above the surface of the surrounding flat mucous membrane. A histopathological classification of polyps is shown in Table 8a. Again, histological examination is the essential investigation but should be after total excision of the polyp, since a forceps biopsy is inadequate.

A carcinoma is usually readily diagnosed as a large, firm, indurated bleeding ulcer or tumour. The diagnosis is confirmed by forceps biopsy.

Rectal biopsy

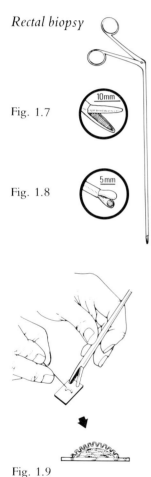

Fig. 1.7

Fig. 1.8

Fig. 1.9

To take a rectal mucosal biopsy without too much trauma, a small pair of biopsy forceps (such as Patterson's, Fig. 1.7 or bronchoscopic, Fig. 1.8) is preferable. Positioning of the biopsy site is important; the rectal mucosa is usually pain insensitive above 5 cm from the anal margin, and the posterior (sacral) aspect of the rectum is the safest site, being extraperitoneal. It is often most convenient to take the biopsy on one of the projecting rectal 'valves'. The site and distance from the anus should always be recorded to make localisation easier in the rare incidence of bleeding or perforation which may follow rectal biopsy. For a mucosal biopsy the jaws are partially opened and a small bit of mucosa is taken and the forceps then twisted 3–4 times until the biopsy separates. Twisting off, rather than cutting through the mucosa reduces the likelihood of bleeding by traumatising the submucosal vessels. The biopsy should then be orientated flat on to a ground glass slide or a piece of filter paper so that the submucosa is on the slide and the mucosa uppermost (Fig. 1.9). It is then placed in formalin for fixing; correct orientation of the specimen enables sections to be cut at right angles to the mucosal surface, which helps histological interpretation. If the specimen is placed directly in formalin it curls up and sections will be cut tangentially. The full thickness rectal biopsy required to make a diagnosis of Hirschsprung's disease is taken as a formal surgical excision procedure under general anaesthetic (see Chapter 2).

Polyps should be totally excised; if they are too big to fit into a pair of biopsy forceps, a more formal approach, using a diathermy snare or a peranal operative technique may be required. In order to establish the diagnosis of carcinoma, a forceps biopsy will suffice.

During sigmoidoscopy samples of stool may be taken for microscopy, microbiological examination and chemical testing for occult blood.

Protoscopy

A proctoscope is used to examine the anal canal and the region of the anorectal junction. A simple tubular instrument such as the Milligan-Morgan instrument is illustrated (Fig. 1.10). Smaller sizes are available, but for patients with severe anal pain and spasm a Lloyd-Davies paediatric sigmoidoscope is particularly useful (Fig. 1.11). A pair of 20 cm Emmett's forceps (Fig. 1.12) are essential for swabbing to obtain a clear view.

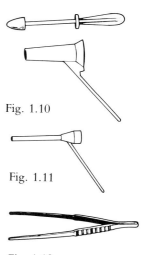

Fig. 1.10

Fig. 1.11

Fig. 1.12

The instrument is lubricated, passed and the obturator removed. The anal canal is inspected as the proctoscope is being withdrawn. Asking the patient simultaneously to strain down may improve the view of anal lesions which will prolapse into the proctoscope. Haemorrhoids, anterior rectal wall mucosal prolapse, fistulous openings and fibrous anal polyps may be diagnosed and certain therapeutic procedures, such as injection sclerotherapy and rubber band ligation of haemorrhoids may be carried out at the same time.

Proctoscopic findings are recorded on a standardised diagram (Fig. 1.13) featuring the line of the anal valves (dentate line) and identifying the anterior aspect; the classical 3, 7, 11 o'clock position of internal haemorrhoids (Fig. 1.14) depend on the 12 o'clock position being anterior.

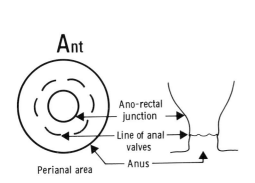

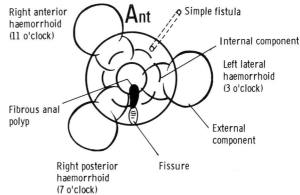

Fig. 1.13 Standard diagram to record proctoscopic findings (left) with anatomical explanation (right).

Fig. 1.14 Common anal conditions represented on standard diagram.

Any colonoscope can be used for limited examination but shorter (60–130 cm) instruments and their accessories are easier to handle and clean. Patients are prepared by the single administration of two warmed phosphate enemas 20 minutes before examination, which will clean the left colon in 90% of cases; the presence of diverticular disease or diarrhoea will cause poor results. No sedation should be required. The operator must have some familiarity with fibre-endoscopic technique to steer around the tight bends of the sigmoid colon and must pull back

Fibre-sigmoidoscopy

to get an accurate view every time he is 'lost'. With a little practice the proximal sigmoid colon will be reached within 3–4 minutes in the majority of cases and a view often obtained of the descending colon. Fibre-sigmoidoscopy is worth the extra time and trouble involved for any patient with rectal bleeding, polyps or a previous history of colon cancer. In a few patients with inflammatory bowel disease fibre-sigmoidoscopy will show the exact upper limit of disease or if there is rectal sparing, may reach to the abnormal area to obtain diagnostic biopsies.

REFERENCES AND FURTHER READING

Gear EV and Dobbins WO. Rectal biopsy: a review of its diagnostic usefulness. *Gastroenterology* 1968; **55:** 522–44.

Lockhart-Mummery HE. Proctoscopy *and* Sigmoidoscopy. In: Todd IP, ed. *Colon, rectum and anus* (3rd ed. Operative Surgery), London and Boston: Butterworths, 1977: 1–3; 4–6.

Marks G, Boggs W, Castro AF, Gathright JB, Ray JE and Salvati E. Sigmoidoscopic examinations with rigid and flexible fibreoptic sigmoidoscopes in the surgeons office. *Diseases of the Colon and Rectum* 1979; **22:** 162–68.

Williams JT and Thomson JPS. Anorectal bleeding: a study of causes and investigative yields. *Practitioner* 1977; **219:** 327–31.

MICROBIOLOGY

THE NORMAL BACTERIAL FLORA OF THE GASTROINTESTINAL TRACT

The fasting normal stomach in man is virtually sterile because of the presence of acid, although after a meal counts of up to 10^5 organisms per ml may be recovered. In the duodenum and upper jejunum there are Gram-positive micro-organisms, mainly streptococci and lactobacilli, in concentrations of up to 10^3–10^4 organisms per ml. In the distal jejunum and ileum, however, the concentration increases and Enterobacteria and Bacteroides species may also be present; there may be 10^6–10^7 organisms per ml in the distal ileum. There are numerous conditions which give rise to small intestinal bacterial overgrowth and to the various metabolic consequences observed in these conditions, the so-called 'stagnant-loop syndrome' (Tabaqchali, 1970).

In the caecum, the composition of the micro-flora is similar to that found in faeces; the non-sporing anaerobic bacteria form the bulk of the flora and aspirates yield up to 10^9 organisms per ml (Gorbach, Plant, Nahas *et al.*, 1967). The total viable bacterial counts obtained from faeces, using very strict anaerobic techniques, are 10^{10}–10^{11} organisms per gram of faeces. Anaerobic bacteria constitute the majority of the faecal flora (98–99% of the total count). The main groups of bacteria and the types commonly isolated, together with the concentrations per gram of faeces are shown in Table 1a.

Table 1a. *Bacteria occurring in the intestine*

Major bacterial groups	Counts/g wet wt faeces	Species often isolated
Enterobacteria	10^7–10^8	*Escherichia coli* *Klebsiella aerogenes* *Proteus mirabilis*
Streptococcus	10^6–10^7	*Streptococcus viridans* *Streptococcus faecalis*
Lactobacillus	10^5–10^6	*Lactobacillus acidophilus* *Lactobacillus casei*
Clostridium	10^3–10^4	*Clostridium perfringens* *Clostridium sporogenes*
Veillonella	10^7–10^8	*Veillonella parvula* *Veillonella alcalesceus*
Bacteroides	10^{10}–10^{11}	*Bacteroides fragilis* group *Bacteroides melaninogenicus*
Bifidobacterium	10^{10}–10^{11}	*Bifidobacterium adolescentis*
Eubacterium	10^{10}–10^{11}	*Eubacterium biforme*

SURGICAL INFECTIONS

Most infections (e.g. wound infection, abscess, peritonitis) following intestinal surgery, particularly if there is spillage of intestinal contents, would involve both aerobic and anaerobic bacteria. The predominant organisms will be *Escherichia coli* and *Bacteroides fragilis* (although many other species may be involved). Therapy should be directed at both groups of organisms.

Laboratory specimens

Because of the presence of the fastidious anaerobes, proper specimen collection and transport are absolutely essential if reliable and meaningful results are to be obtained on culture. Special care has to be taken in the collection of specimens, avoiding contamination with the commensal flora of the mucous surfaces of the oropharynx, the gastrointestinal tract and the genito-urinary tract, as well as the skin. In these areas, the indigenous flora are predominantly anaerobic. This means that specimens such as saliva, throat swabs, sputum, nasotracheal aspirates, faeces, colostomy and ileostomy effluents, vaginal secretions or superficial wound swabs contaminated by skin are inappropriate for anaerobic culture as the results will be difficult to interpret. Acceptable specimens are those derived from normally sterile areas, i.e. blood, peritoneal and joint fluids, bile and surgical specimens of pus and deep wound aspirates. Specimens collected by specialised techniques, i.e. transtracheal aspirates, suprapubic bladder aspirates and culdoscopy aspirates are worthwhile for anaerobic culture. Pus or liquid specimens can also be aspirated by a syringe and kept in oxygen-free conditions by expelling any air and then capping the needle with a rubber stopper (Finegold, 1977). Large amounts of pus can be transported in an ordinary screwcap bottle if sufficient air is displaced from the bottle to ensure anaerobiosis. However, special anaerobic transport bottles should be used whenever possible (Tabaqchali, Fiddian and Atkinson, 1979). Swabs are considered inferior to liquid specimens and should be avoided. However, when a swab is the only available specimen, it should be kept in an anaerobic atmosphere and after collection of the specimen, placed in a second tube containing prereduced semisolid media such as Carey-Blair medium, Amies transport medium or brain-heart infusion.

DIARRHOEA

Not all infective causes of diarrhoea are known. The majority of cases are self-limiting and remain undiagnosed. The microbiological causes of diarrhoea are: bacterial, viral, protozoal and helminthic.

The onset of diarrhoea in a group of people who have recently eaten the same food suggests infection with food poisoning organisms (Salmonella species, *Clostridium welchii*,

Bacillus cereus, Vibrio parahaemolyticus or *Campylobacter jejuni*). If the symptoms are predominantly nausea and vomiting occurring 1–3 hours following the meal, rather than diarrhoea, food poisoning, due to the ingestion of preformed toxin of *Staphylococcus aureus*, is more likely. Outbreaks as well as single cases can be caused by the Shigella group of organisms, by enteropathogenic *Escherichia coli* in neonates and in adults by certain toxin producing or invasive strains of *E. coli*. Enteric fevers caused by *Salmonella typhi* and *paratyphia A, B and C*, cholera, bacillary and amoebic dysentery, giardiasis and other types of protozoal dysentery should also be investigated especially in patients with diarrhoea who have recently returned from parts of the world where endemic tropical diseases occur. Full clinical and epidemiological details should be sent with the specimens as these may affect the type of culture methods used in the laboratory.

Laboratory specimens

Faeces

An adequate specimen of liquid faeces, including any mucus, pus or blood should be sent in a clean screwcapped plastic container. The specimen must not be contaminated with urine or disinfectant and care should be taken not to soil the outside of the container. Stool specimens should be transported to the laboratory without delay. Rectal swabs give inferior results and are only used for emergency screening if faeces are not available. As pathogens may be present in only small numbers compared with the normal flora, it is advisable to send three fresh specimens of faeces on successive days to the laboratory for examination. Stool specimens to be examined for Campylobacter (Skirrow, 1977) should be refrigerated if delay in transit is likely because this organism dies quickly at room temperature. Faeces must be sent for examination if parasites, cysts or ova are suspected; swabs are not suitable. Warm, freshly passed stools should be examined directly for detecting the vegetative forms of *Entamoeba histolytica*. Occasionally sigmoidoscopic specimens may be helpful, particularly in bacillary and amoebic dysentery.

Faeces can also be sent for viral examination by electron microscopy and immuno-electron microscopy to demonstrate the typical rotavirus particles; culture for viruses rarely reveals anything relevant.

Intestinal aspirate and biopsy

Smears of intestinal aspirates or biopsy specimens are helpful in the diagnosis of *Giardia lamblia* (trophozoite form). Rectal biopsies should be examined histologically for ova (amoebiasis and schistosomiasis).

11

Food and fomites

Examination of food and fomites (infectious materials) should also be performed and can be helpful in establishing the causative pathogen or in detecting a toxin.

Serology

Serology is only helpful if a rising titre is demonstrated and in only a few bacterial infections; enteric fevers (Widal), Yersinia infections (Yersinia antibodies) and bacillary dysentery (only *Shigella dysenteriae* type 1). Serology is helpful in the diagnosis of hydatid disease, schistosomiasis and amoebic abscess; the flourescent antibody test is used for the latter.

Blood cultures

Blood should be cultured whenever septicaemia is a possibility. This occurs following enteric fever, and less commonly with *Salmonella typhimurium* and Yersinia. In the postoperative phase, anaerobic blood cultures are as important as the aerobic culture.

OTHER INFECTIONS AND INFESTATIONS

Helminths and protozoa

The diagnosis of threadworms *Enterobius vermicularis* is made by finding the ova. A piece of transparent adhesive tape is placed across the anus first thing in the morning, stuck onto a microscopic slide and sent to the laboratory for examination. Threadworms may also be seen on sigmoidoscopy. Occasionally whole adult worms, e.g. Ascaris, or segments of cestodes are passed in faeces. Stools should be sent for detection of ova of nematodes, trematodes and cestodes and for cysts of protozoa (*Entamoeba histoytica*) and the flagellates (*Giardia lamblia*).

Gastrointestinal tuberculosis

Intestinal tuberculosis can still present, particularly in the non-Europeans where it can mimic Crohn's disease.

Tissue specimens, lymph nodes, or peritoneal biopsy obtained at peritoneoscopy or laparotomy are much more valuable for laboratory examination and culture than peritoneal fluid, although a large amount of the latter should also be sent to the laboratory. A sterile, plain container is used, without fixative.

Culture of faeces for *Mycobacterium tuberculosis* is unsuitable and the results obtained will be difficult to interpret.

Gonorrhoea

If gonococcal proctitis is suspected, rectal swabs for culture should be placed in special transport media (Stuart's) to prevent drying and sent to the laboratory for examination.

The exudate from any syphilitic lesion contains numerous organisms which are highly infectious. If examination of exudate is indicated, it should be handled with extreme care, preferably in a special clinic. A sample of exudate taken in warm saline using a Pasteur pipette is placed on a warmed microscope slide for immediate examination using dark ground or phase contrast illumination in order to visualise the *Treponema pallidum*.

Syphilis

REFERENCES AND FURTHER READING

Cruikshank R, Duguid JP, Marmion BP and Swain RH. *Medical microbiology*, 12th ed. Vol. 2. Edinburgh and London: Churchill Livingstone, 1975.

Finegold SM. *Anaerobic bacteria in human disease.* New York, San Francisco and London: Academic Press, 1977.

Gorbach SL, Plaut AG, Nahas L and Weinstein L. Studies of the intestinal microflora II. Micro-organisms of the small intestine and their relations to oral and fecal flora. *Gastroenterology* 1967; **53:** 856–867.

Skirrow MB. Campylobacter enteritis, a new disease. *British Medical Journal* 1977; **2:** 9–11, 1977.

Tabaqchali S. The pathophysiological role of small intestinal bacterial flora. *Scandinavian Journal of Gastroenterology* 1970; **5:** Supplement **6,** 139–163.

Tabaqchali S, Fiddian AP and Atkinson P. Recent techniques in the investigation and diagnosis of anaerobic infections. *Journal of Infection* 1979; **1:** Supplement **1,** 13–24.

RADIOLOGY

X-rays, with or without contrast medium, provide the ideal means of demonstrating the intestine and its disease processes when these are inaccessible to direct examination. The development of flexible endoscopes brings the colon within the reach of the clinician for inspection and biopsy but radiology scores by its speed, safety and the permanent record provided by x-ray films. Modern equipment ensures that irradiation is minimised but in women of child-bearing age menstrual status must be taken into account, as studies are contraindicated in early pregnancy. Contrast studies are normally contraindicated for two weeks after rectal biopsy and in the acute phase of certain diseases (complicated diverticular disease, toxic megacolon, severe ischaemic colitis) where there is a high risk of bowel perforation.

The clinician decides his own indication for radiography but he must remember that careful studies take time and that each unnecessary examination avoided allows more time to be spent on other patients. Giving the radiologist all relevant clinical detail and the reason for the request will help him to report usefully. When ordering x-rays, as for any other investigation, the rule is 'as little as possible, as much as necessary'.

PLAIN ABDOMINAL X-RAYS

A great deal of information can be obtained from erect and supine plain films and, in some circumstances, they are sufficient for diagnostic purposes without contrast studies – especially if these would be hazardous. Instead of the standard erect view the lateral decubitus film may be asked for if the patient cannot stand.

Normal appearances

Normal appearances of the colon on the plain abdominal radiograph vary greatly both as to the amount of gas (a mixture of air, methane and hydrogen) and faecal residue present in the colon. Gas, when present, provides a natural contrast medium to outline the bowel; prior sigmoidoscopy may account for an apparently large quantity of gas. The upper limit of normal for the diameter of the tranverse colon on a plain film is 5.5 cm. Faecal residue is normally present in the caecum and frequently extends distally into the sigmoid colon. Fluid levels are seen on the normal erect film in the stomach and duodenal cap; although a few short levels may be seen in the small intestine, none occur in the colon.

Obstruction, ileus and volvulus

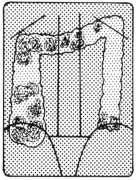

Fig. 1.15

When there is distal obstruction gaseous distension will be seen in the proximal colon, especially in the caecum (Fig. 1.15) with fluid levels in the erect film. The small intestine often appears normal and will only be distended if the ileocaecal valve is incompetent. The appearances in ileus vary, but characteristically involve a degree of distension with fluid levels in either the small or large intestine, or both (Fig. 1.16). Peritonitis is suggested by abnormal separation of loops of bowel (normal upper limit 2 mm) due to the presence of exudate. Volvulus causes obstruction, the involved part being markedly distended and usually assuming a U-shaped configuration. With sigmoid colon volvulus an inverted -U arises from the pelvis (Fig. 1.17), whilst in the caecal volvulus the U-shape points away from the right iliac fossa (Fig. 1.18).

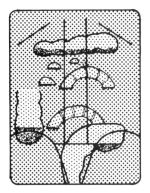

Fig. 1.16 Paralytic ileus.

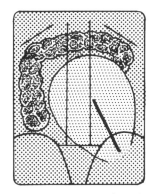

Fig. 1.17 Sigmoid colon volvulus.

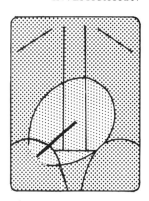

Fig. 1.18 Caecal volvulus.

An abscess often produces a local or generalised ileus. Subphrenic abscess results in splinting of the diaphragm and often causes changes at the lung base. Alternatively, an abscess may be suspected because of a soft-tissue mass, a collection or pattern of extraluminal gas, viscus displacement, loss of normally visualised structures (e.g. psoas outline) or fixation of a normally mobile organ (Meyers, 1976). In appendicitis for

Localisation of abscesses

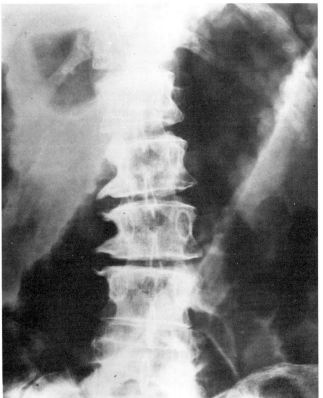

Fig. 1.19 Mucosal islands in 'toxic' dilatation of the colon.

instance, there may be a local small bowel ileus in the right lower quadrant.

Inflammatory bowel disease

The plain film may be particularly useful in assessing the extent, severity or complications of colitis.

Inflamed bowel empties itself, so active disease is associated with absence of faecal residue and the distal extent of residue gives some idea of the proximal extent of active disease. Some normal colons are remarkably empty, but the absence of residue in the caecum is always abnormal and implies total, active colitis.

When gas is present an irregular mucosal outline may be seen; in toxic megacolon the combination of colonic dilatation, loss of normal haustration and the so-called 'mucosal islands' (projecting remnants of colonic mucosa) (Fig. 1.19) are diagnostic and a contraindication to barium enema. Gas may be seen outside the colon or under the diaphragm, indicating perforation, but sealed perforations cannot always be excluded radiologically. If linear tracking of intra-mucosal gas is seen, perforation is imminent.

Pneumatosis coli

This rare and mysterious condition causes numerous cysts, either subserosal or submucosal, readily visible on the plain film, which may be diagnostic (Fig. 1.20). Barium enema simply outlines the luminal surface of the cysts for confirmation

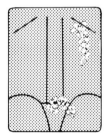

Fig. 1.20

BARIUM ENEMA

There are two methods of examination, the single contrast enema or the double contrast (air contrast) enema.

In the single contrast technique the whole colon is filled with dilute barium suspension, the radiologist watching filling under fluoroscopic control. During filling the radiologist takes films with the patient in various positions with the undercouch x-ray tube (Fig. 1.21) and then a final prone film after the patient has evacuated the barium (after-evacuation or AE film). The mucosa is seen in profile in the filled state and the mucosal fold pattern shown on the AE film.

The double contrast enema was developed in its modern form by Welin in Malmö, Sweden in 1953. In this technique the radiologist fills the colon to the splenic flexure with barium

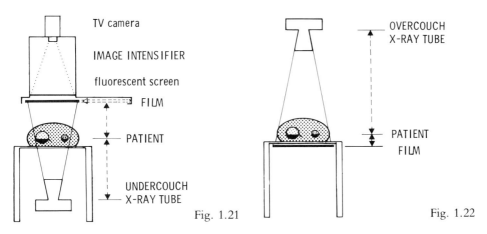

Fig. 1.21   Fig. 1.22

suspension, empties the rectum and then distends the colon with air, rolling the patient round to produce a thin coating of barium over the entire mucosal surface. Films are subsequently taken in various standard positions by the radiographer using the overcouch tube, which produces a sharper image than the undercouch tube, since the patient is closer to the x-ray plate (Fig. 1.22). Detail is also more precise because the mucosal surface is shown both tangentially at the barium/air interface (the mucosal line) and *en face* where the mucosa is visible through the air-filled lumen (Fig. 1.23). The advantages of double over single contrast technique are particularly evident in the demonstration of fine detail, such as inflammatory disease or small polyps. The double contrast technique also makes it easier to distinguish between intra-luminal lesions and any faecal residue, which is seen to move around in the air-filled colon.

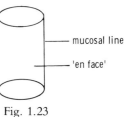

Fig. 1.23

Efficient bowel preparation is of paramount importance, whichever technique is used, and poor preparation is the commonest reason for mistakes in diagnosis on barium enema. A suggested preparation is as follows:

Technical details

Soft diet (excluding meat and vegetables) on the day before and fluids on the day of examination.
Castor oil (30 ml) after lunch on the day before the examination.
Atropine (1 mg) by mouth when the patient arrives unless there are contraindications. This reduces mucus secretion and as an antispasmodic helps administration of cleansing enemas as well as performance of the examination.
Two large-volume water enemas are given immediately before the examination to remove any residue, the second containing a contact laxative (bisacodyl or oxyphenisatin) to stimulate complete colonic emptying

The barium suspension used is also of importance for good double contrast results. It must have the correct viscosity for good coating, be sufficiently dense to show up in a thin layer and not produce artefacts such as bubbles or flocculation.

The standard positions used when taking films are: Preliminary film prone, left lateral pelvis, right and left posterior oblique, AP and PA lateral decubitus (Fig. 1.24). With this standard approach it takes 15 minutes to perform the double contrast barium enema.

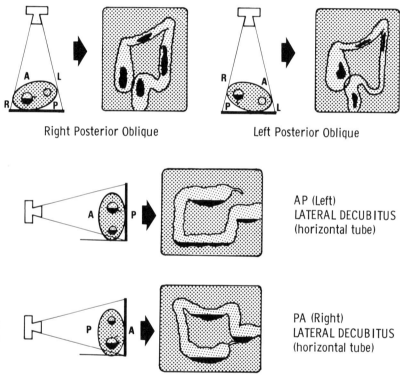

Right Posterior Oblique   Left Posterior Oblique

AP (Left)
LATERAL DECUBITUS
(horizontal tube)

PA (Right)
LATERAL DECUBITUS
(horizontal tube)

Fig. 1.24 Double contrast barium enema—some standard views.

Special techniques

Instant enema

The instant enema is a double contrast barium enema without bowel preparation. It is useful in patients with active ulcerative colitis, since the affected part of the bowel is self-evacuating and adequate mucosal detail is seen in double contrast to allow assessment of severity and extent of the mucosal lesion. It is not usually recommended for assessment of Crohn's colitis where, because of the patchy nature of the disease, residue can accumulate between areas of ulceration.

An instant enema is not sufficiently accurate for the assessment of patients with long-standing ulcerative colitis where there is a possibility of malignancy; in such patients a double contrast enema with full bowel preparation is indicated. The examination is contraindicated if the preliminary film shows evidence of toxic megacolon.

The radiologist's technique is similar to that of the double contrast enema except the air insufflation and rotation are only continued sufficiently to obtain distension and visualisation of the affected region. Four standard views are taken with the overcouch tube: Preliminary film, prone, erect and lateral pelvis.

Water-soluble enema

A water-soluble enema is safe to use in situations where there is a risk of perforation, since the contrast medium used will be absorbed from any site. It may be used to check the anastomotic continuity ten days after large bowel resection. The contrast medium is diluted with water in equal measures. AP and

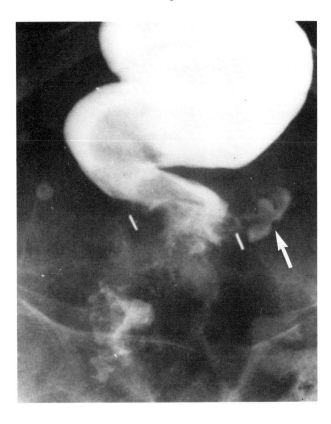

Fig. 1.25 Water-soluble enema showing leak from anastomosis (between clips).

lateral views of the filled anastomotic region are taken. Dehiscence of the anastomosis, identified by clips placed at operation, will be shown by leakage into a cavity, a track (Fig. 1.25) or pouch. Widening of the post-rectal space opposite the anastomosis may indicate an abscess.

Colostomy enema

A large Foley catheter is inserted into the colostomy and the balloon inflated with 10 ml of air and pulled back against the abdominal wall to provide a seal. The barium is injected with a 50 ml syringe until about two-thirds of the remaining colon is filled (usually about 250 ml is needed); air is then insufflated and the patient turned from side to side. Overcouch films are taken as for a double contrast enema, but a supine rather than prone view is used because of the stoma.

Ileostomy enema

An ileostomy enema is similar to a colostomy enema except that less barium is needed. One straight and two oblique views are taken with the undercouch tube to show the distal loops of small intestine.

Clinical significance

Irritable bowel syndrome

The radiologist's main function is to exclude other disease but he should report the occurrence of spasm especially if accompanied by the patient's usual pain. An intravenous anti-spasmodic such as hyoscine-n-butylbromide (Buscopan) or glucagon should be given if the spasm is persistent.

Diverticular disease

There is usually a muscular disorder associated with the diverticula but either abnormality may occur independently.

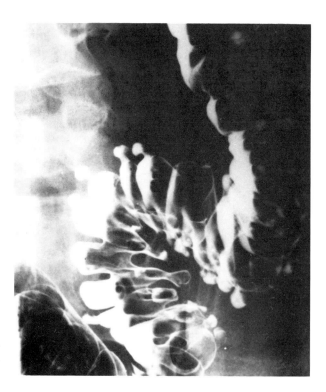

Fig. 1.26 Diverticular disease—out-pouchings and muscle hypertrophy.

Although the sigmoid colon is most commonly affected, in 20% of cases the diverticula are scattered throughout the colon and occasionally are found only on the right side. The muscular abnormality may be seen as apparent stricturing of the lumen, exaggerated by mucosal redundancy and differentation from carcinoma may be difficult. (Fig. 1.26).

The radiologist can demonstrate some of the complications of diverticular disease. When perforation occurs it is often sealed off with the development of an abscess, but free intra-peritoneal air may occur. A definite sign of a pericolic abscess is a track of barium extending outward from a diverticulum into the abscess cavity, which often causes an extrinsic impression – either unilateral or encircling to cause a stricture. The commonest fistulous complication is a colovesical fistula, demonstrated radiologically in about 40% of cases by filling of the bladder with gas on plain films or by contrast at barium enema examinations. Some degree of colonic obstruction is not uncommon; rarely complete large or small bowel obstruction can occur, or localised small bowel ileus can be demonstrated secondary to a pericolic abscess.

Polyps

By definition any projection above the mucosal surface is a polyp. Polyps may be sessile or pedunculated, and radiologically the appearance of a polyp will vary with the angle at which it is viewed (Fig. 1.27), the 'target sign' (Fig. 1.28) being a characteristic of a pedunculated polyp and the 'hat sign' indicating a smaller non-peduncutated polyp. Small polyps may be difficult to differentiate from air bubbles or faecal residue,

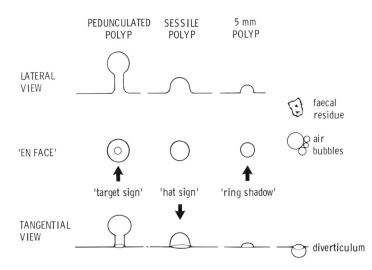

Fig. 1.27 Scheme for radiological interpretation of 'polyps'.

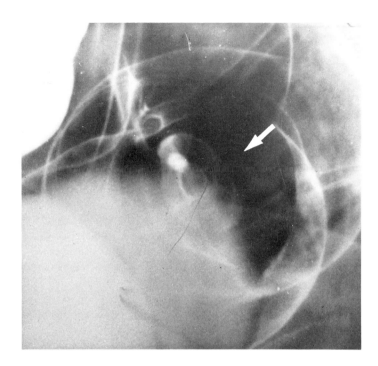

Fig. 1.28 'Target sign'.

and among polyps less than 1 cm diameter there is therefore a significant rate of false negative and positive diagnosis (the double contrast enema being considerably more accurate than the single contrast technique). When the radiologist is in doubt

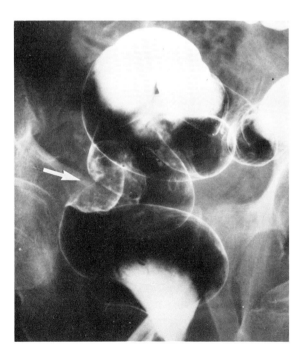

Fig. 1.29 Indurated base suggesting malignancy.

about the significance of what he has demonstrated he may merely report a 'ring shadow'.

The histological nature of a polyp cannot be deduced from its radiological appearance, with the exception of the frond-like postinflammatory polyps after a severe attack of colitis. Radiographic features which suggest possible malignancy in a polyp include indrawing of the outline of the base of a sessile polyp (Fig. 1.29), an irregular surface and large size or evidence of growth between consecutive barium studies. Villous tumours, most common in the rectum and sigmoid colon, may show a radiologically characteristic 'lacework' surface due to barium lying within the frond-like interstices of the tumour; indrawing of the base of a villous tumour is not a reliable index of malignancy.

The importance of radiology nowadays lies in detecting and localising a polyp. The endoscopist will attempt total removal but is helped in his task by having an accurate map. The radiologist will frequently perform the follow-up studies at 2–3 yearly intervals, since barium enema is in most cases an easier procedure than colonoscopy.

The diagnosis of adenomatous polyposis (Chapter 8) is normally made on sigmoidoscopy and biopsy but if operation is to be delayed a double contrast enema is indicated to exclude any large or possibly malignant lesions proximally. The presence of multiple polyps radiologically (Fig. 1.30) does not necessarily indicate adenomatous polyposis; the diagnosis must be confirmed histologically because other polyposis syndromes occur (Chapter 8). The absence of radiologically visible

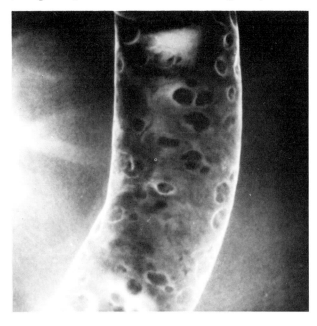

Fig. 1.30 Multiple colonic polyps.

polyps does not necessarily exclude polyposis because in the late teens and early adult life when the polyps are forming, they may be very small.

Carcinoma

The single contrast barium enema has been shown to miss at least 10% of colon cancers on initial examination. When a carcinoma is missed on a good quality double contrast enema this is usually due to observer error and it is, therefore, desirable that films on any high risk patient (e.g. with anorectal bleeding) should be reviewed by a second radiologist.

The radiological appearances of carcinoma may be:

Polypoid – large, irregular sessile mass with 'indrawing' of the base (Fig. 1.29).

Annular – the 'apple-core' lesion with shouldering at each end and an irregular central channel (Fig. 1.31).

Plaque – rare and difficult to detect. Deformity may only be seen in profile.

Linitis plastica – scirrhous intramucosal carcinoma occurs in the colon, producing a narrowed segment with fixed and distorted mucosal pattern.

Calcification – fine punctate calcification in mucinous adeno-carcinoma may be visible in both primary and secondary tumours on the plain films.

Extrinsic carcinoma – cancer may invade from stomach, kidney, pancreas, cervix and ovary and can mimic the appearances of ischaemic colitis or Crohn's disease. Initially there is a fixed deformity of the bowel wall but when the mucosa ulcerates differentiation from colon cancer becomes difficult.

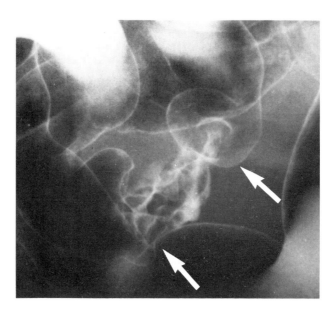

Fig. 1.31 Carcinoma—'apple core' appearance.

Several normal appearances may be mistaken for carcinoma. The ileo-caecal valve (Fig. 1.32) is mistaken for caecal carcinoma with monotonous regularity. 'Physiological sphincters' or areas of spasm, of which the best-known is in the mid-transverse colon, mimic strictures but are smooth with radiating mucosal folds (Fig. 1.33). The contractions are short-lived and abolished by intravenous antispasmodics.

Even though 50% of colorectal cancers are diagnosed on sigmoidoscopy a double contrast enema is mandatory to exclude synchronous cancer (3% incidence) or co-existing adenomas. Once a tumour has been resected the anastomosis must be checked; the presence of any irregularity or nodular mass might be either recurrent carcinoma or stitch granulation tissue and endoscopic biopsy is indicated. Follow up is then indicated, usually by double contrast enema performed every 2–5 years, because of the possibility of subsequent (metachronous) cancer (3.5% incidence) or the development of adenomas.

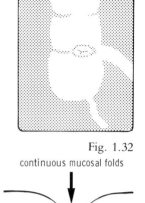

Fig. 1.32
continuous mucosal folds

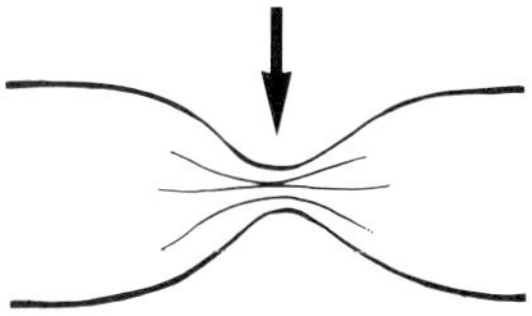

Fig. 1.33

Ulcerative colitis

The use of the plain film and the instant enema in colitis have already been mentioned. Contrast studies are important in assessing the extent, severity and type of colitis and in demonstrating any complications.

The radiological changes in colitis may be considered as being either primary, involving the mucosal surface, or secondary, reflecting the effects of the disease on the musculature of the bowel wall (Fig. 1.34).

The mucosal changes are characterised by:

Granularity which is the earliest radiologically detectable abnormality, in which the normally sharp mucosal line becomes indistinct. Seen 'en face' the barium has a rough stippled appearance.

Ulceration which is shown when the mucosal line is disrupted with barium-filled linear or 'collar-stud' projections. These ulcerated areas are seen 'en face' as irregular tracks or pools.

Inflammatory polyposis which is of two types. In the acute stage 'pseudopolyps' are oedematous mucosal remnants (mucosal islands) between severely ulcerated areas. The mucosal line shows coarse undulation and 'en face' the mucosal remnants are outlined as a series of criss-cross tracks. In the healed stage, the postinflammatory polyps represent frond-like mucosal tags against a background of normal mucosa. Where there has been undermining of the mucosa, characteristic mucosal bridges may form. As well as the fronds, larger rounded polyps are occasionally seen, which may be composed of inflammatory granulation tissue or may uncommonly be co-existing adenomas.

Changes in the bowel wall occur with persistently active

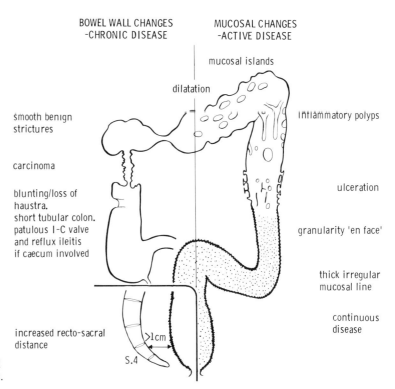

BOWEL WALL CHANGES
-CHRONIC DISEASE

MUCOSAL CHANGES
-ACTIVE DISEASE

mucosal islands

dilatation

smooth benign
strictures

inflammatory polyps

carcinoma

blunting/loss of
haustra.
short tubular colon.
patulous I-C valve
and reflux ileitis
if caecum involved

ulceration

granularity 'en face'

thick irregular
mucosal line

continuous
disease

increased recto-sacral
distance

>1cm

S.4

Fig. 1.34 The radiological
features in ulcerative colitis.

disease – haustration is first blunted, then lost and the bowel
becomes shortened and narrowed. In the rectum this narrowing
is seen as widening of the postrectal space (upper limit of
normal recto-sacral distance is 1 cm at S 4) and the rectal valves
are obliterated. These changes probably reflect changes in
smooth muscle and can occasionally revert to normal but when
the mucosa heals the colon usually remains tubular.

Complications such as toxic megacolon and perforation have
been mentioned. Strictures in chronic colitis are usually benign
and secondary to muscle thickening; the narrowing is symmet-
rical with a mucosal appearance similar to that on either side of
the stricture. A malignant stricture is suggested by irregular
eccentric narrowing and loss of continuity of the mucosal
pattern, but radiological differentiation is difficult and endoscopy with biopsy is indicated.

Carcinoma formation causes concern in the long-term management of patients with chronic extensive ulcerative colitis. It
should be noted that radiology under-estimates the histological

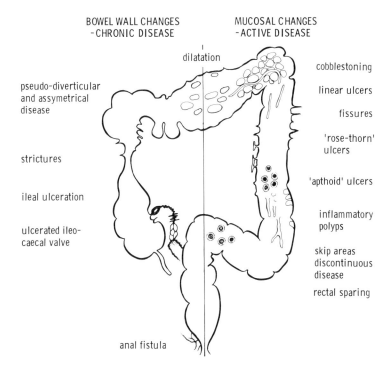

BOWEL WALL CHANGES
- CHRONIC DISEASE

MUCOSAL CHANGES
- ACTIVE DISEASE

dilatation

pseudo-diverticular
and assymetrical
disease

strictures

ileal ulceration

ulcerated ileo-
caecal valve

anal fistula

cobblestoning

linear ulcers

fissures

'rose-thorn'
ulcers

'apthoid' ulcers

inflammatory
polyps

skip areas
discontinuous
disease

rectal sparing

Fig. 1.35 The radiological
features in Crohn's disease.

extent of colitis, so if mucosal changes have been demonstrated to the hepatic flexure the colitis is deemed 'extensive' and the whole colon may be assumed to be abnormal histologically. The formal double contrast enema has some use in delineating the colon and demonstrating any strictures or overt malignancy. Cancers in colitis may, however, be submucosal and may also be preceded by a phase of mucosal dysplasia which cannot always be differentiated radiologically from the already abnormal mucosa. Monitoring of these patients, therefore, requires endoscopic biopsy.

The radiological features that help to distinguish Crohn's disease from ulcerative colitis are shown in Fig. 1.35. Ulceration and asymmetry are the most valuable discriminants, but in some patients Crohn's disease will exactly simulate ulcerative colitis radiologically with a granular mucosa and no discrete ulceration.

Crohn's disease

27

The smallest 'apthoid' ulcers are seen on good quality air contrast films as dark 3–5 mm halos each surrounding a tiny central fleck of barium (Fig. 1.36). Strictures and fissures are common. Small bowel involvement should be determined by barium follow-through. Crohn's disease may co-exist with diverticular disease in the elderly.

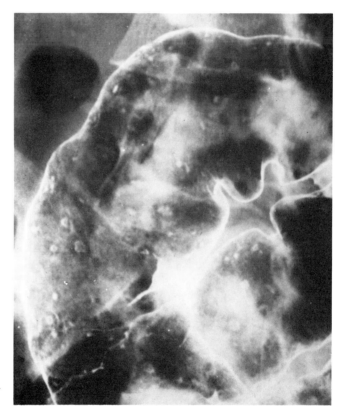

Fig. 1.36 Crohn's disease—multiple 'apthoid' ulcers.

Ischaemic colitis

Ischaemic colitis most commonly involves the splenic flexure but any part of the colon and even the rectum may be affected. The initial radiological findings are of marked spasm and 'thumb-printing' from submucosal haemorrhage or oedema (Fig. 9.9). If the mucosa is further compromised ulceration develops and may simulate other forms of colitis.

Tuberculosis

Tuberculosis may be indistinguishable from Crohn's disease and can produce polypoid lesions and ulcers or result in fibrotic strictures. The ileocaecal canal region is commonly affected; a deformed caecum with a patulous ileocaecal valve and narrowed, ulcerated, terminal ileum are characteristic findings.

Amoebiasis may cause a diffuse colitis with a granular mucosa similar to ulcerative colitis or with discrete ulcers. A characteristic finding is 'funnelling' of the caecum which has a ragged outline due to the ulceration. Amoebomas are commoner in the right colon, and may be found as an irregular filling defect without other changes in the colon, thus simulating carcinoma.

Amoebiasis

Pseudomembranous colitis causes plaques which are seen as small raised areas on double contrast enema; if the membrane is confluent a shaggy, irregular surface is seen. Marked thickening of the haustral clefts with irregularity of the mucosal outline and dilated small bowel have been reported on plain radiographs.

Pseudomembranous colitis

OTHER RADIOLOGICAL STUDIES

The objectives of sinography are to delineate an abscess cavity, fistulous connection or sinus tract, before or after treatment.

Sinography

Precise information should be given to the radiologist as to the location of the sinus, the clinical problem and relevant surgical details (bowel resections etc.).

If the sinus opening is small it should be probed, to show the direction of the pathway and facilitate entry of the catheter. A sterile, thin, soft rubber catheter is introduced as deep as possible without using undue force. If the catheter is left superficially, contrast will reflux on to the skin, rather than penetrate any abscess and so may fail to show a fistula. About 20–50 ml of a sterile, water soluble, contrast medium are injected under steady pressure. Radiographs in the AP and lateral planes are taken to provide a three-dimensional image of the lesion.

The technique of percutaneous femoral catheterisation enables selective arteriography of the coeliac axis, superior and inferior mesenteric arteries to be performed rapidly and safely under local anaesthetic with minimal sedation. The most important application in the colon is in the diagnosis and possible treatment of acute rectal bleeding if the rate of bleeding prevents endoscopic examination.

Arteriography

Providing there is active bleeding at a rate of 1 ml/min or more, extravasation of contrast into the lumen of the bowel should be seen at the site of haemorrhage. Since bleeding from diverticula or vascular lesions (angiodysplasia) is more common in the right colon any abnormality is likely to be shown on the superior mesenteric arteriogram; the inferior mesenteric arteriogram is however performed first so that overlap from contrast medium in the bladder is avoided. Once the bleeding point has been localised a pitressin infusion or embolisation via the catheter may control the haemorrhage.

In patients with repeated rectal bleeding or anaemia of gastrointestinal origin in whom barium and endoscopic studies of the gastrointestinal tract are negative, superior mesenteric arteriography should be performed in the search for angiodysplasia (Chapter 9); the vascular abnormality may be very small and high quality films are essential. Early filling of normal veins or demonstration of venous malformations are important findings during arteriography.

Ultrasound and computerised tomography

Ultrasound and computerised tomography are relatively new methods of scanning the abdomen. They have made a considerable impact due to their ability to visualise soft tissue structures, notably the liver and pancreas, which previously could only be visualised angiographically.

Ultrasound forms a picture from the reflected sound waves at tissue interfaces. Computerised tomography uses computerisation to analyse the absorption of a rotated pencil-thin beam of x-rays as it traverses the body. Each technique shows a slice of the body about 1 cm thick; with ultrasound this may be in any plane, but with computerised tomography it is a transverse cut. The information obtained is different; ultrasound gives a better view of some vascular structures and the texture of the internal organs. Unfortunately the ultrasonic beam is completely reflected by air, so that large areas of the abdomen cannot be seen. There is no such limitation for computerised tomography which can visualise any part of the abdominal or pelvic cavity; structures are clearly defined and each cut gives a complete anatomical cross section that is easier to interpret than ultrasound.

Computerised tomography is particularly useful to demonstrate the extraluminal component of tumours, especially pelvic masses such as a recurrence after resection. Ultrasound will demonstrate larger pelvic masses displacing the bladder; the development of rectal probes may make it more useful. Both techniques may be used to demonstrate liver metastases and define palpable intra-abdominal abscesses, but computerised tomography will demonstrate smaller lesions and give a more accurate anatomical picture of their situation and extent.

Isotope scanning

Isotope scanning is less accurate than the above methods in detecting liver metastases but the gamma camera will diagnose bone metastases at an early stage. 99 m Technetium will sometimes concentrate in the gastric mucosa of a Meckel's diverticulum and has also been used (with a wide field gamma camera) to localise the source of active colonic bleeding. Being quick, safe and non-invasive this technique may prove to have an important role in the assessment of patients with bleeding.

REFERENCES AND FURTHER READING

Bartram CI. Radiology in the current assessment of ulcerative colitis. *Gastrointestinal Radiology* 1977; **1:** 383–92.

Laufer I. *Double contrast gastrointestinal radiology*. Philadelphia: Saunders, 1976.

Meyers MA. *Dynamic radiology of the abdomen. Normal and pathological anatomy*. Berlin: Springer-Verlag, 1976.

Thomas BM. The instant enema in inflammatory disease of the colon. *Clinical Radiology* 1979; **30:** 165–73.

COLONOSCOPY

The use of fibre-sigmoidoscopy or limited colonoscopy has already been described. More extensive or total colonoscopy has been made much easier by recent instruments which are very flexible and acutely-angling and also more durable than early instruments. These improvements are due mainly to the development of finer glass-fibres; these are less liable to break, permit smaller fibre-bundles and therefore a larger suction and instrument channel within the standard 15 mm diameter colonoscope shaft and a wide-angle view (100° or more) because of the high resolving power of small fibres.

Nonetheless colonoscopy remains an unpredictable procedure since each patient's bowel varies in length, elasticity, attachments and adhesions. Individuals also vary in pain sensibility to stretching of the colon or its mesenteries. Previous surgery, sepsis or diverticular abscesses may create fixed bends which are difficult or impossible to pass; the most acute flexures or marked haustral folds can be extremely difficult to examine completely. Often colonoscopy provides a highly accurate close-up colour view, with the added advantage of biopsies, but examinations can be tedious or painful and may not always visualise the whole colon.

For these reasons colonoscopy should follow and complement a good quality double contrast barium enema, the radiographs providing overall view and permanent records and selecting patients with possible abnormalities who merit colonoscopy. The endoscopist can take photographs, film or a colour video-tape recording of areas of interest.

TECHNIQUE

Bowel preparation

No bowel preparation regime is always effective in every patient. In giving instructions attention should be paid to the patient's normal bowel habit (constipation necessitates extra preparation, but diarrhoea less) and to the results of previous preparation for barium enema.

Limited colonoscopy can be performed in patients with normal bowel habit (no diverticular disease) following only two warmed disposable hypertonic phosphate enemas (Fleet's, Fletcher's) given together 20–30 minutes before examination; the colon is usually clean to the splenic flexure.

The most widely used regimes for whole bowel preparation are the conventional combination of diet, purgation and enema, as used before barium enema. One day of low-residue diet is followed by fluids and a dose of castor oil (30 ml) or senna syrup (80 ml) on the afternoon before colonoscopy. The purgative may take between 2–12 hours to work and the patient must realise that profuse diarrhoea is necessary for a good result. One hour before examination large volume tap-water enemas are given as necessary until the returns are clear and without solid matter. Patients with diverticular disease or colon spasm can be given an intramuscular antispasmodic (hyoscine-n-butyl bromide 20 mg) if administration of the enema proves painful or difficult.

The alternative preparation regime is by an osmotic or isotonic peroral purge. Magnesium salts (sulphate or citrate) must be given in repeated large quantities and the results are unpredictable. The nasal tube saline lavage method produces excellent results but may require up to 10–12 litres administered over 4–5 hours spent sitting on a padded lavatory seat; this is impracticable as a routine without suitable facilities and nursing supervision. Drinking isotonic saline (3–4 litres) or 10% mannitol solution (1 litre) will cause diarrhoea within an hour and produce a reasonably clean colon by 4–5 hours although there may be residual fluid and some patients are nauseated. There is a theoretical risk of colonic bacteria fermenting mannitol, a non-absorbed sugar, to form hydrogen; carbon dioxide insufflation should be used for the examination if electrosurgery is intended.

Medication

Limited colonoscopy is rarely painful except in the presence of adhesions or diverticular disease and therefore needs no sedation. Many total colonoscopies are also well tolerated without sedation but some can be extremely painful due to loop formation which stretches the mesentery of the sigmoid colon or the visceral peritoneum. Whether sedation is required depends on the character and pain threshold of the individual patient and the technical performance of the endoscopist and his instrument. The combination of intravenous diazepam (Valium) 5–10 mg with pethidine (meperidine) 25–50 mg will give 5–10 minutes of analgesia and a useful degree of amnesia for the difficult part of a colonoscopy which is usually during passage through the left colon and into the tranverse colon. After examination the patient is normally fit to be escorted home but should not drive or work for 24 hours. Children can be given an oral or intramuscular premedication one hour beforehand followed by a reduced dose of diazepam and pethidine intravenously. Naloxone (Narcan) 0.2–0.4 mg is given intravenously for immediate effect if there is respiratory depression or can be given intramuscularly towards the end of the procedures if the patient appears oversedated. There is no medical indication for general anaesthesia which deprives the endoscopist of the valuable early-warning sign of pain and may increase the risk of complications.

The need to use sedation will be markedly reduced if the endoscopist talks to the patient reassuringly before and during the procedure. The best policy may be to start the procedure without sedation and in many cases it will prove unnecessary.

Anti-spasmodics (hyoscine-n-butylbromide 40 mg or glucagon 1 mg) are given intravenously if circular muscle contractions interfere with inspection. Since their duration of action is only about 5 minutes they are normally only given as the instrument is withdrawn; trials have shown no benefit of anti-spasmodics in speeding insertion.

Choice of instrument

Any colonoscope can be used for limited examination or polypectomy but only a long (165–185 cm) instrument will always reach the caecum and is thus the best all-purpose

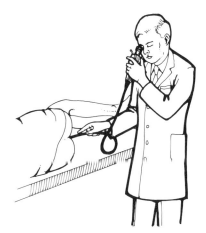

Fig. 1.37 'Single-handed'. manipulation of the colonoscope.

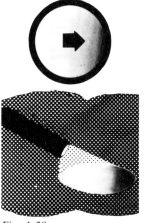

Fig. 1.38

Manipulation

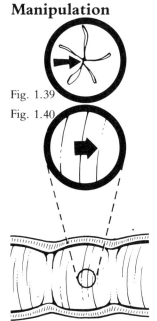

Fig. 1.39

Fig. 1.40

instrument. Medium or intermediate-length instruments (110–150 cm) are slightly easier to handle and clean in routine sessions or clinics; the only advantage of a 60–70 cm instrument is that it must be quick to use since it cannot be inserted far.

Children over 2–3 years can be examined with an adult instrument, but a small-diameter paediatric colonoscope (floppier than the paediatric gastroscope) is useful for babies, small children and limited examination in some adults, such as those with strictures or adhesions. Large diameter two-channel instruments are clumsy except for special circumstances (bleeding, multiple polyps).

The so-called 'one-handed' technique of holding and managing the colonoscope has proved best, the left hand holding the control section and knobs and the right pushing, pulling or rotating the shaft (Fig. 1.37). It requires a little practice and self-discipline to master this technique and to develop relaxed and logical co-ordination of eye and hand; at least 2–3 examinations a week are needed to speed up the process. An assistant is useful to steady the instrument shaft from time to time. Fluoroscopy is helpful during the learning phase and for occasional difficult cases thereafter in order to explain and help to unravel the variable loops that may form.

The basis of efficient colonoscopy (Cotton and Williams, 1980) is to observe accurately so as always to know in which direction the lumen lies, even if the colon is very tortuous. When manoeuvring in a confined space and in bowel which may contract or flop about over the moving instrument it is easy to make steering errors; the lumen is usually towards the dark side of the field of view (Fig. 1.38), at the convergance of folds (Fig. 1.39) or on the concave side of a circular-muscle arc (Fig. 1.40). Each time direction is lost in spite of these clues or

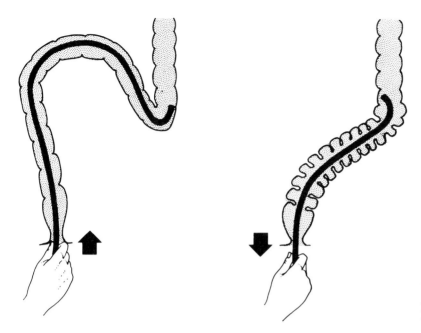

Fig. 1.41 Pulling-back the colonoscope to straighten a loop.

the lens is so close to the mucosa as to cause a 'red-out' the quickest and best course is to *pull-back*, which simultaneously disengages the tip, improves the view, and tends to straighten out the shaft of the instrument (Fig. 1.41) making it easier to handle.

The further in the instrument passes the more likely it is to loop (loops being almost always in the sigmoid colon) and if a loop is hurting the patient unduly or reducing angulation through friction on the control wires the shaft is pulled-back as far as possible until the tip starts to slide back. If possible, such a pull-back attempt is made after the tip has passed around an acute bend, which results in it being 'hooked' and fixed. When the colonoscope is fully straightened the colon becomes amazingly shortened, the caecum being at only 70–80 cm from the anus and the splenic flexure at 50 cm (Fig. 1.42). Conversely, when there are loops the tip of a fully inserted 110 cm colonoscope may only have reached the descending colon. The need for repeated pull-back is the fundamental difference in the handling of a flexible compared to a rigid endoscope and the commonest failing is not to pull back enough.

With modern acutely-angling and flexible instruments formal procedures such as the 'alpha-manoeuvre' are no longer necessary. The colon is considered simply as a series of bends and straights to be negotiated as quickly and gently as possible.

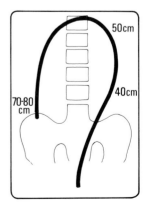

Fig. 1.42

35

Exact location is of no great importance during insertion but is usually quite adequately assessed during withdrawal by a combination of distance on the straightened shaft and seeing the tip transilluminating the abdominal wall in the transverse colon or caecum.

In reaching to the right colon various manoeuvres may be helpful, particularly those which prevent or reduce looping of the sigmoid colon; the assistant can press firmly in the left iliac fossa or a stiffening tube may be passed over the colonoscope under fluoroscopic control. Aspiration of excess air shortens the voluminous caecum and ascending colon. Changes of patient position are also sometimes effective.

Successful colonoscopy requires determination and adaptability; very small adjustments may be needed at one place and then massive looping or withdrawal at another. It takes 50–100 examinations to become confident with the procedure and its variations. By that time total colonoscopy should be feasible in 90% of patients and should take on average about 30 minutes, although sometimes much less. The technical unpredictability of colonoscopy from patient to patient is its main limitation.

INDICATIONS

Abnormal barium enema

Doubtful abnormalities or obvious abnormalities of uncertain cause can be inspected or biopsied. Some strictures may be too narrow to pass without a paediatric instrument and in them the cytology brush can be more effective than the biopsy forceps. Even severe diverticular disease can usually be traversed and inspected, avoiding the need for resection in many cases.

Rectal bleeding

Older patients referred for colonoscopy with unexplained and persistent red or dark-red rectal bleeding but a normal barium enema are found to have hidden pathology in 30–40% of cases (Hunt, 1978) including missed carcinomas in 10%, and polyps, colitis or angiodysplasia. Children and patients under 40 rarely show any obvious abnormality. The yield in unexplained iron-deficiency anaemia is also low, but worthwhile in some patients to exclude the possibility of a missed caecal carcinoma or angiodysplasia. Angiodysplasia (Chapter 9) can be safely electrocoagulated by pulling up the abnormal mucosa in electrically insulted 'hot-biopsy' forceps; the wall of the right colon is too thin to coagulate safely with the conventional button electrode.

In selected patients the extra accuracy of colonoscopy is useful (Williams and Waye, 1978) in showing the exact extent of colitis, obtaining biopsies from the terminal ileum or proximal colon or checking for recurrent disease. In occasional patients, especially children, colonoscopy will demonstrate extensive mild colitis or Crohn's disease not seen on barium enema. In chronic and extensive colitis biopsies of the colon help to identify patients at risk for cancer.

Inflammatory bowel disease

Over 95% of polyps can be removed by colonoscopic polypectomy. Colonoscopy is also very accurate for diagnosis; either limited or total colonoscopy may be indicated in high-risk patients (adenomatous polyposis families) or for follow-up after polypectomy or cancer surgery.

Polyps

The smallest polyps (1–2 mm diameter) may only be shown up by the 'dye-spray' technique in which a dilute blue dye is washed over the surface, the tiny polyps projecting as pale islands which are biopsied. Providing that they are not so numerous as to justify surgery, small polyps are easily destroyed by the 'hot-biopsy' technique in which the polyp is grasped and pulled up on a 'pseudo-pedicle' which, being the narrowest part, is selectively electrocoagulated whereas the biopsy is by-passed and not heated at all (Fig. 1.43).

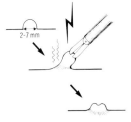

Fig. 1.43

Snare polypectomy is considered in Chapter 8. Careful electrocoagulation is essential before severance, especially in thick stalked polyps where haemorrhage can occur. Patients with larger polyps are admitted afterwards but most polypectomies are rapid and easy and are managed on a day-case basis.

LIMITATIONS AND COMPLICATIONS

It takes more time and skill to perform colonoscopy than to fill the colon with barium and some sedation is usually required, making total colonoscopy not well suited as a first-line or screening examination for the whole colon. The adhesions, strictures or diverticular disease which may make colonscopy impossible and the potential blind-spots have been mentioned (Fig. 1.44).

The complication rate of colonoscopy (usually perforation resulting from instrument trauma or air pressure) should be less than one in 500 examinations. Complications are most likely in the learning phase, especially with a stiffer (two-channel) or older instrument. Haemorrhage is rare except after polypectomy (one in 50 polypectomies). Bacteraemia has been shown to occur during colonoscopy; consideration should be

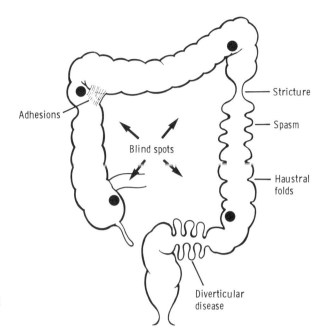

Fig. 1.44 Blind spots and difficulties in colonoscopy.

given to antibiotic cover (ampicillin, gentamycin and metronidazole) in immunosuppressed patients and those with heart valve disease. The mortality of colonoscopy (1 in 5000) is low compared to the potential mortality of the operations avoided. The possible hazards of colonoscopy are, however, enough to restrict total colonoscopy to patients with sufficient clinical indication and to make it desirable to have 'informed consent' beforehand.

REFERENCES AND FURTHER READING

Cotton PB and Williams CB. *Practical gastrointestinal endoscopy*. Oxford: Blackwell Scientific, 1980.

Hunt RH. Rectal bleeding. *Clinics in Gastroenterology* 1978; **7**: 719–40.

Rogers BHG, Silvis SE, Nebel OT, Sugawa C and Mandelstam P. Complications of fibreoptic colonoscopy and polypectomy. *Gastrointestinal Endoscopy* 1975; **22**: 73–77.

Williams CB and Waye JD. Colonoscopy in inflammatory bowel disease. *Clinics in Gastroenterology* 1978; **7**: 701–17.

ANAL MANOMETRY AND ELECTROMYOGRAPHY

Physiology studies are helpful in assessing the normality or abnormality of the muscles of the pelvic floor. The two methods most commonly used are anal manometry and electromyography. Radiological studies to assess the site of the anal canal relative to the bony landmarks of the pelvis may be helpful, as also is a defaecating proctogram. In general, the tests are useful in the assessment of a patient with a deficiency of part of the sphincter or with an intrinsic abnormality of the muscle itself.

ANAL MANOMETRY

The methods used for measuring intra-luminal pressures have been standardised for many years. An open-ended, perfused tube can be used or a miniature balloon connected to a transducer head by a fine catheter. Pressure recorded along the anal canal at rest is mainly due to the internal sphincter and this can be measured by withdrawing the probe through the anal canal from the rectum, taking readings at intervals of 0.5 cm or 1.0 cm (Fig. 3.3). The resulting trace indicates not only the pressure profile but also the length of the functioning anal canal. A low-pressure tracing indicates abnormality in the internal sphincter. Distention of the rectum with a balloon results in a transient relaxation of the internal sphincter. This response is absent in Hirschsprung's disease and the test is a simple and helpful way of differentiating between Hirschsprung's disease and other varieties of megacolon.

The maximum resting anal canal pressure is in the region of 70 to 80 cm of water. With voluntary contraction of the external sphincter muscle, a pressure of 150 cm of water can be achieved. This increment is a useful indication of the functional state of the external sphincter mass. It does not however, differentiate between the various abnormalities which can affect the skeletal muscles.

ELECTROMYOGRAPHY

Simple electromyography using a concentric needle electrode will detect the presence of electrical activity in any of the skeletal muscles of the pelvic floor, or total absence of activity as, for instance, in damage to the cauda equina. It is chiefly useful in those cases where there is a defect in the muscle ring

39

due, for instance, to agenesis or trauma and will delineate the extent. It is of limited value only in detecting intrinsic abnormality of the muscle.

A somewhat more sophisticated investigation is the measurement of reflex latency, assessed by measuring the time interval between an electrical stimulus applied to the perianal skin and the muscle response (anal reflex). This provides some information regarding the state of the nerves supplying the muscles. In the normal it is in the region of 8–10 msec but can rise to 20 msec or above when gross neuropathic change is present. Single fibre electromyography gives even more precise information and is the best method of detecting neuropathic or myopathic change of the pelvic floor, but is a much more difficult technique.

Though it is possible to make a reasonably accurate assessment of the various deficiencies in the pelvic floor muscles by clinical means, physiological studies are helpful in confirming a clinical impression and occasionally in revealing a situation previously unsuspected.

REFERENCES AND FURTHER READING

Lane RH. Clinical application of anorectal physiology. *Proceedings of the Royal Society of Medicine* 1975; **68:** 28–30.

Henry MM and Swash M. Assessment of pelvic floor disorders and incontinence by electrophysiological recording of the anal reflex. *Lancet* 1978; **1:** 1290–91.

Henry MM and Parks AG. The investigation of anorectal function. *Hospital Update* 1980; **6:** 29–41.

2. Normal and Disordered Function of the Colon

PHYSIOLOGY

The essential function of the colon is to receive the fluid contents from the small intestine and, by extracting water, prepare faeces suitable for defaecation at a socially acceptable time at the discretion of the individual. In the course of this preparation electrolyte exchanges occur, and the motor activities of the colon may affect and be affected by other areas of the gastrointestinal tract and even other body systems. As an organ of social comfort, its functions have attracted rather more than their share of interest and knowledge of its physiological activity has often been clouded by unguarded and ill-informed folklore and even professional prejudice.

THE COLONIC MUCOSA

Structure

The normal colonic mucosa presents a smooth surface perforated only by the openings of the crypts of Lieberkuhn. These are remarkably straight and parallel tubules which in the rectum attain a length of 0.07 mm although they are rather shorter in the colon. The mucosa comprises a columnar epithelium with a thin striated border and goblet cells which are more numerous at the mouth than in the depths of the crypt. Electron microscopic studies suggest that many potential mechanisms for defence against mechanical and toxic insult are concentrated at the surface of the colonic mucosal cell, important amongst these being the microvilli with their extended tiny 'hairs'.

The lamina propria is thin but is believed by many authors to be an active part of the reticulo-endothelial system as it is active in phagocytosis, having a high content of histiocytes, reticulin

41

fibres, plasma cells and lymphocytes. The cell content, too, varies with alterations in the bacterial flora.

Mast cells, which store histamine, heparin and 5-hydroxy-tryptamine, are common in the submucosa of the normal colon and their numbers increase greatly in ulcerative colitis. Paneth cells are relatively rare in the normal bowel but increase some 200 times in ulcerative colitis. They contain easily recognisable granules which probably represent proteolytic enzymes.

Mucosal regeneration

Colonic mucosal cells have proliferation rates of 1–2 cells per 100 cells per hour. As crypt columns have, on average, 100 cells, the whole crypt will be replaced in 3–4 days. However, these data have been obtained from terminal patients with malignant disease so that results may be atypical. In animals there is a wide variation in cell turnover rates in the large intestine; variables include the method of study, the use of either colchicine or tritium labelled thymidine, the age of the animal, the state of nutrition and the area of colon studied. In rats the descending colon has three times the proliferation rate of the ascending colon.

The growth of the colonic mucosa may be influenced by gastrointestinal hormones, especially gastrin.

Lesions produced by biopsies of normal human colon, approximately 0.5 cm in diameter and including muscularis mucosae, heal by mucosal regeneration from the periphery, spreading over the base. New crypt formation at the periphery can be recognised in 7–9 days after injury and the lesion is usually completely covered in 21 days. These healing processes are associated with changes in mucosal enzyme activity.

HANDLING OF FLUID BY THE COLON

The colon transforms the fluid chyme accepted from the ileum into a semi-solid mass, faeces, suitable for defaecation. A person with an ileostomy will discharge each day approximately 600 ml of fluid containing 75 mmol of sodium and 5 mmol of potassium. The content of the faeces can be estimated either by direct analysis of the homogenised stool or, more conveniently, by obtaining a dialysate following ingestion of a semi-permeable bag. The daily faecal volume is approximately 100 ml, containing 5 mmol of sodium and 10 mmol of potassium per day. Thus, the activity of the colon results in a net absorption of water and sodium and excretion of potassium. It is probable, however, that the ileum of normal subjects delivers much larger volumes of fluid to the colon than are lost by the ileostomy patient and that the normal colon, therefore, absorbs larger quantities than are suggested by studies on ileostomy subjects. Sodium is absorbed from both proximal and distal colon, but potassium is secreted only in the distal segment, in response to aldosterone. The movement of water and electrolytes is bidirectional and in humans the net exchanges are the resultant of this rapid two way traffic across the mucosa. The colon has a considerable reserve capacity and it is probable that in health it can reabsorb between 2 and 7 litres of fluid. There is a definite limit to the extent to which it can handle electrolytes. If the amount of fluid presented to the colon by the small intestine is greater than this reserve capacity, even if only the small intestine is diseased, the body will lose fluid and electrolytes. The colon also absorbs chloride but excretes bicarbonate; the transport of sodium and water across the colonic mucosa seems to be an active process while that of chloride is passive. Active transport in the colon is associated with lower sodium concentrations in the cell than in the lumen, a potential difference being generated across the cell membrane so that the lumen of the bowel is electrically negative in relation to the intracellular potential. Unlike the small intestine where sodium interacts with glucose in absorption the colon seems to have only a sodium facilitating mechanism and there is no definite evidence of exchange of sodium ions for hydrogen ions by the colonic mucosa.

The absorptive function of the colon can be modified by the general electrolyte control of the body. During salt deprivation, sodium disappears almost entirely from the faeces and such conservation may be at the expense of an increased secretion of potassium. In normal subjects under experimental conditions treatment with d-aldosterone or 9-α-fluorohydrocortisone increases the sodium and water absorption from the colon, demonstrating yet another extra-renal site for the action of mineralocorticoids. Aldosterone also enhances the negative luminal potential difference in the colon. Potassium secretion is not affected by the mineralocorticoids.

It has been estimated that the concentration of stool sodium is 40 mmol per l and of stool potassium 90 mmol per l. The chloride concentration in stool water is only 15 mmol per l and stool bicarbonate about 30 mmol per l. There is, thus an anion gap which is balanced by organic anions, including lactate derived from bacterial fermentation of food residues.

Bile acids are absorbed from the colon by passive diffusion which may be critical in maintaining homeostasis if the terminal ileum has been resected or is affected by disease. Estimates suggest that 5 to 10% of the total body pool of bile acids are absorbed daily from the colon.

The transport of water and electrolyte in the colon is markedly affected by the presence in the lumen of unconjugated bile acids or conjugated dihydroxy bile acids. The mechanism of these effects is not established but both tissue damage and increase of mucosal cyclic AMP have been incriminated. These effects can be significant in disorders of the terminal ileum where the greater quantities of bile acids discharged into the colon can result in severe diarrhoeal states, sometimes termed cholereic enteropathy.

Stool also contains quantities of short chain volatile fatty acids, mainly acetate, proprionate and butyrate. High concentrations of volatile fatty acids can cause diarrhoea and non-volatile fatty acids, especially hydroxy acids, cause water and electrolyte to be secreted by the colon.

COLONIC BACTERIA

Contrary to belief, the majority of colonic bacteria are viable in the stool. Not surprisingly, studies have focused mainly on the aerobic organisms because of the ease with which they can be cultured and isolated, although they account for only a small proportion of the total, as Bacterioides and anaerobic Streptococci may be present in large numbers (see Chapter 1). Lactobacilli of various groups may also exist in numbers exceeding 10^6 viable bacteria per g of stool and large numbers of other bacteria are present but have never been satisfactorily classified or enumerated for lack of suitable culture techniques.

Wide variations in bacterial types and counts occur, but there are no consistent data about the influence of geography or climate on the intestinal flora. The relative proportions of bacteria in the colon are altered by antimicrobial agents and by diet. Non-absorbed sugars passing unsplit into the colon (disaccharidase deficiency: alactasia) may promote a relative overgrowth of lactose fermenting organisms resulting in reduction in stool pH and frequency of defaecation.

The quantity and type of dietary fibre has marked effects on the bulk and nature of the stool (See Constipation). The ingestion of certain fibres results in a stool 2 to 3 times normal weight. Lignins and certain celluloses probably have the greatest effect; hemi-celluloses, which are largely digested in the human gastrointestinal tract, also have some effect. The bacterial composition of the stool is quite different in populations ingesting high fibre diets from populations with lower fibre intake.

Less well understood are the subtle effects of general environmental factors on the microbial population of the colon. Such alterations can cause histological damage and allow the establishment of intestinal pathogens or favour the multiplication of microbial species which, though not truly virulent, have undesirable chemical activities such as the production of ammonia or of biologically active amines. Other environmental agents may have toxic effects on the colonic mucosa. Agents including cadmium and asbestos have been suggested as contributing to the increased incidence of colon cancer. Similarly, lithocholic acid produced by bacterial action on the primary bile acids in the colon has been shown to be carcinogenic in high concentrations. Much interest has centred around the possible protection against these agents provided by binding materials such as fibre but the significance of this is not yet defined.

The importance of colonic bacteria to the host has become more obvious following the observation of anatomical and physiological alterations which occur in the gastointestinal tract of germ-free animals. In these animals the caecum, for example, becomes enormous but its wall is hypotonic, probably due to the abnormal presence of musculotropic bioactive materials; the mucosa is viliform and the content much more fluid than expected. The haemoconcentration suffered by such animals is thought to be due to alterations in absorption from the large bowel.

INTESTINAL GAS

All normal persons pass gas (flatus). The amount passed ranges widely from about 200 to 2000 ml per day. The amounts are influenced by diet; the effect of beans in increasing the quantities passed has been well studied. Most swallowed air is belched up but some probably passes through the intestine to be passed *per rectum*. Ninety-nine per cent of the gas passed *per rectum* is a mixture of nitrogen, carbon dioxide, hydrogen, oxygen and methane. Oxygen is present only in small amounts, most of the nitrogen is swallowed, hydrogen and methane are produced entirely by bacterial action and the carbon dioxide is probably also a metabolic product.

Most of the hydrogen produced in the colon is absorbed and excreted by the lungs and a good correlation exists between simultaneous measurements of breath hydrogen excretion and hydrogen production in the colon. Breath hydrogen has, therefore, been used as an estimate of colonic hydrogen production and thus indirectly of colonic bacterial activity. Agents known to change colonic bacterial composition, such as non-absorbed sugars (sorbitol, mannitol, lactulose) result in increases in breath hydrogen output.

NEUROMUSCULAR FUNCTION OF THE COLON

Transit

Transit through the alimentary tract is relatively slow. Studies with glass beads have shown that a considerable percentage of normal subjects retain 30 or 40% of the beads ingested for as

45

long as nine days. Using the non-absorbed marker chromic oxide labelled with Cr^{51}, three quarters of the radioactivity is excreted in 96 hours but there is wide variation between subjects, and in the same subject on different occasions (Fig. 2.1). Transit through the colon accounts for the greater part of

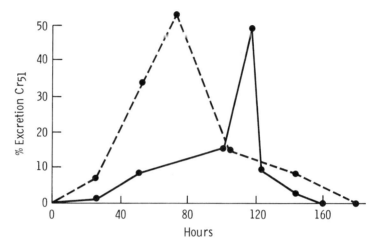

Fig. 2.1 Different faecal excretion rates of Cr^{51}.

the total time of passage. Free mixing of content occurs in the colon so that material may be passed from the anus earlier than similar substances ingested previously; barium discs or pellets ingested 12 hours before radiography arrive in the distal colon before others taken 24 hours previously.

Alvarez (1948) has likened transit through the colon to a railway siding on which are standing three trucks:

'Every day a new one arrives and bumps off the end one so that three remain. Occasionally one arrives with such force that it bumps all three off, and then three days have to elapse before the siding is full enough so that a truck arriving at one end can push one out at the other. Some normal persons are found to have seven trucks on the siding, and some constipated patients who become bloated and uncomfortable when they are put on the usual bulky diet have perhaps ten trucks on the siding'.

This analogy is useful provided it is also appreciated that some mixing takes place between each day's ileal discharge and material previously in the colon.

Following the taking of laxatives the colon may be completely emptied and thus the bowel will not and, indeed, cannot act until refilling occurs, which may take 3–4 days. The constant administration of a laxative is thus illogical.

The movements of the colon can be studied radiologically or by measuring the pressure generated within the bowel.

The study of movements of the colon

Radiology

Radiology has been used to study motility since the turn of the present century and pioneer radiologists including Cannon, Hurst and Holznecht, made large contributions to our understanding of colon function. Radiology gives useful information about the change in contour of the colon and the movement of its content, but the usefulness of the technique is limited on account of the radiation hazard, particularly in view of the fact that colonic movements are slow and thus only a small number of complete cycles of activity can be recorded within the permitted exposure time.

Pressure recordings

Balloon studies introduce a foreign body into the lumen of the bowel but are a simple, reliable and inexpensive method of recording comparative data. Miniature balloons record pressure changes reflecting intraluminal activity and large balloons measure pressure/volume relationships approximating to wall 'tone'.

Open ended tubes with a suitable transducer and recording system measure the pressure in the lumen of the colon. Blockage of the tube by mucosa or faeces can be overcome by having multiple holes near the tip and by constantly perfusing fluid through the tube at a slow rate to maintain patency.

Radiotelemetry capsules are small pressure-sensitive radio transmitters that are swallowed by the subject and pass freely through the intestine. They may remain relatively immobile in the caecum for long periods of time, recording the intraluminal pressure in their vicinity. They are specially indicated in studies in the right of the colon.

Description of movements

Radiological appearances

The movements of the colon are so slow that Barclay thought that the colon presented a picture of still life. However, as early as 1911, Schwartz made repeated tracings of the image of the bismuth filled colon on the x-ray screen and found that slow contractions were constantly occurring, and this has been repeatedly confirmed by cineradiographic studies.

Haustrations

The normal colon is partially or completely divided into segments by so-called haustrations. This appearance is the result of three factors. Some of the sacculations and contraction rings are permanent and persist after death. At the sites of these rings there is a concentration of thickened muscle and they are probably pivotal points of colonic muscular activity. Mucosal folding also contributes to the haustral appearance. The third component is provided by the intermittent muscular activity of the colonic wall. These segmenting contractions do not normally result in transit of the colonic content but in to-and-fro movements over a short distance.

Mass movements

From the early days of radiology it became clear that occasionally the content of the colon is transported rapidly over considerable lengths. Holznecht saw this twice in one-thousand examinations. He described this as

> 'a widespread and vehement act, consisting in a sudden shift in a volume of faeces filling about one-third of the colon to the next empty section of the colon of somewhat similar length. This shift is preceded by a sudden disappearance of the haustral segmentation. The wall of the lower receiving sector shows the same behaviour which, however, is immediately replaced by a quick return to haustral segmentation'.

It is likely that these mass movements occur by the fortunate association of a powerful but otherwise normal segmenting wave (see below) associated with extensive distal relaxation. Whatever the exact mechanism, these movements are the main factors resulting in the passage of faeces along the colon.

Intraluminal pressure records

Various attempts have been made to classify the variable patterns of activity that can be recorded from the intestine. No fully adequate classification of colonic motility has yet been devised, although the application of computer techniques has resulted in a clearer understanding of the underlying physiological processes.

Segmentation

The most common waves recorded from the sigmoid colon have the simple form illustrated in Fig. 2.2. The principal waves represent slow pressure changes, waxing and waning over approximately half a minute. The pressure varies from less than 5 to more than 100 cm of water. The distribution of activity is irregular and phases of activity alternate with phases of relative inactivity. The duration and proportion of the active and inactive periods vary widely from subject to subject and in the same subject from time to time. Periods of complete quiescence of up to one and a half hours have been observed.

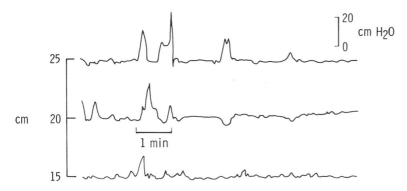

Fig. 2.2 Principal pressure waves recorded simultaneously at different distances from the anus.

Waves may occur singly, in small groups, or in rhythmic sequences lasting many minutes.

Duration of activity

The left colon is a relatively active organ and pressure changes occur for a high proportion of the recording time.

The right colon has been studied less intensively than the left but the total duration of its activity is less and the pressure waves are more often single and are less frequent. Because the motility of the right colon is less, the caecal content is retained for long periods allowing ample time for absorption.

Motility in diarrhoea and constipation

Pressure studies have been useful in the study of the mechanics of diarrhoea and constipation. The common impression among clinicians is that diarrhoea is a hypermotile state while constipation is a hypomotile state. However, paradoxically, in patients with diarrhoea there is usually a great decrease in the degree of pressure activity recorded, while in persons with constipation activity is often normal or increased. When intraluminal pressures are present, resistance to passage is great and transit is restricted; whereas when intraluminal pressures are low, resistance is low and transit is facilitated.

Myoelectric control

Electrical activity exists in the colon, as in other areas of the gastrointestinal tract. Slow waves of action potential occur but their configuration and time course is less regular than in the small intestine, electrical activity being interspersed with electrical silence. From time to time rapid or more prolonged spike bursts occur.

In isolated colon preparations of the cat, the frequency of the slow wave gradually increases from the ileocaecal junction with a marked increase in the frequency in the distal colon; in man the situation is less clear possibly because of the inadequacies and inaccuracies of available recording methods. How these electrical potential changes relate to mechanical activity in man is also not yet clear.

Slow wave activity and spike bursts have been shown to be altered by autonomic drugs, for example carbachol prolongs slow wave activity and increases the frequency of spike bursts; neostigmine produces a greater percentage of motor activity in the rectosigmoid as does morphine, serotonin, pentagastrin and ouabain.

Factors affecting the movements of the colon

There is a large day to day variation in the motility recorded from the colon of any given individual and possibly the main factor responsible for this variation is the difference in the state of mental activity. Sleep can depress the motility of the colon and noxious stimuli may result in large alterations. Some of the factors influencing the movements of the colon are illustrated in Fig. 2.3.

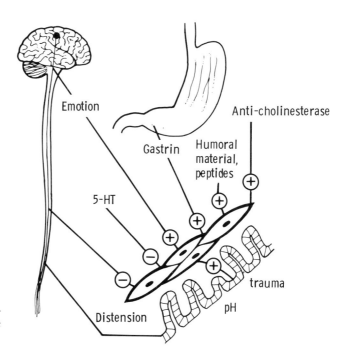

Fig. 2.3 Some factors influencing movements of the colon.

Emotion

Many claims have been made that life stress affects colonic motility and experimentally it has been shown that the discussion of emotional experiences can result in changes in colonic activity. Approximately the same proportion (one-quarter) of normal subjects, persons suffering from irritable bowel syndrome or ulcerative colitis studied manometrically showed a colonic response to emotional interview. However, attempts to establish causal relationships between emotion and physical changes in the colon are difficult to interpret.

Changes in posture, such as standing up or lying down, or pressure on the abdominal wall can affect the motility recorded from the colon. Physical activity increases the rate of transit along the colon, particularly after meals. *Physical activity*

Eating is probably the most important physiological stimulus which affects changes in the secretion and motility of the alimentary tract. Since the turn of the century it has been known that eating results in an increase in the 'writhing movements' of the terminal ileum and caecum and that at this time the ileum may discharge its contents into the colon. At the same time, there is an increased chance that the contents of the colon will be propelled in a mass movement. *Food*

After eating there is an augmentation of the segmenting activity of the colon, most marked in the sigmoid region. In man and animals, this response can be elicited by the sight or smell of the meal and the degree of the response may be related to the subject's relish for eating.

The term 'gastro-colic reflex' is an imprecise one and should be dropped. It has been used to refer to the mass movement which occurs more frequently after eating, to the increase in segmenting activity with food and to the frequency of defaecation after eating. These phenomena, though related, are distinct. The term is also unhelpful as there is doubt whether the events it describes are nervous reflexes.

Experimental studies in animals conflict about the possible pathways for the gastro-colic responses and in man increased segmentation after eating has been shown to persist after vagotomy, after transection of the spinal cord at different levels, and following complete destruction of the lumbo-sacral cord. Evidence that this response is conducted along the plexuses of the gut is based on a single series of animal experiments and has never been confirmed in man. The response may be mediated by hormones and cross-circulation experiments have shown that a humoral substance is released after eating which can result in changes in colonic motor activity. The exact nature of this hormone is not clear but various candidates have been considered. Cholecystokinin increases colonic segmenting activity whereas glucagon and secretin decrease it. The probability is

51

that the colonic response to eating is the result of the effects of the several gastrointestinal hormones released by eating.

This response to eating is probably one of the most important co-ordinating mechanisms of the gastro-intestinal tract, and disturbance of it may be the basis of a number of clinical syndromes.

Nerve supply to the colon

The large bowel is innervated by sympathetic and para-sympathetic nerves (See Chapter 4).

The intrinsic plexuses

Classically divided into the condensations of Meissner's and Auerbach's plexuses, it is clear that an abundant network of ganglia and nerve cells is present throughout the submucosa and muscularis propria of the bowel. These plexuses are responsible for the intrinsic activity of the gut. Bayliss and Starling, at the end of the last century, enunciated their law of the intestine, stating 'Excitation at any point of the gut excites contraction above, inhibition below'. This response occurs after all cerebrospinal connections to the gut have been excised and even after removal of Meissner's plexus. In animals the colonic muscle can be stimulated mechanically or chemically through the mucosa, a response that can be blocked by local administration of hexamethonium or by cocainisation of the mucosa.

Autonomic control

The classical description of the parasympathetic system as motor to the colon and the sympathetic system as inhibitory is unhelpful since the response of the muscle of the intestine varies according to the nature of the applied stimulus. It is more likely that the function of autonomic nerves is to provide fine control over the local reflex and intrinsic muscular mechanisms.

In the distal colon of man the main extrinsic nerve supply may be inhibitory. An inhibitory centre for colonic movements exists in the lumbar region of cats, and paraplegic patients with complete destruction of the lumbo-sacral cord have more irregular activity than normal, associated clinically with gross constipation (Fig. 2.4). Spinal cord transection above T.10 without major destruction of the lumbo-sacral region does not result in any marked change in colonic segmenting activity.

Reflexes elicited by distension

It is difficult in the normal subject to demonstrate any marked change in the segmenting activity of the colon in response to a distending bolus, but in paraplegic patients with complete transection of the cord in the cervical or thoracic region, who have intact somatic reflex activity in the segments

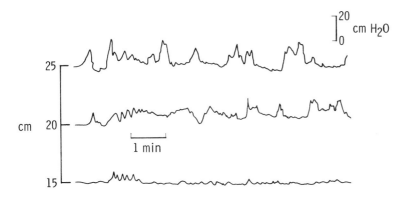

Fig. 2.4 Irregular pressure waves recorded in a patient with complete destruction of the lumbo-sacral cord.

below the level of the lesion, a definite response to distension can be elicited.

Balloon distension in the sigmoid colon results in local reflex inhibition of segmenting activity with movement of bowel content distally and also an increase of segmenting activity in the duodenum and terminal ileum. Motor activity of the colon can have profound effects on.other areas of the body (e.g. sweating) via pathways of the autonomic nervous system. Rectal distension results in a prompt and complete relaxation of the anus, although normally defaecation does not occur.

The effect on the colon of a number of physiological agents has been studied. 5-hydroxytryptamine, which stimulates the small intestine, inhibits segmentation in the colon and in excess causes diarrhoea.

Cholinergic agents in general stimulate colonic motility although the response to methacholine or acetylcholine can be variable. Prostigmine results in a 300–400% increase in sigmoid motor activity in normal persons although the response of the right side of the colon is less marked than that of the left, the response being even greater in persons who have the irritable colon syndrome or a postdysenteric irritable bowel.

The response to belladonna type alkaloids is also variable. Atropine in high doses usually inhibits all colonic activity but in the usual therapeutic doses the results are decidedly variable.

Opiates, particularly morphine, given intravenously or intramuscularly increase intraluminal pressures recorded from the colon, the effect being exaggerated in segments of colon bearing diverticula. In contrast, pethidine may diminish the number of phasic contractions. The effects of other pharmacologic agents including barbiturates, benzodiazepines and other tranquillisers and sedatives have not been defined.

Effect of drugs

53

The role of prostaglandins on colonic function is also un-defined, but probably significant. *In vitro* prostaglandin F contracts both muscle layers of the colon, whereas prostaglandin E contracts the longitudinal muscle but relaxes the circular muscle. Given orally in man, prostaglandin E_1 increases transit along the colon with expulsion of gas and faeces. Intravenous administration also produces an effect, but only in higher doses suggesting that the diarrhoea noted after oral administration may be related to the presence of a metabolite. Some of the effects of prostaglandins registered in studies on the colon may be related to the increased rate of flow of ileal fluid resulting from the increased small intestinal secretion stimulated by prostaglandins.

NORMAL BOWEL HABIT

It is sometimes implied that anything goes for normal bowel habit and that failure of the bowel to act for 2 or 3 weeks is normal. However, the great majority of persons evacuate their bowel approximately once per day and in any normal population more than 99 per cent will have bowel actions between the limits of three per day and three per week. More than three bowel actions per day for any length of time should be regarded as abnormal until proved otherwise.

Defaecation

The mechanism of defaecation is now reasonably clear. The initiating stimulus is still not fully defined, but it is related to a critical threshold of sigmoid (and possibly descending colon) distension. Both the area of bowel distended and the pressure per unit area are probably important.

Subsequently haustrations disappear and the bolus begins to move forwards. The length of the bolus varies from time to time and may include the content of the lower sigmoid and upper rectum only, or the whole content of the descending colon. With the subject in the squatting position, the bolus, lubricated by rectal mucus, moves largely under the influence of gravity. It is followed by a single peristaltic wave (mass movement) but, as in the case of the oesophagus, this wave does not so much force the bolus forwards as sweep clean the sigmoid and rectum.

On reaching the upper rectum the bolus induces afferent impulses thought to be due to stimulation of stretch receptors in the pelvic floor, which initiate the defaecation reflex (see Chapter 3). At this stage the subject gives conscious consent to the act and relaxes the voluntary component of the anal sphincter mechanism. The further movement of stool into the rectum, possibly aided by some rise in intra-abdominal pressure due to straining, distends it and establishes the full recto-anal reflex. The anus dilates widely and the bolus is discharged.

The whole defaecation mechanism is dependent on the integrity of the lumbo-sacral cord and the pelvic and pudendal nerves, although it can be elicited in subjects with complete transection of the spinal cord at higher levels; in some of these paraplegic persons the defaecation mechanism can be triggered by a stimulus to the somatic innervation such as stroking the thigh or the peri-anal region.

REGULATORY PEPTIDES

Several regulatory peptides are known to be present in the muscle and mucosa of the colon. Two of these, somatostatin and enteroglucagon, are localised to endocrine cells in the mucosa. Enteroglucagon is released by luminal nutriments and is thought to act mainly on the small intestine, slowing transit and increasing mucosal cell growth. It thus acts as a feed-back to prevent unabsorbed nutriments from escaping into the colon. Somatostatin on the other hand, probably acts locally (paracrine or local hormone) exercising an inhibitory influence on colonic mucosal growth and secretion.

Other peptides, including encephalin, vasoactive intestinal peptide (VIP), bombesin and substance P are localised to the neural elements. They are thus synthesised in the neurones of Auerbach's and Meissner's plexuses and released locally to affect smooth muscle contraction, blood flow and secretion. They probably play an important role in control of the ileocaecal valve and anal sphincter.

REFERENCES AND FURTHER READING

Alvarez WC. *An introduction to gastroenterology*. London: Heinemann, 1948.

Bloom SR. ed. *Gut hormones*. Edinburgh: Churchill Livingstone, 1978.

Connell AM. The motor action of the large bowel. In: Code CF, ed. *Handbook of physiology—alimentary canal, 4, motility*. Washington: American Physiological Society, 1968: 2075–91.

Duthie HL, ed. *Gastrointestinal motility in health and disease*. Lancaster: MTP Press, 1978.

Mekhjian HS, Phillips SF and Hofmann AF. Colonic secretion of water and electrolytes induced by bile acids: perfusion studies in man. *Journal of Clinical Investigation* 1971; **50:** 1569–77.

Schuster MM, Hookman P, Hendrix TR and Mendeloff AI. Simultaneous manometric recording of internal and external anal sphincteric reflexes. *Bulletin of Johns Hopkins Hospital* 1965; **116:** 79–88.

Truelove SC. Movements of the large intestine. *Physiology Review* 1966; **46:** 457–512.

DRUGS FOR DISORDERED MOTILITY

Accounts of the drugs used in treating disordered motility of all regions of the alimentary tract have been written by Bennett and Misiewicz (1973) and Greenberger, Arvanitakis and Hurwitz (1978); Binder (1977) has reviewed the pharmacology of laxatives. This chapter describes the drugs available to treat diarrhoea, constipation or muscle spasm, and discusses their modes of action, but details of adverse effects are mainly omitted. Reference to original publications can be found in the reviews cited above.

DIARRHOEA

Most drugs used to treat diarrhoea act non-selectively to cause slow transit. Although generally safe these drugs can be harmful, for example in inflammatory or infective bowel disease such as ulcerative colitis and antibiotic-associated colitis. In most cases, there has been little or no investigation of the mechanism of action in man, so that animal data are included.

Antidiarrhoeal drugs which slow transit

Morphine

Morphine in low non-analgesic doses is useful for treating acute diarrhoea, and is often given mixed with kaolin. Its mode of action is not entirely clear, but seems to result from decreased propulsion in both the small and large intestine, accompanied by increased muscle tone and raised intraluminal pressure; the stomach is similarly affected. It seems likely that morphine acts on receptors for enkephalins. The increase of non-propulsive muscle activity in human intestine may involve a cholinergic mechanism, since atropine inhibits morphine-induced spasm of the terminal ileum. Guinea-pig ileum is often used as a laboratory model of the human intestine, but this is not entirely appropriate as numerous species-differences occur. For example, morphine reduces the output of acetylcholine from intramural nerves in guinea-pig ileum at low rates of stimulation, but such a mechanism seems contrary to the atropine-sensitive stimulation of human intestine by morphine. Furthermore guinea-pig colon does not respond like the ileum, since morphine does not affect colonic acetycholine output. Studies in dogs indicate that morphine acts on intramural cholinergic nerves and not directly on the muscle, since the drug was effective when it was perfused through the blood vessels of the gut but not when it bathed strips of isolated muscle. An additional mechanism in dog intestine is probably the release of 5-hydroxytryptamine but not of histamine. Other possibilities, such as a blocking action on inhibitory nerve pathways in the gut, have not been examined, but in rats there is evidence that morphine acts centrally to cause constipation: intracerebroventricular injection of morphine slowed the intestinal passage of a charcoal meal given orally, but the systemic dose needed to produce this effect was about 200 times greater. The morphine antagonist naloxone given intracerebroventricularly blocked the effect of morphine given by either route.

Codeine (methyl morphine) and similar derivatives presumably act like the parent compound to produce constipation. Codeine has an extremely low potential for addiction, and is therefore preferable to most of the others in this class for treating chronic diarrhoea.

Codeine and other morphine-like drugs

Diphenoxylate (Lomotil) resembles pethidine chemically but it is not analgesic. Prolonged administration may produce dependence of the morphine type but short-term administration in recommended doses carries negligible risk. However, to make drug abuse even less likely diphenoxylate is mixed with a sub-therapeutic amount of atropine. On the rabbit isolated ileum the pure drug has 1% of the anticholinergic activity of atropine, and similar antispasmodic activity to papaverine. Studies in guinea-pig ileum show diphenoxylate to be more potent than morphine in reducing the circular muscle peristaltic contractions but less potent in reducing the longitudinal muscle activity. Diphenoxylate may act on intramural ganglia and its mode of action in reducing the peristaltic response may be intermediate in type between those of morphine and of ganglion-blocking drugs. However, the available data do not exclude other actions such as stimulation of postganglionic nerves, inhibition of a non-cholinergic excitatory transmitter, or a direct action on the muscle. It is again difficult to relate these data to man in whom diphenoxylate usually increases segmenting pressure waves in the small intestine, perhaps acting like morphine.

Diphenoxylate

Loperamide (Imodium) is structurally related to diphenoxylate but has different pharmacological characteristics and a long plasma half-life (about 40 hours). It does not constrict the pupil, unlike the drugs discussed so far, and may therefore lack the

Loperamide

57

central effects which can cause other drugs to be abused. No narcotic effects occur in man and the morphine antagonist naloxone does not cause symptoms or signs of withdrawal. However, loperamide binds to narcotic receptors *in vitro* and can inhibit the signs of morphine withdrawal in monkeys. Again, guinea-pig intestine has been used for pharmacological studies. *In vitro*, loperamide reduces the frequency and amplitude of ileal peristaltic waves; the mechanism of action is not entirely clear but may involve block of acetylcholine release within guinea-pig intestine. However, the earlier discussion on species differences casts doubt on whether this mechanism occurs in man. Some drug is excreted in the faeces so that there may be a local action, but it is also possible that the drug acts after reaching the intestine through the circulation. Because of its effectiveness, the mild and infrequent side effects, and the apparent lack of central action, loperamide seems preferable to the other drugs discussed so far for treatment of chronic diarrhoea.

Antidiarrhoeal drugs with different actions

5-hydroxytryptamine antagonists

Methysergide is useful in the treatment of diarrhoea in the carcinoid syndrome, but it has no effect on the flushes which may have a different aetiology. The drug antagonises the effect of 5-hydroxytryptamine which acts in man at intestinal receptors located on the muscle cells.

Aspirin

References relating to aspirin, prostaglandins and diarrhoea can be found in the review by Bennett (1978). Uterine cervical irradiation for cancer can produce diarrhoea resistant to usual forms of therapy but which responds to the prostaglandin synthesis inhibitor aspirin. Presumably incidental irradiation damages the bowel and releases prostaglandins which have various effects including a strong stimulation of ileal secretion. Prostaglandins may be involved in diarrhoea associated with some endocrine tumours and in some diarrhoeas due to intestinal infection. In some species indomethacin, an inhibitor of prostaglandin synthesis, reduces the diarrhoea caused by cholera toxin, and *Escherchia coli* endotoxin can stimulate prostaglandin synthesis in rabbit intestine. It remains to be seen whether or not inhibitors of prostaglandin synthesis are of value in human infective diarrhoeas. Since prostaglandins are formed in human intestinal mucosa their normal release may also increase the effect of diarrhoeogenic stimuli which may act by non–prostaglandin mechanisms. If so, inhibitors of prostaglandin synthesis may have a wider usefulness.

This strongly basic ion-exchange resin is not absorbed when taken orally, and binds acidic substances within the gut. Cholestyramine is therefore used to bind bile acids in various conditions including the watery diarrhoea induced by excessive amounts of bile salts reaching the colon in ileal dysfunction, ileal resection or after vagotomy.

Cholestyramine

Nutmeg is commonly used in India to treat diarrhoea but this use is not widely known in the West. Various reports have indicated the value of nutmeg in treating severe diarrhoea, and the action possibly involves inhibition of prostaglandin synthesis or action. Thus minute amounts of powdered nutmeg inhibited synthesis of prostaglandin-like material when human colonic mucosa was homogenised, and nutmeg non-selectively inhibited prostaglandin E_2-induced contractions of rat stomach. However, we do not know if either of these mechanisms contribute to the therapeutic effect, since the active ingredient(s) may be metabolised *in vivo*.

Nutmeg

A problem with nutmeg in man is its toxicity, since symptoms can occur which are similar to those produced by toxic amounts of amphetamine and atropine. The value of nutmeg may therefore be in diarrhoea resistant to conventional treatment. Investigators have used several grams daily in divided doses, but no experiments have been reported on the effect of lower doses.

The uses and actions of bulk expanders in both diarrhoea and constipation are discussed later in this Chapter.

Bulk expanders

CONSTIPATION

Constipation is probably the most common disturbance of gut motility, and many drugs are available to treat it. Although laxatives relieve trivial constipation, they are generally unsatisfactory in the management of severe and chronic disorders. In simple constipation, where there is no underlying organic disease, excessive segmental contractions of the colon occur which delay the transit of faeces (the reverse of diarrhoea). Consequently, more water is absorbed, the stools become small and hard, and the reduced distension of the colon diminishes the stimulus to defaecate. The pathophysiology of constipation is not fully understood, but poor toilet training and a low-residue diet can be contributory factors.

Various names are given to drugs used in constipation: purgatives, laxatives, cathartics and aperients. Some use a name to indicate the efficacy and the type of stool produced, whereas others use the terms interchangeably. The drugs which stimulate the gut in constipation have been described as 'irritant' but with many drugs this term is inaccurate and the term 'stimulant' is preferable.

Some discussions on the mechanisms by which laxatives act have concentrated on the stimulation of gut muscle. In his review Binder (1977) concentrated mainly on stimulation of water secretion by laxatives. Both mechanisms can probably be important as primary events in laxation, but presumably in some cases the increased motility results mainly from distension by the increased intraluminal content.

Laxatives

Anthraquinone derivatives

The anthraquinone (anthracene) group includes senna, cascara, aloes and rhubarb, and contains oxymethyl-anthraquinones mostly as their glycosides. The glycosides are inactive but they are converted in the intestine to the active aglycones emodin and chrysophanic acid (tri- and di-oxymethyl-anthraquinone, respectively) partly by bacterial action; danthron, a constituent of Dorbanex, is a synthetic dihydroxyanthraquinone laxative chemically related to emodin. The aglycones are thought to stimulate Auerbach's plexus in the colon (not in the stomach or small intestine), but this mode of action has not been proved. Furthermore, senna, aloes and cascara have some effect when administered parenterally. Senna inhibits water absorption in the cat large intestine and, as with other laxatives, this is probably an important part of the drug's action in man. The additional intraluminal fluid softens the faeces, and the increased bulk stimulates bowel motility.

Diphenylmethane derivatives

This group includes phenolphthalein and bisacodyl. Since phenolphthalein turns red in alkaline solution, its presence can easily be detected in the stool. This is a useful test in patients with diarrhoea due to phenolphthalein abuse.

Bisacodyl (Dulcolax) is irritating and is therefore administered as enteric-coated tablets, which should not be chewed or given with antacids that cause tablet disintegration in the stomach, or as suppositories. Another member of the group, oxyphenisatin (Veripaque) is no longer used orally as it may cause jaundice, particularly when given with dioctyl sodium sulphosuccinate; Veripaque enemas appear to be safe. These diphenylmethane derivatives have been called 'contact' laxatives since bisacodyl acts on the human or cat colon by stimulating sensory nerves which can be blocked by local anaesthetic drugs.

Bisacodyl introduced into the rectum of anaesthetised cats activates mucosal sensory nerves which reflexly stimulate the proximal colon, with little effect on the distal colon.

Further evidence in cats for a contact action of bisacodyl is that the dose has to be increased 8 times for an effect with parenteral adminisration, and the drug is ineffective if the bile duct or small intestine is ligated. Studies with rabbit isolated intestine show that the colon is more sensitive than the ileum.

In man only small amounts of orally administered bisacodyl are absorbed so that at least 95% of the drug reaches the colon. Up to 15% of phenolphthalein may be absorbed and then partly excreted in the bile, thus prolonging the effect of the drug.

The diphenylmethane drugs undoubtedly have a strong stimulant effect on colonic motility, but they also affect fluid transport. Thus bisacodyl increased the output of ileostomy fluid in patients; in rat gut it increased the net flux of water and sodium into the lumen, the colon being 40 times more sensitive than rat jejunum.

Saline purgatives are poorly absorbed salts of magnesium, usually magnesium sulphate (Epsom salts) or phosphate. Previously they were thought to act by retaining intraluminal fluid, but this is only part of the explanation. Cholecystokinin released by magnesium sulphate probably stimulates motility of the small intestine and colon, and magnesium sulphate increases the intraluminal content of water and sodium.

Saline purgatives

Bulk expanders may be used in the management of both constipation and diarrhoea since by retaining water they 'average out' stool consistency. Unprocessed bran is the most natural way of increasing bulk in the stool, and its use is described later in this chapter.

Other agents may be used, and they include methyl cellulose (Celevac), ispaghula (Isogel) and sterculia (Normacol Special). Sterculia is also marketed combined with the contact laxative frangula (Normacol Standard) which is unsuitable for many patients with bowel frequency or pain of colonic origin.

Bulk expanders

Liquid paraffin is a mild laxative which is poorly absorbed. It therefore lubricates the colon and it softens the stools in various ways which are not fully understood.

Mineral oil

Dioctyl sodium sulphosuccinate is an anionic detergent which has previously been classified as a surfactant (i.e. a substance which increases the faecal penetration and retention of

Dioctyl sodium sulphosuccinate

water). However, in human jejunum the drug decreases water absorption, and in rat caecum it increases the net secretion of water and electrolytes probably due to an increase in mucosal cyclic AMP.

Castor oil

Castor oil is a triglyceride of ricinoleic acid which is hydrolysed in the small intestine to the free acid. Unlike the drugs mentioned previously, the cathartic action is due to a stimulant effect on the small bowel, and semi-fluid stools are produced within 1–6 hours. Recent evidence suggests that the action may involve stimulation of prostaglandin synthesis; some prostaglandins strongly stimulate fluid secretion in the small intestine.

Bile salts

Bile salts are anionic detergents included in some proprietary laxatives. They presumably act by increasing the amount of fluid in the intestinal lumen and by stimulating colonic motility (see previously under cholestyramine).

Lactulose

Lactulose (Duphalac) is a synthetic disaccharide (beta-galactosidofructose) which is poorly absorbed because the intestine does not contain the appropriate disaccharidase. Lactulose itself has no primary action on gut mosility, and although it retains water in the small intestine this seems of importance only with large doses. Colonic bacteria break the drug down into lactic acid and other poorly absorbed products which increase the osmolarity of the colonic contents and increase their water content; the effect on pH may also be important. Intraluminal acidification of isolated guinea-pig ileum or colon increases the peristaltic activity and the propulsion of fluid. In man, the faeces are acidified to pH 4–5 within 4 days following the administration of lactulose, and elevated faecal excretion of organic acids occurs in diarrhoea accompanying malabsorption. Furthermore the lower pH may reduce sodium and water absorption, as occurs in rat intestine.

Resins

Resins such as podophyllum, jalap, ipomoea, colocynth, elaterin and gamboge produce copious fluid stools, but are irritant, produce griping and have systemic side effects. They are therefore rarely used and have no place in modern medicine.

SPASMOLYTIC DRUGS

Drugs which inhibit spasm of colonic muscle are used to treat the painful contractions that occur in the irritable bowel syndrome and in diverticular disease.

Cholinergic antagonists

Acetylcholine contracts almost all regions of the human

gastrointestinal tract, and this effect can be antagonised by drugs which block acetylcholine receptors. Cholinergic antagonists such as atropine, glycopyrronium, poldine (Nacton) and propantheline (Probanthine) block the receptors on the muscle cells (muscarinic receptors). Propantheline also blocks the cholinergic receptors in the ganglia of parasympathetic nerves (nicotinic receptors), and so inhibits the stimulus to release acetylcholine from the post-ganglionic nerves supplying the muscle cells.

Drugs which are not pimarily anticholinergic

The side effects of parasympathetic blockade such as a dry mouth and blurred vision limit the usefulness of anticholinergic therapy. Drugs which relieve spasm by another action on the muscle include mebeverine (Colofac) which in guinea-pig and rabbits is substantially more potent than papaverine as a spasmolytic. Dicyclomine (Merbentyl) is an anti-spasmodic drug with low anticholinergic activity.

No other newer agents have been reported to be useful as spasmolytics although it has been suggested that peppermint oil (in enteric-coated capsules) may give symptomatic improvement in patients with the irritable bowel syndrome.

REFERENCES AND FURTHER READING

Bennett A. Prostaglandins. In: Turner P, Shand DG, eds. *Recent Advances in Clinical Pharmacology*. Edinburgh: Churchill Livingstone, 1978: 17–30.

Bennett A, Misiewicz JJ. Drugs used in treating disordered motility of the alimentary tract. In: Holton P, ed. *Encyclopaedia of Pharmacology*. New York: Pergamon Press, 1973: **39a,** 433–55.

Binder HJ. Pharmacology of laxatives. *Annual Review of Pharmacology and Toxicology* 1977; **17:** 355–67.

Greenberger NJ, Arvanitakis C, Hurwitz A. *Drug Treatment of Gastrointestinal Disorders: Basic and Practical Principles*. New York: Churchill Livingstone, 1978.

IRRITABLE BOWEL SYNDROME

In a large number of patients with gastrointestinal disorders a definite diagnosis is never reached, despite thorough clinical and laboratory investigation. Many of these patients suffer from a disordered bowel habit and abdominal pain, but their general health and nutrition remains good and they are usually diagnosed as having the irritable bowel syndrome. The term irritable bowel syndrome is to be preferred to others such as mucous colitis or spastic colon, because it implies no preconceived ideas regarding the aetiology of the syndrome, but it makes the point that disturbance of function with irritability of either the large or the small bowel (or both) may play a part in the mechanism of the symptoms.

Irritable bowel syndrome is one of the commonest disorders of the gut encountered in clinical practice and has been estimated to account for approximately one third to one half of all patients presenting with digestive complaints. In the absence of objective diagnostic tests there are no reliable epidemiological data about the prevalence, or the incidence of irritable bowel syndrome in the community, but the number of patients in whom this diagnosis is made appears to be rising; whether this reflects a true increase in numbers, or an increased frequency with which the diagnosis is made by doctors, is not known.

Irritable bowel syndrome is commoner among women than men. Most patients develop symptoms in the second to fourth decade, although irritable bowel syndrome of childhood is well recognised and may persist into adult life.

PATHOGENESIS

Colonic motility

Much attention has been focussed on abnormalities of colonic motility in the pathogenesis of irritable bowel syndrome. Normal colonic motility can be divided into two modes; the segmenting contractions which are non-propulsive in nature and the mass movements, which are the main effectors of colonic transit. This subject is considered in detail earlier in this chapter.

Most of the data on human colonic segmental contractions have been obtained with intraluminal manometry using a multi-lumen assembly of polyethylene tubes through a sigmoidoscope, which is then withdrawn leaving the tubes in the distal 25–30 cm of the large bowel. Very few studies have been done in normal subjects. Moreover, the analysis of colonic intraluminal pressure tracings is unsatisfactory and no generally accepted method has been evolved. The wide between- and within-subject variations in the level of colonic segmentation have prevented the establishment of a normal range of values. Colonic segmentation and mass movements are greatly affected by physiological, psychological and pharmacological stimuli; they are diminished or abolished by sleep and increased by ingestion of food. Many hormones (e.g. glucagon, cholescysto-kinin), neurotransmitters, (acetylcholine, 5-hydroxytryptamine) and biogenic substances (prostaglandins, polypeptides) can be shown to alter motility.

Motility is also affected both by the extrinsic and intrinsic innervation of the bowel. The innervation comprises at least two types of excitatory neurones (cholinergic and non-cholinergic) and at least two types of inhibitory nerves (adrenergic and non-adrenergic). The relative importance of all these various factors and the way they are altered in the irritable bowel syndrome is not clear.

In general, colonic segmentation is decreased and mass movement activity increased in diarrhoea, while the reverse is found in constipation. The relative absence of segmental contractions in diarrhoea diminishes the resistance offered to propulsive colonic activity, allowing mass movements to move the colonic contents faster and along longer sections of the large bowel than normally. Excessive segmentation in constipation slows down the passage of faeces and may eventually result in the pellety or rabbity stools which are characteristic of the irritable bowel syndrome.

Abdominal pain experienced by patients suffering from the irritable bowel syndrome is generally considered to originate in the colon. In some patients correlation between episodes of pain and pressure events in the bowel lumen can be demonstrated and intense hypersegmentation may be recorded from the distal colon during episodes of abdominal symptoms. Parenteral administration of drugs that inhibit smooth muscle contractions simultaneously abolishes both the pain and the motor activity. The mechanism through which strong colonic segmental contractions produce pain is not certain and the correlation between hypersegmentation and pain cannot always be demonstrated. In some cases hypersegmentation is recorded with the patient symptom free while in others the reverse is true. There are several reasons for these discrepancies. One is that the segmentation may be focal in character and out of reach of the pressure sensors. Another is the variation in the pain threshold of the colon to distension; patients with irritable bowel syndrome have been shown to have a lower threshold than control subjects to colonic pain produced by a distending balloon.

Measurements of colonic myoelectrical activity in irritable bowel syndrome are different from controls. There is evidence in some cases that intestinal motility may also be abnormal.

Unfortunately studies of colonic motility in irritable bowel syndrome have not so far demonstrated clear cut differences from the normal, either in the basal state, or after physiological or pharmacological stimuli; abnormalities of colonic motility may be present during exacerbations and absent during remissions of irritable bowel syndrome. The abnormal myoelectrical activity, however, remains unaffected by the clinical state of the patient and thus may provide a basis for the chronic, relapsing nature of irritable bowel syndrome. In its present stage of development, measurement of colonic motility has no place in the routine investigation of patients and is of no value in establishing the diagnosis of irritable bowel syndrome.

Postinfective diarrhoea

Gastro-intestinal infections such as bacillary or amoebic dysentery may leave patients with symptoms resembling those of irritable bowel syndrome at a time when all laboratory evidence of infection has disappeared. These post-dysenteric symptoms can persist for long periods and are common in areas where enteric infections are endemic. The mechanism by which the symptoms of post-dysenteric bowel are produced is not clear and few patients with the irritable bowel syndrome give any history of a preceding diarrhoeal illness.

Hypolactasia

Patients with hypolactasia (lactose intolerance) may have some symptoms of the irritable bowel syndrome following the ingestion of a lactose load. There is no evidence to suggest however, that hypolactasia is more common in irritable bowel syndrome patients than in other groups, and in general symptoms of irritable bowel syndrome do not respond to a lactose-free diet.

Psychological factors

Psychological factors are generally accepted to be important and remissions or exacerbations of the syndrome can often be correlated with periods of tranquility or stress, respectively. Studies using personality index profiles show that patients with irritable bowel syndrome include a high proportion with marked neurotic traits. Measurements of the state of background activity of the autonomic nervous system, for example by the rate of forearm blood flow, also suggest that patients with irritable bowel syndrome differ from the normal population, although in general abnormalities of personality and of other variables are not as marked as in patients with a formal diagnosis of neurotic illness. Attempts to produce characteristic abnormal patterns of colonic motility during acute stress induced experimentally have not been entirely convincing, because very similar changes can be shown to occur in normal subjects under similar circumstances. Furthermore, it is not at all clear why one person should respond to stress by developing bowel symptoms, while another responds in a different way. Stress is a non-specific, not easily quantifiable stimulus which evokes a wide range of somatic reactions; the effects of chronic or repeated stress are probably quite different from those of acute stress, which is what is usually experimentally studied in man. A proportion of patients (perhaps 20%) with the irritable bowel syndrome have no apparent neurotic personality traits and do not associate worsening of their symptoms with psychological upsets. The incidence of clinical depression in patients with the irritable bowel syndrome is difficult to define; uncontrolled series report encouraging results in the therapy of some symptoms of the irritable bowel syndrome with tricyclic antidepressants, but there have been no controlled clinical trials. Moreover, tricyclic antidepressants have atropine-like effects, so that they may be acting directly on the colon. Although stress, anxiety, depression and tension undoubtedly play an important role in irritable bowel syndrome, they should not be overemphasised to the exclusion of other factors.

CLINICAL FEATURES

As there is no specific test for the irritable bowel syndrome, the clinical features are important in making the correct diagnosis and in planning treatment. The commonest clinical features of the irritable bowel syndrome are abdominal pain with an abnormal and irregular bowel habit. A number of other, less easily defined symptoms are often present in addition and these include epigastric discomfort (dyspepsia), flatulence, bloating, distension, excessive borborygmi or wind and a sense of incomplete evacuation after defaecation. Patients suffering from the irritable bowel syndrome can be broadly classified into three types:

> *Colonic spasm.* In patients with colonic spasm abdominal pain is most prominent, bowel habit often alternating between constipation and diarrhoea. This category is the most frequent clinical type of the irritable bowel syndrome.
> *Diarrhoea.* The patients have a chronic, often relentless, watery diarrhoea, which is usually painless. This clinical picture is relatively uncommon.
> *Abdominal pain.* In this category are the patients whose predominant complaint is abdominal pain, often related to meals, but the irregular bowel habit is less marked.

All of these symptoms may be continuous, but they are more often intermittent. Studies of patients with the irritable bowel syndrome show that although the symptoms may appear somewhat vague and diffuse, follow-up demonstrates that the pattern remains fairly characteristic in each individual. It is uncommon for the symptoms to alter extensively and should they do so, this should alert the doctor to the possibility of alternative diagnoses.

The male:female ratio is 2:3 in most series. There are no reliable data regarding the socio-economic distribution, but the clinical impression is that the middle class professional person is more liable to develop the irritable bowel syndrome than the manual worker; the stressed executive and the lonely, frustrated, or dissatisfied housewife are frequently seen. Cultural differences may determine to some extent the presentation of the syndrome. Patients of Italian or French extraction may interpret their symptoms as arising from the liver or the biliary tract, while Anglo-Saxons or Jews tend to somatise their symptoms via the colon.

Abdominal pain

Abdominal pain can vary in severity from mild discomfort to an intensity severe enough to be disabling, or to interrupt sleep (although this is uncommon). There is often a relationship to defaecation and to meals. The pain may be made either better or worse by defaecation, and it may be improved or worsened by the ingestion of food. In some patients, however, the pain is not substantially altered by either. Some patients experience post-defaecation pain which they describe as a burning, or a hot uncomfortable sensation in the region of the descending colon; this post-defaecation pain proves to be quite common if the patient is asked about it.

The meal-related pain is usually characterised by distension or a sense of epigastric or subcostal fullness and may be so marked that the patient cannot tolerate any tight garments around the abdomen. The symptoms tend to get progressively worse during the day.

An important feature of the meal-related pain of the irritable bowel syndrome is its poor response to antacids, cimetidine or other anti-ulcer drugs. There may be associations between certain items of diet and the occurrence of pain; onions, beans, cabbage or cauliflower are frequently implicated.

The usual descriptions of the abdominal pain in the irritable bowel syndrome locate it mainly in the left iliac fossa but the distribution is very variable. In addition, the pain may be felt in the suprapubic region, in the right iliac fossa, in the back, upper thighs or, indeed, at several sites simultaneously. The upper abdominal meal-related pain is often described by the patient as transverse in distribution, in marked distinction to the pain of peptic ulcer which is usually sharply localised to the epigastrium. If the pain of peptic ulcer can be said to produce the 'pointing sign', the patient's finger being directed inwards and at right angles to the abdominal wall, the meal-related pain of the irritable bowel syndrome may be said to produce the 'rubbing sign', the palm of the hand being passed to-and-fro transversely across the upper abdomen, to indicate the distribution of the discomfort.

Bowel habit

In some patients constipation predominates and at the other end of the scale others complain of diarrhoea which is usually painless. In most, the bowel habit alternates between diarrhoea and constipation. Bowel frequency is often worst in the morning and subsides during the day. The stools do not have the characteristic of steatorrhoea but defaecation may be urgent and accompanied by excessive flatus. The shape of the formed stool is often abnormal and may be ribbon or pencil-like, rabbity, or pellety, due to excessive moulding of the bowel contents by abnormal motor activity.

DIAGNOSIS

Since there is no pathognomonic sign or specific diagnostic test for the irritable bowel syndrome, the diagnosis is based on the clinical assessment of the patient in which irritable bowel syndrome is suspected and on the exclusion of organic pathology.

A detailed history of symptoms and their relationship to the various triggering factors should be taken. A history of symptoms along the entire length of the gastro-intestinal tract (nausea – upper tract, distension and gurgling – small intestine, left-sided pain and constipation – colon) makes organic disease most unlikely. Urinary symptoms with frequency or discomfort frequently co-exist (the irritable bladder) and the patient may complain of feeling faint and looking grey and ill during attacks; this has been called dysautonomia.

The relationship to psychological stresses should be explored and the existence of such stresses and psychological problems identified. It is worth making a direct enquiry regarding past formal psychiatric treatment. A dietary history and questions regarding previous or present medication, and gastrointestinal infections are important.

Many patients with the irritable bowel syndrome have had numerous previous consultations and these repay careful documentation. Surveys of patients with the syndrome show an increased incidence of previous radiological investigations such as intravenous urogram, cholecystogram, barium meal and enema (often repeated several times and all usually normal) as well as appendicectomies done for 'chronic appendicitis' and, in females, various gynaecological operations. There may be a history of cholecystectomy, vagotomy, or even of an exploratory laparatomy for abdominal pain. All of these surgical procedures will have left the patient no better, the symptoms returning soon after the operation.

Clear definition of what the patient means by diarrhoea or constipation is important; the complaint of constipation may mean the regular passage of a hard, uncomfortable stool, or the patient may be describing decreased frequency of defaecation. Similarly the patient complaining of diarrhoea may be referring to the frequent passage of small volumes of loose stool and/or mucus, or the symptoms may relate to large bulk of soft or liquid faeces. In patients in hospital the best measurement of the severity of diarrhoea is the 24 hr faecal weight: in adults on a normal diet this should not exceed 200 g per day. Higher weights mean true diarrhoea and suggest an organic cause.

On physical examination signs of diabetes, alcoholism, thyrotoxicosis or recent weight loss should be carefully looked for. The abdomen should be palpated and percussed; the caecum, descending and sigmoid colon are often palpable in normal subjects and may be tender in the irritable bowel syndrome. Patients complaining of abdominal distension sometimes unconsciously accentuate the lumbar lordosis of the spine and this is worth looking for.

Rectal examination is preceded by careful inspection of the anus for tags, fissures or perianal lesions. Any patient who complains of a sense of incomplete evacuation should be asked to bear down or strain, in order to look for rectal mucosal prolapse or an abnormal degree of perineal descent (Chapter 3).

Digital rectal examination, proctoscopy and sigmoidoscopy should always be performed. The rectal and lower sigmoid mucosa are examined for normality of vascular pattern and the absence of granularity, friability or blood in the lumen. If in doubt a rectal biopsy should be taken. Manipulation of the bowel and distension by insufflated air at sigmoidoscopy may reproduce the patient's pain, especially if it is predominantly localised to the left iliac fossa; this is suggestive but not diagnostic of the irritable bowel syndrome. The passage of the sigmoidoscope may be arrested by colonic contractions but such spasm can be a normal finding.

Further investigations that must be done in each new case include a full blood count, sedimentation rate, bacteriological examination of the faeces and a double-contrast barium enema. The results should all be normal.

The typical history, the lack of evidence of organic disease, constant weight, psychologically associated remissions and relapses with normal laboratory and radiological findings should all allow the clinician to make the diagnosis of irritable bowel syndrome.

DIFFERENTIAL DIAGNOSIS

It is unusual for the irritable bowel syndrome to present for the first time after the fifth decade and in such patients organic colonic disease should be rigorously excluded, before the diagnosis of irritable bowel syndrome can be accepted. In all cases, intrinsic colonic pathology, such as inflammatory bowel disease, carcinoma, diverticular disease or polyposis must be excluded by appropriate investigations: the diagnosis of these conditions is discussed elsewhere in this book.

The differential diagnosis of irritable bowel syndrome unfortunately covers a very wide field. The doctor must decide after initial clinical evaluation of the patient if further investigations are indicated; if so, it is best to get them done at the beginning of management, rather than to do them piecemeal, which may suggest lack of confidence in the diagnosis.

The onset of ischaemic colitis is usually acute with severe pain and rectal bleeding. Generalised arteriopathy may be present. Barium enema may show a localised lesion and typical thumbprinting appearances.

Ischaemic colitis

Blood and mucus will be present in the diarrhoea stool. History of travel to areas where amoebiasis is endemic may be present. Abnormal laboratory tests, sigmoidoscopy, biopsy, examination of a fresh stool for motile amoebae and of the blood for amoebic CFT will establish the diagnosis.

Amoebiasis

Pneumatosis is a rare and mysterious condition of uncertain aetiology which may affect the small or large intestine (pneumatosis coli). The patients usually present with pain or other functional symptoms but sometimes with bleeding from the haemorrhagic mucosal covering of the gas cysts which characterise the condition. The diagnosis may be made on sigmoidoscopy or plain abdominal x-ray (Chapter 1). The condition is harmless but if treatment is indicated the patient is admitted for oxygen therapy (Wyatt, 1975). Relapses may occur at infrequent intervals.

Pneumatosis cystoides intestinalis

Patients with the irritable bowel syndrome who have meal-related pain may be mistakenly suspected to have duodenal or gastric ulceration, or cholelithiasis. The symptoms of these conditions are usually quite distinct from those of the irritable bowel syndrome but if uncertainty exists, appropriate radiological and/or endoscopic examination should be done. The presence of gallstones does not necessarily mean that they are causing the symptoms and in the absence of a typical history, it is better to leave the gallstones alone. Carcinoma of the pancreas may deceive the physician by the absence of abnormal laboratory and radiographic findings but the relentless nature of the pain, radiating to the back, progressive weight loss and lack of response to medication should suggest the diagnosis.

Abdominal pain

Other important causes of lower abdominal pain arising in the colon are initially ruled out by the barium enema, since for any colonic disease to cause pain it must be sufficiently advanced to be obstructing the lumen or have caused obvious ulceration. Ureteric, bladder and gynaecological pains are different in quality and not associated with bowel symptoms.

Diarrhoea

The investigation and differential diagnosis of diarrhoea is a very large subject, and cannot be comprehensively covered here. The diarrhoea of the irritable bowel syndrome never produces malabsorption so evidence of malabsorption of fat, iron, vitamin B_{12} or folic acid negates the diagnosis of irritable bowel syndrome. If the stools are suggestive of steatorrhoea, faecal fat is estimated in a 3-day collection of stool (normal upper limit/24 hours: 20 mmol): further tests might include jejunal biopsy for the diagnosis of coeliac disease or tropical sprue, and/or tests of pancreatic function (chronic pancreatitis). A macrocytic blood picture might indicate malabsorption of vitamin B_{12} or folic acid and the need for further investigation. Diarrhoea in the presence of B_{12} malabsorption is suggestive of bacterial colonisation of small intestinal blind-loops which would be seen on barium follow-through. Infestation with *Giardia lamblia* can be diagnosed by microscopy of stools, but exclusion of this diagnosis requires duodenal aspirate or peroral jejunal biopsy.

Thyrotoxicosis should be considered as a cause of diarrhoea. Diarrhoea due to lactose intolerance may be suspected on careful dietary history and confirmed by lactose-free diet or a lactose tolerance test.

A rare, but difficult to diagnose, cause of diarrhoea is concealed self-medication with laxatives. Some patients habitually take large quantities of laxatives and conceal the habit for complicated psychological reasons. They complain of diarrhoea or, paradoxically, constipation. The diagnosis is often difficult owing to the skill with which the deception is done. High index of suspicion in patients with diarrhoea for no apparent cause, especially in women working in the paramedical professions is needed. Sigmoidoscopy and rectal mucosal biopsy may show pseudomelanosis coli, stool or urine tests for phenolphthalein-containing laxatives may be positive and a cache of laxatives can sometimes be discovered in the patient's bedside locker. Hypokalaemia is a frequent laboratory finding.

TREATMENT

Drugs and diet

The treatment of the irritable bowel syndrome is highly unsatisfactory, partly because the underlying pathophysiology of the large and small intestine is imperfectly understood, and partly because the drugs available for pharmacological control of intestinal motility are far from perfect. The difficulties of assessing the efficacy of a particular treatment are increased by the marked tendency to spontaneous remissions and relapses in irritable bowel syndrome. This, and the need to use the largely subjective symptomatic assessments to measure the effects of therapy, make controlled therapeutic trials difficult. The lack of positive diagnostic tests to identify patients with the irritable bowel syndrome and the sheer impossibility of finally excluding organic disease in everybody leads to poor standardisation of treatment groups. To this must be added the unpredictable and capricious nature of individual responses to therapeutic agents in the irritable bowel syndrome. This means that a number of drugs may have to be tried in the hope that – for no clear reason – one with beneficial actions will be found: or else spontaneous remission of the irritable bowel syndrome will supervene. It is interesting that many of the drugs for disorders of motility are promoted as acting specifically on the large bowel; such specificity of action has not in most cases been adequately confirmed in human subjects.

Anticholinergics, such as atropine or propantheline, inhibit smooth muscle contractions throughout the alimentary tract. The unwanted effects of cholinergic blockade, however, limit acceptable dosage and it is doubtful whether these agents have any part to play in the treatment of the irritable bowel syndrome. Hyoscine–n–butylbromide (Buscopan) inhibits gut motility when given parenterally; it is not absorbed from the gut and should not be prescribed by the oral route.

The drugs most commonly used for the treatment of diarrhoea in the irritable bowel syndrome are codeine phosphate, diphenoxylate (Lomotil) and loperamide (Imodium). All of these have been reported to slow intestinal transit after oral administration, although stool frequency or weight, rather than transit, have been measured in most studies. Codeine is a derivative of morphine and probably acts on the human gut in a manner similar to its parent substance, i.e. by increasing intestinal tone, narrowing the calibre of the gut lumen and stimulating non-propulsive segmental contractions in both the small and the large intestine. Although the detailed effects are difficult to demonstrate experimentally in man, there is little doubt that it is an effective drug and valuable in the treatment of diarrhoea in the irritable bowel syndrome. Occasionally abdominal pain is made worse by codeine, and other drugs may have to be used instead.

Diphenoxylate and loperamide are smooth muscle inhibitors that can be used for the treatment of diarrhoea and the abdominal pain of irritable bowel syndrome. Mebeverine (Colofac) is another spasmolytic which acts similarly to papaverine, but is substantially more potent than the latter – at least in laboratory animals. It is widely used in the irritable bowel syndrome as an anti-spasmodic. Adequately controlled comparisons between these agents do not show one to be markedly better than another, but idiosyncratic responses have to be allowed for in prescribing. In many patients two or more of these drugs may have to be tried before adequate therapy can be established.

Constipation and pain in the irritable bowel syndrome have recently been frequently treated by increasing the amount of vegetable fibre in the diet and by supplementing the dietary content of fibre with added bran. There is little doubt that bulking the stools with dietary fibre will speed up transit through the gut and relieve constipation in many patients. The use of high fibre diets in the management of irritable bowel syndrome however does not rest on evidence from extensive controlled trials and the results of some studies have shown no benefit. This may be due to inadequate dosage, or to faulty selection of patients. Some patients with the irritable bowel syndrome feel worse on a high fibre diet and are thankful when it is abandoned. The place of bran in the management of the irritable bowel syndrome needs further study before it can be properly defined but in the meantime the treatment should certainly be tried on an empirical basis.

Some patients with the irritable bowel syndrome in whom constipation is the main symptom may need treatment with laxatives. Whichever laxative is selected, it should be used intermittently, with the aim of avoiding habituation and loss of efficacy. Standard senna tablets are probably preferable in the anthraquinone group. These glycosides are degraded in the alimentary tract, probably by bacterial action, to oxymethyl-anthraquinones which may act by stimulating the intrinsic myenteric plexus of the large bowel. Other useful laxatives are lactulose and magnesium sulphate. Lactulose is a synthetic unabsorbable disaccharide which is utilised by colonic bacteria, with the production of osmotically active substances and lactic acid; the increased osmotic pressure and lowered pH increase the plasma-to-lumen flux of water and electrolytes, with consequent relief of constipation. Magnesium sulphate may act partially as an osmotic laxative but may also work by releasing cholecystokinin, which increases colonic motility. Apart from the systemically administered laxatives, glycerine suppositories are sometimes useful and certainly harmless. The main clinical problem in treating constipation in the irritable bowel syndrome is to persuade the patient to use laxatives sensibly and to get away from the idea that a daily bowel action is necessary for health.

PSYCHOLOGICAL ASPECTS

The psychological aspects of the irritable bowel syndrome need as much careful attention as drug therapy. Unhurried history taking should include sympathetic enquiry into circumstances in the home and at work that may affect the patient. Careful and gentle physical examination will gain the patient's confidence. When the diagnosis of the irritable bowel syndrome is reached, time spent on explaining the mechanism of symptoms is time well spent. Many patients with irritable bowel syndrome carry a considerable load of guilt, or frustration, produced by being told that there is nothing seriously wrong, that all the tests are normal and that it is 'all due to nerves'. Patients may need help to talk about these feelings, while the clinician needs not to feel guilt (and therefore anger), at not being able to relieve the symptoms of irritable bowel syndrome completely. Prospective follow-up studies suggest that sympathetic support enables the patient to cope with the symptoms better, even though drug therapy is not very effective.

Anxiolytics such as diazepam are very useful where anxiety is a marked symptom. The irritable bowel syndrome may be a symptom of depression and this possibility should be borne in mind; treatment with tricyclic antidepressants, best taken as a single dose at night, can be very helpful in some patients. There is seldom any need for formal psychiatric therapy, although the occasional patient may require it.

REFERENCES AND FURTHER READING

Holdstock DJ, Misiewicz JJ, Waller SL. Observations on the mechanisms of abdominal pain. *Gut* 1969; **10:** 19–31.

Misiewicz JJ, Colonic motility. In: Sircus W, Smith AN, eds. *Scientific Foundations of Gastroenterology*. London: Heinemann, 1980: 483–91.

Thomson WG. *The Irritable Gut. Functional Disorders of the Alimentary Canal*. Baltimore: University Park Press, 1979.

Wyatt, AP. Prolonged symptomatic and radiological remission of colonic gas cysts after oxygen therapy. *British Journal of Surgery* 1975; **62:** 837–9.

DIVERTICULAR DISEASE

True diverticula containing all coats of the colon are extremely rare and for all practical purposes colonic diverticula are 'false' diverticula which are acquired. They consist of herniations of the mucous membrane through the colonic musculature. As they enlarge their muscle covering atrophies so that fully developed diverticula consist of mucous membrane, connective tissue and peritoneum.

It was once assumed that colonic pain and other abdominal symptoms in patients with diverticular disease were always the result of inflammation, but it is now realised that excessive muscular segmentation of the colon alone may cause recurrent pain or colic. This has led to a reappraisal of the time-honoured terms diverticulosis and diverticulitis. The term diverticular disease of the colon is now used to shift attention away from the mucosal herniations and towards the colonic muscle and its abnormal behaviour.

PATHOLOGY

The muscle abnormality in the sigmoid region is the most consistent and striking abnormality. The taeniae coli appear thick, assuming an almost cartilaginous consistency. The circular muscle is thick and has a corrugated or concertina-like appearance. The diverticula lie between these muscular corrugations where they herniate through the bowel wall to enter the pericolic fat (Fig. 2.5). This herniation occurs mostly at the weakest points, namely the sites of entry of the colonic vessels. Inflammation in diverticular disease (diverticulitis) is the result of infection around diverticula which spreads within the pericolic fat to form a dissecting abscess. Involvement of the peritoneum results in local peritonitis which may become generalised in the event of perforation. Faecoliths predispose to the development of pericolic abscesses. Usually, a single diverticulum is the source of the inflammation even when this is very extensive.

Bleeding in diverticular disease often can be traced to an infected diverticulum. This may cause either the erosion of a vessel in its wall or the formation of vascular granulation tissue inside the diverticulum.

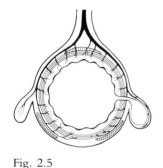

Fig. 2.5

The pathogenesis of colonic diverticula

As diverticula are hernias, they must be caused either by weakness of the colonic wall or abnormal intracolonic pressure, or by both. Intracolonic pressures have been found to be the same in health and diverticular disease under basal conditions so that at first sight it would appear that diverticula are not caused by intracolonic 'hypertension'. When, however, the diseased sigmoid colon is activated by emotion, eating or certain mechanical stimuli, or drugs such as morphine and prostigmine, it generates very high intracolonic pressures in those segments which bear diverticula. These pressures are greater

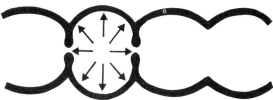

Pressure is normally generated in contracting segment, separated from its neighbours by contraction rings.

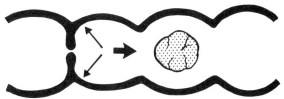

Relaxation of one of these contraction rings allows the contents to be propelled into next segment where pressure is lower.

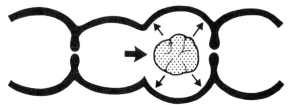

Material moving through the colon can be halted by segmentation and pressure is produced.

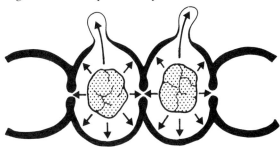

Segmented colon acts as a series of 'little bladders'. Further contraction generates pressure and the mucosa is driven through the colonic wall.

Fig. 2.6 Diagram to show role of segmentation in formation of diverticula.

than those in the normal colon or those generated in apparently normal segments in a colon that bears diverticula elsewhere. This differential response is present in the earliest stage of the disease and may account for the fact that once it appears diverticular disease tends to progress.

Simultaneous cineradiology and pressure recording have shown that the colon produces these pressures by segmenting so that it acts as a series of 'little bladders' whose outflow is obstructed at both ends by contraction rings (Fig. 2.6). Segmentation is increased by prostigmine and by morphine which increase intracolonic pressure, and is lessened by pethidine which decreases both the intracolonic pressure and the colonic motility. Propantheline, which paralyses the colonic musculature, abolishes pressure production in the colon. Diverticula are almost certainly caused by excessive segmentation of the colonic musculature which causes abnormally high intracolonic pressures.

AETIOLOGY

The exact incidence is unknown but can be estimated from necropsy or radiological studies. In western industrialised countries the disease was almost unknown in 1900; since then it has become the commonest affliction of the colon. Today one-third of patients over 60 years old have diverticula and two-thirds at age 80. By contrast the disease is still rare or unknown in rural Africans and Asians.

This geographical distribution is not due to race; American negroes and West Indians and Asians living in Britain, and Japanese reared in Hawaii or on the mainland of the United States are just as prone to the disease as Caucasians in these countries. There are few diseases which vary in incidence so much throughout the world, namely from nil to nearly 30% of a population. This appears to be related to the level of economic development and to the degree to which the diet has altered due to the processing of foodstuffs. The disease appears to be extremely common in those countries where food is processed and refined. In Britain there is a correlation between the rising incidence of diverticular disease during the last century and an increased consumption of refined flour and sugar. Sugar contains no fibre and its consumption has almost trebled since 1860. During the years 1870–1880, the stonegrinding of flour was replaced by roller milling which crushes the grain and removes more fibre. Modern white and most brown breads contain little fibre compared with the amount in wholemeal bread which was previously a staple part of the diet. The consumption of cereal fibre has fallen to between 1/5th and 1/10th of that eaten by our recent ancestors. Their unrefined diet containing plenty of fibre produced swiftly passed soft stools that subjected the sigmoid to little strain. By contrast our modern fibre-deficient diet leads to stiff viscous stools that need high intracolonic pressures to propel them. These cause the sigmoid to overwork and hypertrophy, and lead to herniation of the mucosa. A return to a high fibre diet should prevent the appearance of the disease in later generations.

CLINICAL FEATURES

A clinical classification of the manifestations of diverticular disease is shown in Fig. 2.7.

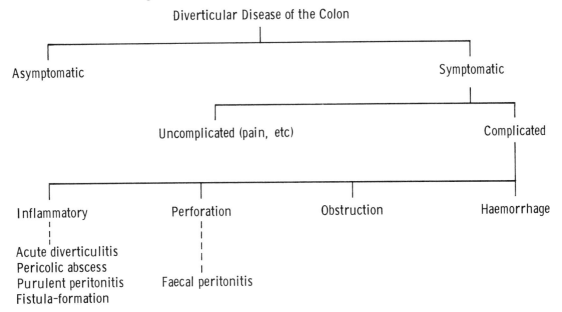

Fig. 2.7

Asymptomatic diverticular disease. Since diverticula are so common in people over the age of 65, it is not surprising that many are asymptomatic. It is probable that over 80–90% of patients who have diverticula suffer no symptoms from them and the lesions may be discovered incidentally by a barium enema or meal examination or by colonoscopy. The nature of the condition should be explained with the aid of a diagram to the patient who should be reassured that only 10% of people with colonic diverticula develop symptoms and that only 1% ever require surgery. New symptoms, such as the passage of blood with mucus, or alteration of the bowel habit, should be reported, since the patient is as liable to develop carcinoma or other colonic disease as anyone else. Dietary advice is the only active measure necessary at this time.

Symptomatic diverticular disease. In only a minority of patients are symptoms due to secondary complications of the disease. Most have uncomplicated disease in which symptoms result from abnormal colonic muscle motility.

Uncomplicated diverticular disease

The symptoms include anorexia, flatulence, a sensation of fullness, abdominal distension, discomfort or pain. Discomfort may be referred to the epigastrium but usually to the lower abdomen. The bowel habit is variable; most patients are not constipated but pass one motion a day. Some pass several hard stools a day and these 'sheep droppings' are voided only after considerable straining. Many complain that their rectum never feels empty. The patient may in addition complain of lower abdominal pain, usually referred to the left iliac fossa. It is described as cramp-like or colicky in nature and may be severe. Examination reveals tenderness in the left iliac fossa or suprapubic region and a tense firm sigmoid colon is often felt. The symptoms are caused by the abnormal colonic muscle motility, certainly the diverticula are not responsible for them since they can be relieved by a high fibre diet while the diverticula remain *in situ*.

Management

All patients should be examined by the rigid or flexible sigmoidoscope in addition to having a barium enema to exclude a rectal or rectosigmoid carcinoma. The hallowed regime of a low residue diet and liquid paraffin should be abandoned; a low residue diet is the cause of the disease and so is contra-indicated. The prolonged use of paraffin theoretically may cause vitamin deficiency. The patient should be advised how to take a 'high fibre diet' with added bran and should eat wholemeal bread, wholewheat breakfast cereals, rough porridge or muesli, together with fresh fruit and vegetables daily. Patients should understand that the colon has to struggle with the stiff stools that result from a fibre-deficient diet. Bran lowers the intracolonic pressures and returns the electrical activity of the colon beset with diverticula to normal, increases the stool weight and reduces the transit time (Srivastava, Smith and Painter, 1976; Taylor and Duthie, 1976). In patients with pain, antispasmodics such as propantheline or mebeverine may be found useful but, as yet, no controlled trial has proved their efficacy. The patient may be helped by small doses of phenobarbitone or a tranquilliser. Pain may be severe enough to warrant admission to hospital since it may not be possible to exclude acute diverticulitis or other abdominal conditions.

Despite these measures, recurrent episodes of pain at frequent intervals may make the patient's life a misery. Elective resection of the sigmoid colon, or possibly myotomy, is then indicated. Timely surgery will relieve pain and prevent more serious complications occurring when the patient is older and less fit to withstand an operation. The reduction in intracolonic pressures that follows sigmoid myotomy or resection is not permanent however, unless the patient changes to a high-fibre diet with added bran.

How to prescribe bran

Each patient is given a packet of millers' unprocessed bran together with a sheet of instructions. These explain that bran is difficult to swallow because it is dry. Hence it should be washed down with water or fruit juice or mixed with bran-containing breakfast cereals such as All Bran, Weetabix or Shredded Wheat. It can be added to porridge oats or muesli and to soup, particularly pea soup. Bran can be added to wholemeal flour, one part in five, by those who bake their own bread, to make a 'bran-plus' loaf. Wherever possible patients should eat 100% wholemeal bread and the difference between this and refined bread coloured brown should be explained to them. They should choose wholewheat or bran-containing cereals, coarse porridge as opposed to 'instant' porridge, unpolished rice instead of white rice and wholemeal pasta products instead of white spaghetti. They should eat plenty of fruit and vegetables, especially cabbage, and should restrict their intake of refined sugar whether brown or white.

Initially they should take 2 teaspoonsfuls of bran with every meal and after two weeks, this amount should be slowly increased until they open their bowels once or, better still, twice a day without straining. Patients understand readily that if they do not strain to defaecate then their bowel has not had to overwork and produce symptoms as it struggles with abnormal contents. Nearly half those who change to a high-fibre diet, including bran, experience flatulence or a feeling of distension. They must be warned of this otherwise they may stop taking bran, whereas if they persevere with it these symptoms disappear in about a month.

All patients should be seen after a month to ensure that they have followed the instructions. Some will not have done so and will need further advice. They should be seen at monthly intervals until they void soft stools without any effort and should then continue taking this amount of bran for life.

Many people have to eat at work or away from home when they are forced to eat refined cereals and when it is difficult to take bran. They should be given bran in the form of tablets (Fybranta), each of which contains about a teaspoonful of bran. These can be carried easily and should be chewed and washed down with fluids. They can be taken in hotels, when on holiday or wherever unprocessed bran is not available.

Reilly introduced sigmoid myotomy as an alterative to resection for diverticular disease in 1966. The narrowed sigmoid is widened by dividing the circular muscle with a longitudinal incision after the manner of Rammstedt's operation. The incision is made through a taenia so as to avoid opening diverticula and is deepened until the mucosa is seen.

The operation lowers the sigmoid intraluminal pressures and abolishes symptoms but after three years the pressures rise

Sigmoid myotomy

again. However the pressures remain normal if myotomy is followed by the patient changing to a high fibre diet for life. The need for myotomy has lessened since the adoption of the high fibre diet, but it may still have a place in the treatment of frail and obese patients.

Sigmoid myotomy may be complicated by perforation and peritonitis post-operatively, following damage to the mucosa at operation. This is usually caused by the zealous division of every strand of circular muscle. The author aims to divide only about three-quarters of the circular muscle thickness. This results in symptomatic improvement and radiological widening of the sigmoid lumen and increases the safety of the operation.

Complicated diverticular disease

Inflammation of one or more diverticula may resolve spontaneously with minimal symptoms and signs. On the other hand, the inflammatory process may spread to involve several centimetres of the sigmoid colon, the mesocolon and surrounding tissues. The disease process may progress to abscess formation or generalised peritonitis.

Acute diverticulitis and pericolic abscess

The presentation of acute diverticulitis has been likened to a 'left-sided acute appendicitis'. Pain is felt over the affected colon, which usually lies in the left iliac fossa but may curve into the right iliac fossa. Fever, malaise, anorexia and nausea are experienced. If adjacent small gut becomes involved, it may obstruct. Occasionally, loose motions are passed. Tenderness in the lower abdomen maximal over the sigmoid colon is due to local peritonitis and a mass indicates abscess formation. There is often tenderness on rectal examination and the affected bowel or a pelvic abscess may be felt. Local ileus due to involvement of small or large bowel may lead to obstruction. The white cell count is raised.

Even when an abscess is localised, the condition remains dangerous as at any time the abscess may rupture into the peritoneal cavity causing a rapidly spreading peritonitis. Alternatively, it may burst through the skin or into the bladder, vagina, another part of the bowel or rarely into the ischiorectal fossa, forming a fistula.

Management

The patient should be treated with rest, antibiotics and analgesics. Pethidine lessens intracolonic pressures and decreases colonic motility and appears to be the analgesic of choice. Enemas are contra-indicated. Occasionally the condition does not settle, in which case early operation is necessary, but the majority of patients never require surgery. It is therefore best not to make any decision about this until the patient has recovered and has tried the effect of high fibre diet. Barium enema should be carried out after recovery, especially if a carcinoma cannot be excluded. Colonoscopy will usually resolve the matter. If episodes of severe pain occur so frequently as to make life intolerable, resection should be performed when the disease is quiescent.

An abscess should be drained through the overlying skin and a proximal colostomy fashioned prior to resection of the sigmoid at a later date. Some surgeons prefer not to drain an abscess at once, but to observe it in the hope that it will resolve, avoiding thereby a cutaneous fistula. However, abscesses treated conservatively can rupture suddenly causing a fatal peritonitis; earlier intervention may prevent this catastrophe. A cutaneous fistula due to drainage of an abscess will heal only after the diseased colon has been removed.

Peritonitis

Peritonitis due to diverticular disease may be purulent or faecal. Purulent peritonitis presents as 'left-sided appendicitis' whereas faecal peritonitis is usually generalised and its onset catastrophic. Generalised boardlike rigidity occurs early and the patient is usually shocked. The former is due to rupture of a pericolic abscess. the latter to the perforation of a diverticulum which is usually not apparently inflamed.

Management

Initially some patients appear too ill for surgery. Their condition may improve with conservative measures. Broad spectrum antibiotics should be given intravenously at once and a drip started. Time spent improving the patient's condition before operation is never wasted. The patient will often continue to improve when anaesthetised partly because ventilation is no longer restricted by pain. The surgeon should always be prepared to operate on these very shocked patients; they will otherwise die.

After peritoneal toilet has been completed a choice between the following procedures must be made:

Closure of perforation, if found, and drainage of the abdomen.
Closure of performation, drainage of abdomen and proximal colostomy.
Exteriorisation of the affected bowel with drainage of the abdomen.
Resection of the affected bowel followed by proximal terminal colostomy and closure of the rectal stump and drainage of the abdomen or immediate end-to-end anastomosis with drainage of the abdomen.

The choice of which procedure to use is a vexed question. Purulent peritonitis carries a mortality of about 15%. Before the introduction of antibacterial agents and the better understanding of electrolyte and water balance, the mortality was nearer 40% and in faecal peritonitis almost 50%. The problem has been discussed more fully by Painter (1975).

Simple drainage

Purulent peritonitis may respond to simple drainage and peritoneal toilet together with supportive therapy.

Drainage with proximal colostomy

It has been shown that adding a proximal colostomy in the right half of the transverse colon to simple drainage and peritoneal toilet adds nothing to the operative risk and improves the prognosis. This emergency operation thus becomes the first stage of a three-stage curative procedure, followed later by resection and, finally, by closure of the colostomy. The operation has the disadvantage of leaving behind the diseased bowel in the acute stage. It is also less effective in faecal peritonitis probably because it is still possible for faeces between the colostomy and the perforation to empty into the peritoneum after the abdomen has been closed. To avoid this, exteriorisation of the affected colon is practised by many surgeons both in purulent and faecal peritonitis.

Exteriorisation of the affected colon

In faecal peritonitis the mortality is less if the bowel is exteriorised. The diseased segment, usually the sigmoid colon, can almost always be mobilised sufficiently for it to be brought to the surface and further contamination of the peritoneal cavity is prevented. The diseased bowel can usually be resected within a few weeks. Exteriorisation with resection of the part of the inflamed colon which lies outside the abdomen immediately following closure of the abdomen is a compromise between exteriorisation alone and primary resection that is well within the capabilities of young registrars.

Emergency resection of the diseased colon

All the above procedures leave the infected bowel to discharge toxic products into the circulation and this may contribute to the high mortality. Emergency resection of the diseased sigmoid has been practised, therefore, in the belief that it is not the operation but the disease that kills these very ill patients. There may be rapid clinical improvement following resection of the affected bowel.

After resection of the sigmoid colon, three procedures are available:

Creation of a double-barrelled colostomy (Paul–Mikulicz operation).

Exteriorisation of the proximal colon as a terminal colostomy with closure of the distal stump or

Immediate end-to-end anastomosis.

All should be accompanied by peritoneal toilet and drainage of the pelvis. The technique chosen depends on the experience of the surgeon.

Emergency resection and immediate anastomosis, with or without a protecting proximal colostomy, can be performed with a mortality of about 7%. It must be emphasised that these results were obtained by surgeons with a special interest in the large bowel and those with limited experience would be ill-advised to attempt this operation. A temporary proximal colostomy is necessary in at least a quarter of cases.

In those treated without resection, a barium enema examination and sigmoidoscopy should be performed after recovery is complete to assess the extent of the disease and to exclude carcinoma. Patients who survive this emergency and have not had their sigmoid colon resected are almost certainly fit for this operation after an interval of about three months. A colostomy should never be closed without resection of the diseased sigmoid as past experience has shown that this leads to a recurrence of complications and these may be fatal.

It should be emphasised that drainage and proximal colostomy is the most widely practised emergency operation, but since our treatment of peritonitis due to diverticulitis remains so unsatisfactory, there is no reason to believe that it is the best procedure.

Laparotomy and drainage, with or without colostomy, was followed by a mortality of 38% in a large series; exteriorisation lowered this to 15% while emergency resections with and without immediate anastomosis resulted in a mortality of 7% and 5% respectively (Painter, 1975).

Fistula formation

Recurrent attacks of inflammation may cause the sigmoid colon to adhere to neighbouring structures, and if a pericolic abscess forms it may burst into them so that a fistula connects the colonic lumen with another epithelial surface.

Fistulae may form between the colon and the skin, bladder, vagina or neighbouring gut and may even extend from the colon through the pelvic peritoneum to the ischiorectal space and thence to the surface of the buttock. They do not heal unless the primary source of infection, the sigmoid colon, is removed. The underlying pathology must be determined as fistulae may be caused not only by diverticular disease, but also by carcinoma of the colon or cervix, Crohn's disease or by irradiation.

A colo-vesical fistula occurs more commonly in men than in women as the uterus tends to keep the colon and bladder apart. The fistula results in urinary infection and the passage of wind or even faeces in the urine. Barium studies and endoscopy of colon and bladder may not demonstrate the track but the presence of these symptoms is sufficient to make the diagnosis.

A colo-vaginal fistula results in the passage of air, faeces or pus *per vaginam* as the presenting symptoms. Sometimes the fistula involves the uterus.

A colo-enteric fistula may form between the colon and adherent small gut and, rarely, the large bowel. Internal fistulae may be demonstrated by barium enema but on occasions have only been found by cineradiographic studies of barium followed through the small bowel.

A colo-cutaneous fistula may follow the rupture of a pericolic abscess through the abdominal wall or the buttock via the ischiorectal fossa, but more often is the sequel to surgical drainage of an abscess.

Obstruction of the large bowel

The symptoms of obstruction in either the small or large bowel have been frequently reported. Usually the obstruction is due to ileus caused by local or general peritonitis. Mechanical obstruction of the small bowel by adhesions due to diverticular disease is a rare occurrence and for all practical purposes mechanical obstruction in diverticular disease occurs only in the sigmoid colon. The differential diagnosis is between diverticular disease and carcinoma. Sigmoidoscopy and barium enema must be performed and be repeated in patients who are known to have diverticular disease and a recent change in bowel habit. Colonoscopy should settle the diagnosis if doubt remains. Stenosis due to diverticular disease is uncommon, and requires surgical resection.

Haemorrhage

The blood passed is usually dark red and small in amount. Sometimes bleeding may be massive. The patient should be nursed in hospital. In over 80% of cases the bleeding stops spontaneously and the colon may then be examined radiologically and endoscopically. In the remainder selective angiography will localise the site of bleeding and an infusion of pitressin or embolisation will stop it in most cases. Often bleeding occurs in the caecum or ascending colon even when the sigmoid colon is most affected by diverticula. The cause is said to be infection of the mucosal pouches affecting the segmental artery which is in close proximity.

Surgery is indicated only if massive bleeding continues. Usually the site of the bleeding point is not known and a sub-total colectomy with immediate ileo-rectal anastomosis will remove all diverticula and stop the haemorrhage.

In conclusion, diverticular disease of the colon is a deficiency disease which like scurvy is preventable. It develops through lack of roughage in our modern diet. The symptoms can be relieved in almost every patient by adding bran to the diet, eating non-refined foods and avoiding refined flour and sugar, whether brown or white. Surgeons may relieve the complications and symptoms of the disease; only a change in diet will remove the underlying cause. A return to a high fibre diet containing plenty of cereal fibre should lessen the incidence of the disease and possibly prevent its appearance in future generations.

REFERENCES AND FURTHER READING

Edwards HC. Diverticula of the colon and vermiform appendix. *Lancet* 1934; **1**: 221–6.

Painter NS. The aetiology of diverticulosis of the colon with special reference to the action of certain drugs on the behaviour of the colon. *Annals of the Royal College of Surgeons of England* 1964; **38**: 98–119.

Painter NS. *Diverticular Disease of the Colon*. London: Heinemann, 1975.

Painter NS, Almedia AZ and Colbourne KW. Unprocessed bran in treatment of diverticular disease of the colon. *British Medical Journal* 1972; **2**: 137–9.

Painter NS and Burkitt DP. Diverticular disease of the colon: A deficiency disease of western civilisation. *British Medical Journal* 1971; **2**: 450–4.

Painter NS, Truelove SC, Ardran GM and Tuckey M. Segmentation and the localisation of intraluminal pressures in the human colon with special reference to the pathogenesis of colonic diverticula. *Gastroenterology* 1965; **49**: 169–77.

Reilly M. Sigmoid myotomy. *Clinics in Gastroenterology* 1975; **4**: 121–45.

Taylor I and Duthie HL. Bran tablets and diverticular disease. *British Medical Journal* 1976; **1**: 988–90.

Srivastava GS, Smith AN and Painter NS. Sterculia bulk-forming agent with smooth-muscle relaxant versus bran in diverticular disease. *British Medical Journal* 1976; **1**: 315–18.

CONSTIPATION

Constipation implies irregular, infrequent defaecation and passage of hard motions which are passed with difficulty, discomfort and even pain. The term is used much more widely by some patients who may attribute general symptoms to constipation, even though their bowels are moving normally every day. The first essential is to interpret the patient's true complaint and to achieve a good doctor-patient relationship. Patients may feel they are wasting their doctors' time and such thoughts must be immediately dispelled. Constipation is a basic symptom which may reflect so many causes but, nevertheless, a few simple checks and simple advice can greatly help the majority.

CLASSIFICATION

Simple constipation

In the absence of a primary cause constipation may be self-induced, with low intake of food, particularly fibre-containing foods, lack of exercise, or ignoring the call to stool. There may be environmental factors such as poor toilet facilities, unfavourable working conditions, change of daily routine, particularly with travel or admission to hospital.

Constipation secondary to motility disorders

There is a group of disorders characterised by alteration in the motility pattern of the colon. There may be slow transit, so that at any one time there are several days' faeces still in the colon (slow transit constipation). There may be an irritable colon characterised by cramping pain and a varying bowel rhythm – sometimes constipated but sometimes normal or loose (the irritable bowel syndrome). There may be a disturbance of the circular smooth muscle mainly in the distal colon, giving rise to delayed transit and often pain, resulting ultimately in diverticular disease. With idiopathic megacolon there may be prolonged transit, rectal inertia and an overloaded bowel, but here the disorder may be due to disturbance of the sensory mechanisms or to a localised zone of failure of relaxation. Many factors – hormonal, electrolytic, metabolic, biliary and nervous – may affect colonic muscle activity, and there is no doubt that these unpleasant, rather vague, conditions will be much better defined in the future.

Constipation due to psychiatric states

There appear to be motility disorders, particularly associated with depressive states, chronic psychoses and anorexia nervosa; obsessional states, such as purgative addiction, come into this group and there is also a small curious group of patients who deny bowel action, but who in transit studies show no abnormality.

Constipation secondary to known causes

Constipation may result from a wide group of disorders; colonic, rectal and anal, neurological, endocrine and metabolic. Local causes include diseases giving rise to obstruction or pain or interference with the defaecation reflex. These can be largely sorted out by simple examinations. The condition of the descending perineum syndrome, particularly in women, may cause pseudo-stimulation to defaecation and simulates constipation. Hirschsprung's disease, Chagas' disease, systemic sclerosis, disseminated sclerosis and spinal injuries are occasional neurogenic causes. Important endocrine disorders always to be kept in mind, include hypothyroidism (skin and hair changes, sensitivity to cold), hypercalcaemia (thirst, polyuria and weakness) and diabetes (thirst and polyuria). Rarities such as porphyria and lead poisoning are examples of metabolic and toxic causes.

Drug-induced constipation is relatively common and easily forgotten. Immobilisation both in medical and surgical illnesses is particularly liable to slow down colon activity and may result in chronic constipation or other disturbances of bowel function.

Constipation secondary to treatment

CLINICAL APPROACH TO CONSTIPATION

In the management of constipation the initial history must consider dietary fibre intake, medical treatment and the possibility of endocrine, metabolic and psychiatric disorders; appropriate leading questions should be asked. A general examination including rectal examination, sigmoidoscopy and proctoscopy should be performed; if there is rectal inertia the rectum is characteristically full of stool. In the majority of patients the answer will turn out to be one of the mechanisms of simple constipation, particularly inadequate fibre intake, and a therapeutic trial of bran may be indicated without further investigation. If the response is inadequate, it is then reasonable to consider a barium enema, always performed if the history of constipation is short, especially in patients in the cancer age group. A further possible investigation is to check the transit time by giving 20 radio-opaque markers by mouth (Hinton, Lennard-Jones and Young, 1969). These may be conveniently taken in jam and a plain film four days later will give an indication of the site of delay, if any; normally not more than four markers should remain. A further film can be taken a few days later. There is delayed passage of markers in slow transit constipation. There is some rationale to the treatment of constipation but it is difficult to systematise when individual response is so variable and the underlying mechanisms poorly understood. Simple constipation usually responds to an increase of dietary fibre in the form of bran and secondary constipation to management of the underlying disorder. It is the patients with idiopathic slow transit constipation who are particularly difficult to treat; bulky agents invariably make them uncomfortable. If palpable stool is demonstrated in the rectum it is logical to try the effect of glycerine suppositories or disposable enemas. The alternatives are then either to accept the passage of fewer stools than normal (whilst keeping the motions soft with lubricants or saline purgatives) or to use purgatives to stimulate the colon. Various purgatives may need to be continued indefinitely.

DIETARY FIBRE

The most important development in the management of constipation has been the better appreciation of the role of dietary fibre. There is nothing new about the idea and, indeed, voices have been raised against white bread over the centuries ever since Greek and Roman times. Now the scientific basis of dietary fibre has been studied and there are very clear explanations of why extra dietary fibre can be so beneficial in relation to bowel function, particularly for constipation and for diverticular disease. Dietary fibre consists of a number of different macro-molecules which make up the structure of a plant:

> *Cellulose* consists of unbranched polysaccharide chains of 3000 or more glucose molecules which form strong elastic fibres with the capacity to take up water and swell.
> *Hemicelluloses* are entirely different chemically, consisting of branched polysaccharides, composed of different sugars and uronic acid, which is important for its high water-binding and ion exchange properties.
> *Pectins* are present in cell walls and intracellular layers and have a particular ability for forming gels; they also tend to bind minerals such as calcium.
> *Gums, mucilages, and storage polysaccharides* are present between the cells and form the sticky exudates seen at the site of injury to plants; they are a complex group of finely branched uronic acid-containing polymers with an ion-binding capacity which may influence cholesterol and bile salt metabolism.
> *Lignin* is also entirely different chemically, consisting of phenol-propane polymers.

Other fibre-associated chemical factors include phytic acid, silica, lipids, waxes and proteins. Not only are there big chemical differences, but each sub-group has particular physico-chemical properties and between different food sources there are wide variations in the relative amounts of these substances.

It has long been known that low fibre diets produce small, hard stools which pass through the gut slowly and high fibre diets produce large, soft motions which pass more quickly (Cowgill and Anderson, 1932). A rural African with his very high fibre intake may pass approximately 500 grams of stool daily, in contrast to a European with a much lower fibre-containing diet producing daily stools of about 100 grams. Fibre provides substrate for the normally present bacteria in the colon, stimulating their growth. The breakdown products of fibre include the volatile fatty acids which have a mild stimulant effect on colonic motility and carbon dioxide, hydrogen and methane, which contribute towards the softening of the stool. There are other important physico-chemical activities; the absorption of bile salts for example may actually reduce bowel frequency. The effect of dietary fibre on alimentation can be summarised as follows:

The effects of dietary fibre on colonic function

Faecal weight increased
Transit time reduced
Colonic pressure lowered
Bacterial metabolism increased
Lipid metabolism modified
Bile salt excretion increased
Energy intake reduced (there is a satisfying volume but with fewer calories)
Delayed absorption from the small intestine
Absorption of bile salts, calcium, iron, zinc and vitamins reduced.

The potential of dietary fibre to alter colonic metabolism, to dilute colonic contents and also to absorb toxic materials means that it may have great therapeutic importance.

In clinical practice bran is assuming a major role in increasing intake of dietary fibre. It is a by-product of the flour milling process for making white bread and comprises all the outer layers of the wheat grain. Bran is the material left after flour has been separated from the grain. Studies have shown that bran is more efficacious than vegetable and fruit fibres; bran has the greatest laxative action, followed by cabbage, whereas lettuce and celery have no significant effect. The stools from subjects on cereal supplements have been shown to be heavier than those on vegetable or fruit supplements. The addition of 30 grams of bran daily can approximately double the weight of stool.

Bran

Payler, Pomare, Heaton *et al.* (1975) showed that a bran supplement can have a regulatory effect on both constipation and diarrhoea. Kirwan, Smith, McConnell *et al.* (1974) found that giving the coarser bran had a greater effect than using fine bran; there was also a significantly greater water-holding capacity, the coarse and fine bran holding 6 grams and 2 grams of water per gram of bran respectively. Furthermore, fine bran failed completely at a dose of 20 grams a day to produce significant changes in colonic motility or transit time.

A final note of caution must be added about the clinical use of dietary fibre. If there is any intestinal obstruction increasing the dietary fibre can expose the patient to the risk of colonic impaction. There may be possible hazards relating to the absorption of minerals and vitamins associated with the phytic acid content. There are also a significant number of patients whose intestinal symptoms are actually worsened by taking bran and who may be much improved by stopping it.

MELANOSIS COLI AND CATHARTIC COLON

Mottled grey-brown mucosal pigmentation is a commonly seen side-effect of anthracene purgatives taken over a long period. The coloration is due to the degenerative pigment lipofuchsin and has no particular significance, although it is useful in patients with adenomas, which show up as non-pigmented areas.

Chronic and high-dose purgative addiction has been shown to cause neural changes and the dangers of purgation have rightly been given wide publicity, although the clinical condition of *cathartic colon* is rarely seen. Affected patients may complain of diarrhoea due to the purgatives and their now functionless colon, but the primary features are of weakness due to potassium loss and thirst due to dehydration and hypokalaemic renal damage. Barium enema shows a characteristically dilated and featureless colon with slowly-changing pseudo-strictures.

Having thought of this diagnosis the stool can be tested for purgatives and the patients' self-medication investigated. Patients not infrequently deny that they are constipated and that they are taking aperients. This is often a psychological quirk but may occasionally be true as with patients taking 'health salts'. Potassium replacement and attempts at purgative withdrawal will usually save the situation, although irreversible damage may have occurred.

REFERENCES AND FURTHER READING

Cowgill GR and Anderson WE. Laxative effect of wheat bran and washed bran in healthy man. *Journal of the American Medical Association* 1932; **98:** 1866–8.

Hinton JM, Lennard-Jones JE and Young AC. A new method for studying gut transit times using radio-opaque markers. *Gut* 1969; **10:** 842–7.

Kirwan WO, Smith AN, McConnell AA, Mitchell WD and East-wood MA. Action of different bran preparations on colonic function. *British Medical Journal* 1974; **4:** 187–9.

Jones FA and Godding EN. *Management of constipation.* Oxford: Blackwell Scientific, 1972.

Payler DK, Pomare EW, Heaton KW and Harvey RF. The effect of wheat bran on intestinal transit. *Gut* 1975; **16:** 209–13.

MEGACOLON AND MEGARECTUM IN THE ADULT

Megacolon and megarectum can be defined as conditions in which the diameter of the intestine is considerably increased, more or less permanently. The term indicates the state of the bowel and not the cause of the abnormality, the word 'idiopathic' often being used to imply our lack of understanding of the aetiology. If sought for, however, a cause is often apparent, even if ill understood.

The 'mega' condition may arise as a result of long standing and persistent distal obstruction resulting from damage to the large bowel's nerve supply, inadequate contractile potential, or possibly abuse of drugs. Relatively acute conditions such as neoplastic strictures, diverticular disease and ischaemia may cause slight proximal dilatation and even a little hypertrophy, but never to the same degree as in true megacolon. Volvulus may occasionally be considered in differential diagnosis but should not be included under the same heading since it is seldom a long standing condition and is primarily a closed loop obstruction with dilatation.

CLASSIFICATION

Megacolon and its causes can be considered under the following broad headlines:

Mechanical obstruction
Neurological causes
Muscular abnormalities
Connective tissue defects
Rare and unclassified disorders

Some of these conditions are well understood, some are controversial and some not understood at all: In each case, however, the symptoms are essentially the same, with prolonged constipation and no bowel action for weeks or months (even up to a year). Distension is a frequent complaint, with a bearing down sensation or 'weight' in the perineum. Spurious diarrhoea may occur due to impaction. It is important to find out whether or not the symptoms have been present from birth, if and when laxatives were first taken, including the type and amount used, whether enemas have been used regularly or whether soiling or incontinence have ever been features.

The clinical signs vary to some extent in each condition. Those of special note are a splayed rib margin, the presence of faecalomas in the colon or rectum, rectal ampullary dilatation, ease of sigmoidoscopy and the presence of a lax anal sphincter.

A plain x-ray of the abdomen can demonstrate the colon outlined by gas or its vast faecal content. Contrast studies may also be of value. If the plain film shows uniform faecal retention throughout the colon, a double contrast barium enema should be carried out with full bowel preparation. If there is gross faecal retention in the rectum a water-soluble enema, without preparation, is prefered to outline the rectum and exclude a short aganglionic segment – anteroposterior and lateral views should be obtained.

Electromyography and sensory studies of rectal, anal and sphincteric function are helpful. Motility and transit studies rarely help, but a full thickness rectal biopsy should probably be carried out as the final investigation in all cases where conservative management has failed.

MECHANICAL OBSTRUCTION

Perhaps the most important cause of mechanical obstruction is the missed minor congenital abnormality of the anorectum, where the anus opens in the wrong site and is stenotic. Correction of the abnormality may not relieve the constipation or improve the secondary megarectum and megacolon if the deformity is discovered at a late stage, but should nonetheless be attempted. It has been mentioned that sigmoid colon volvulus is not a cause of generalised megacolon and before making this diagnosis it is important to decide whether the dilatation is confined to the sigmoid colon. If the transverse colon is markedly distended the diagnosis of 'volvulus' is probably incorrect and, therefore, sigmoid colectomy will not be permanently curative.

NEUROLOGICAL CAUSES

Ganglionic disorders may be either congenital or acquired, the resultant change in the wall of the intestine differing remarkably. Hirschsprung's disease and Chagas' disease are the classic models of each type. Congenital disorders of ganglia may be classified as being due to immature ganglia (as found in a premature infant) oligoganglionosis and lastly true Hirschsprung's disease (congenital aganglionosis), which is the only form found in the adult, in which the abnormal segment may be short or long. Unfortunately many conditions are incorrectly given this or a similar name, varying from country to country, and this leads to a great deal of misunderstanding. The term 'pseudo-Hirschsprung's disease' as used in Sweden, South Africa and Brazil means different things in each country and should be abandoned therefore. Hyperganglionosis has now been recognised.

In Hirschsprung's disease the ganglia of the submucosal and myenteric plexuses are apparently absent from the anorectal ring proximally for a variable distance. Most commonly the absence of ganglia extends for some 10 to 15 cm but there may be ultra-short or longer segments, involving even the whole colon or rarely the whole intestine. The lowermost rectum immediately above the anorectal ring is, however, always aganglionic. The affected segment does not transmit progressive peristaltic activity and remains unrelaxing. The intestine proximal to this functional obstruction then gradually dilates and hypertrophies. Normally the internal sphincter region has no ganglia. Isolated colonic aganglionic segments do not occur.

Hirschsprung's disease

Hirschsprung's disease may occur in more than one sibling. The vast majority of cases present in infancy, but the disease may also present in adolescence and older age. Usually there is a history of constipation dating more or less from birth, but without soiling or incontinence. Rarely disorders of micturition occur as well, possibly related to ganglionic abnormality at the lower end of the ureters, or in association with the bladder.

Clinical features

Distension may be alarming, the rib margin bends outwards and respiration becomes embarrassed. Unless active measures are taken, pneumonia and death may occur. Washouts may relieve the condition temporarily but in the neonate urgent surgical intervention may be needed (Chapter 10). Under these circumstances, other conditions such as 'meconium ileus' or 'meconium plug' must be borne in mind. Rectal examination reveals an empty ampulla and no dilatation.

Barium enema examination may show the diagnostic features of proximal distension, a coned area (in which a few abnormal ganglia will be present) and a narrowed (distal) segment usually

Investigations

down to the anal canal (in which no ganglia are found) (Fig. 10.1).

In the older patient the coned area is less obvious, fore-shortened and often aganglionic. This is presumably due to prolonged impaction of faeces causing some degree of enlargement. Lateral films of the pelvis must be taken to show the short segment Hirschsprung's disease or the narrowed segment may not be seen behind the hugely dilated rectum or sigmoid.

In the infant the x-ray appearance and a rectal biopsy including mucosa and submucosa showing abnormal nerves may be sufficiently diagnostic to enable surgery to be undertaken without further investigation. In theory a diagnosis may be made on a biopsy which shows only the submucosa in which ganglia are absent and the nerve plexus is grossly distorted, appearing as wavy hypertrophic nerve bundles. However, in the adult, few pathologists would be prepared to commit themselves without a more extensive piece of tissue which incorporates the myenteric plexus. A full thickness biopsy of the rectal wall is, therefore, taken as a strip from just above the anorectal ring; this requires general anaesthesia (Todd, 1977).

Rectal sensation studies with an intrarectal balloon and electromyography can be helpful. The anal pressure profile may be diagnostic; this tests the internal sphincter response, the sphincter failing to relax as the rectum is distended.

Treatment

The treatment of Hirschsprung's disease is to remove as much as possible of the obstructive aganglionic segment whilst retaining the rectal and pelvic floor sensory area to preserve continence. The Swenson pull-through procedure is often the operation of choice for the very young. Depending on age and the severity of symptoms, this may be preceded by a colostomy. It must be carefully placed in a portion of the colon containing ganglia but leaving sufficient normal ganglionic bowel distal to it for subsequent anastomosis after resection of the aganglionic portion. In younger patients part of the dilated hypertrophic ganglionic bowel should also be removed, since it is liable to contract poorly after anastomosis, being shown by Smith (1972) to contain atypical or degenerate ganglia. It is usual to preserve between 1–3 cm of aganglionic rectum to help retain full sensation.

In the adult the dilated proximal bowel will preclude an eversion pull-through procedure and some authorities advocate a low anterior resection (State procedure), because it is unlikely to damage the pelvic autonomic nerves or interfere with sex function. However, a Duhamel operation seems preferable as this removes more of the aganglionic segment, pelvic nerve damage is minimal, the operation is technically easy and complications are rare (Chapter 10).

Chagas' disease is only found in parts of Central and South America and is due to infection by *Trypanosoma cruzi*. It provides a model of what happens when intestinal ganglia or neurones degenerate. The affected intestine becomes less efficient, initially hypertrophies as it tries to push material along and then becomes decompensated and dilates. The vector is an infected triatomal fly which bites the patient, causing a brief acute pyrexial illness (Fig. 2.8). Ganglionic degeneration, probably due to a toxin, takes place slowly in a quantitative manner throughout the body. The effect of this is greatest on those organs which are subjected to most work, the heart, oesophagus and distal large intestine, giving rise to cardiomegaly, megaoesophagus and megacolon and megarectum respectively. Resection of the whole decompensated portion of the large intestine is required when constipation, distension and obstruction become intolerable. There is a difference of opinion as to

Chagas' disease

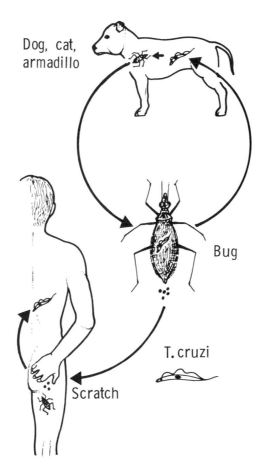

Dog, cat, armadillo

Bug

T. cruzi

Scratch

Fig. 2.8 Chagas' disease – the life cycle of *Trypanosoma cruzi*.

the best surgical procedure in Chagas' disease: the choice is between a very low anterior resection, a Cutait-Turnbull pull-through procedure (Cutait, 1977) and a modified Duhamel operation. It should be remembered when deciding which procedure to adopt that the sphincters have been subjected to the effect of prolonged straining and the inhibitory and closing reflexes may have been impaired.

Drugs

Changes similar to those of Chagas' disease can be caused by certain substances which are neurotoxic and may damage the neural plexus (Smith, 1972). In some susceptible people administration of anthracene derivatives – aloes in the South African Bantu, senna in western civilisation – and some tranquillisers and anticholinergic agents can be associated with these changes and the development of megacolon. However, it cannot be proved that the laxatives are the cause of the changes demonstrated as they may have been taken because of a real problem of bowel function.

The extreme example of this condition is cathartic colon, though this can exist without enlargement of the bowel. If symptoms are severe, colectomy with ileo or caecorectal anastomosis is required. Retention of the ileocaecal valve improves bowel function and gives rise to a lower frequency of defaecation than follows ileorectal anastomosis.

MUSCULAR ABNORMALITIES

Two poorly defined conditions occur for which no aetiology is known; neither can be diagnosed with certainty except at laparotomy when the true state of the intestine can be seen.

Paper-thin colon presents most frequently in females between the ages of 15–25. The condition is suspected if constipation occurs which worsens over a period of a few years in spite of using increasing doses of laxatives. Whether the taking of laxatives precedes the colonic wall abnormality, is not known. Distension and upper abdominal discomfort across the whole hypochondrium, particularly after meals, can be so marked that pregnancy may be suggested. There is frequently an inability to pass wind freely; the abdomen is usually tympanitic but may contain a large faecaloma in the sigmoid colon. A plain x-ray often shows air in the transverse colon. A double contrast barium enema shows a long redundant hypotonic colon which may appear to contract in the post-evacuation film, but can easily be blown up to a very large diameter, the haustral pattern being maintained but uniformly enlarged.

These patients can respond to medical treatment in the form of Epsom salts (magnesium sulphate) or Rae's mixture (liquid paraffin, magnesium sulphate and neostigmine), but stimulant laxatives such as the anthraquinone group should be avoided. If conservative methods are unsuccessful, surgery may have a place but resection of the redundant thin sigmoid colon alone seldom helps for more than a few months since the remaining colon is thin and has inadequate musculature. The preferred procedure is colectomy and caecorectal anastomosis (Lane and Todd, 1977). After this the retained caecum may blow up with gas on occasions, although passage of a finger or a flatus tube through the anus will relieve this at once. No abnormality of the sphincter inhibitory reflexes has been shown and unfortunately anal dilatation has not helped.

Hypertrophic colon and rectum is exceedingly rare. Distal obstruction is postulated but none is found. On occasions a colostomy may be needed but there is no logical surgical procedure to help this condition. Internal sphincterotomy has not proved to be beneficial.

CONNECTIVE TISSUE DEFECTS

Connective tissue disorders such as scleroderma and Ehlers-Danlos syndrome can cause megacolon. Treatment should be conservative except when colonic rupture occurs, when colectomy and ileorectal anastomosis is carried out.

RARE AND UNCLASSIFIED DISORDERS

Rare causes of megacolon include disorders of endocrine function such as myxoedema and cretinism, mental retardation (failure to appreciate normal defaecatory sensations) and unclassified paralytic problems.

Drugs seem to have excessive effects in some people who may be unduly sensitive to them. Most tranquillisers and antidepressants are also smooth muscle relaxants and problems already present may be accentuated by their use.

RECTAL INERTIA

The term dyschezia, first used by Hurst, is synonomous with rectal inertia and can give rise to secondary enlargement of the rectum. It results from persistent failure to respond to the normal call to stool, either because of laziness or failure of appreciation, as occurs in the mentally retarded. The constipation is primarily due to rectal overloading with the colon becoming secondarily distended as the rectum decompensates. The recto-sphincteric inhibitory reflex is initially normal and soiling and incontinence will occur. Later as rectal volume enlarges sensation becomes dulled. The changes finally become irreversible.

The most common presenting symptoms are overflow incontinence or spurious diarrhoea. Though rectal sensation is poor in these cases, anal canal sensation is retained so the semi-fluid stool impinging upon the anal papillae (the area where differentiation of solid, fluid and gas takes place) provides an urgent call to stool. On investigation the barium enema shows dilatation in both antero-posterior and lateral films down to the anorectal ring. Transit time of ingested radio-opaque markers may be normal to the sigmoid colon, but then there is a failure of evacuation.

Treatment is mainly directed towards emptying the rectum completely and keeping it empty in the hope that the rectal ampulla may regain its tone and sensation, the latter being a muscle-stretch phenomenon. The patient is told to answer any call to stool immediately. Initially laxatives must not be given until the bowel has been emptied by suppositories or washouts, otherwise more and more faeces will be forced into an already overloaded rectum. Glycerine or bisacodyl suppositories, two to six at a time, may be needed to initiate defaecation. Later on laxatives are used to keep the stool almost liquid for many months until the rectal tone has recovered. The most satisfactory laxatives to use in dyschezia are once again Epsom salts or Rae's mixture. An adequate dose to produce the desired effect must be used and continued. Early weaning off the drug is unwise and results in a relapse.

Dyschezic constipation with secondary bowel distension will also occur in most varieties of imperforate anus if the orifice is not kept adequate from birth. Even if definitive surgery is to be delayed, an adequate anus, which will admit an average index finger, must be surgically fashioned, since the results are better than those of simple dilatation (Chapter 10).

SIGMOID VOLVULUS

The long term effects of volvulus in a redundant sigmoid colon may be very similar to those of segmental idiopathic megacolon, although the cause is quite different. If the diagnosis is correct, the condition will be cured by a localised resection providing it is undertaken early rather than late. Persistent medical treatment will clearly not alleviate the condition. The colon does not show gross muscle hypertrophy, as the symptoms are due to the twisted (and thus 'closed') loop distending rather than to distal organic obstruction.

Clinical presentation is with pain of a colicky nature associated with gross distension and constipation. The onset of symptoms may be sudden or indefinite and recurrent episodes can occur. The distended sigmoid colon may often be palpated or seen on plain x-ray in the right upper quadrant of the abdomen (Fig. 1.17).

The volvulus can often be reduced and the acute condition overcome by passing a soft large bore tube through a sigmoidoscope. However, gangrene can occur and in this case excision of the devascularised segment with exteriorisation of the ends is probably the safest procedure to adopt. As volvulus tends to recur, it should be resected once diagnosed.

REFERENCES AND FURTHER READING

Cutait DE. Endo-anal abdominal perineal pull-through resection with colorectal anastomosis. In: Todd IP, ed. *Colon, rectum and anus.* (3rd ed. Operative surgery). London and Boston: Butterworths, 1977: 168–77.

Duhamel B. Historical investigations into idiopathic megacolon. *Archives of Diseases of Childhood* 1966; **41:** 150–1.

Ferrera-Santos R. Megacolon and megarectum in Chagas' disease. *Proceedings of the Royal Society of Medicine* 1961; **54:** 1047–53.

Lane RHS and Todd IP. Idiopathic megacolon: A review of 42 cases. *British Journal of Surgery* 1977; **64:** 305–10.

Nixon HH. Hirschsprung's disease. In: Todd IP, ed. *Colon, rectum and anus.* (3rd ed. Operative surgery). London and Boston: Butterworths, 1977: 271–82.

Smith B. *The neuropathology of the alimentary tract.* London: Arnold, 1972.

Todd IP. Intractible constipation and adult megacolon. In: Todd IP, ed. *Colon, rectum and anus.* (3rd ed. Operative surgery). London and Boston: Butterworths, 1977: 268–70.

3. Normal and Disordered Function of the Rectum and Pelvic Floor

ANATOMY AND PHYSIOLOGY

ANATOMY

Developmentally the anorectal region is composite in structure, consisting of two tube-like components, one within the other. The inner visceral component consists of the termination of the alimentary tract, and contains only smooth muscle innervated by the autonomic nervous system. The outer (somatic) component is composed of skeletal muscle which forms the external sphincter (Fig. 3.1). The muscle is mainly under reflex

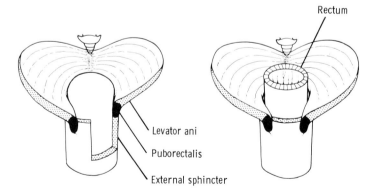

Fig. 3.1 The anal canal – the somatic muscle tube enclosing the visceral muscle tube.

control, but is also influenced by conscious motivation. This component not only has a sphincteric action, but its upper part is continuous with the levator ani muscles which fan out to close the pelvic hiatus.

The visceral component of the anal canal has a longitudinal layer of muscle, a circular layer (the internal sphincter), submucosa and mucosa. The internal sphincter is a fairly large muscle mass which superficially resembles the thickened segment of the circular muscle of the lower rectum. There are, however, profound functional and anatomical differences between them. The upper half of the anal canal is lined by columnar, mucus-secreting epithelium identical with that of the rectum. In the course of development ectoderm migrates into the lower half of the anal canal which is lined by squamous epithelium as a result. The importance of this is that it is dry and does not secrete mucus; it is also richly innervated by the pudendal nerve and plays an important part in the maintenance of continence. The muco-cutaneous junction, about half way along the anal canal, is fixed to the underlying internal sphincter so that columnar epithelium cannot prolapse externally. The somatic or skeletal muscle component of the pelvic floor comprises the external sphincter, the puborectalis and the levator ani muscles (pubo-coccygeus and ileococcygeus). The external sphincter is usually divided into three parts, but functionally it is a unit. The innervation is derived from the inferior haemorrhoidal nerve.

The puborectalis muscle, probably the most powerful, arises from the pubic ramus near the mid line anteriorly and passes behind the upper anal canal as a sling. It therefore has a sphincteric action on all the viscera of the pelvic hiatus and at the same time has the important task of maintaining the angulation between the lower rectum and the anal canal (Fig. 3.2).

The levator ani muscles have no sphincteric activity but have an antigravity function, preventing herniation of the viscera

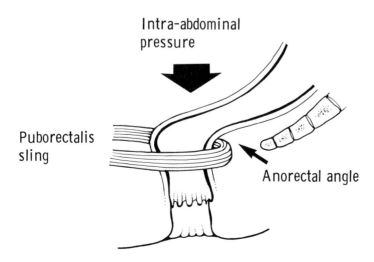

Fig. 3.2 The anorectal angle.

through the pelvis. Innervation of the levator ani muscles, and probably the puborectalis, comes from the branch of S4 which descends on their internal surface. The blood supply to the skeletal muscles of the pelvic floor, on the other hand, enters via their external aspect.

In between the two components of the pelvic floor there is an embryonic plane of fusion. In the normal person very few blood vessels cross this plane and practically no nervous structures. It is of practical importance in as much as fistula tracks tend to spread within it. In addition it is a useful plane of dissection for certain operative procedures, as no important structures are encountered.

PHYSIOLOGY

The visceral component

The importance of the squamous mucosa of the lower 2 cm of the anal canal has been mentioned. Its rich innervation gives rise to conscious sensory information. If flatus or faeces enter the anal canal stimulation of the receptors causes immediate contraction of the external sphincter. The internal sphincter itself maintains closure of the anal canal in the resting state. The effective length of the sphincter can be observed by inserting a pressure probe into the lower rectum and drawing it down through the canal, recording the pressure changes 'en route' (Fig. 3.3). The length (about 3.5 cm) is greater in men than

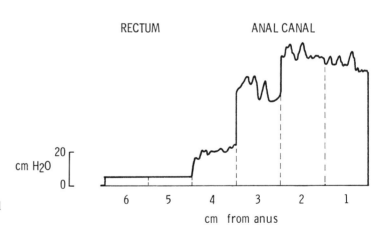

Fig. 3.3 Normal anal canal pressure tracing.

women by about half a centimetre and is unrelated to age or parity. The resting pressure is the same for men and women and diminishes with increasing age in both sexes. The maximal pressure is found half way along the internal sphincter; this is also observed in patients with a cauda equina lesion, a lesion of the sacral nerve roots and after transection of the spinal cord.

Serial distension of the rectum with small volumes produces transient relaxation of internal sphincter after each increment (Fig. 3.4). With each increment the base line pressure falls and

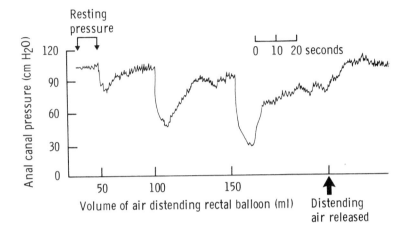

Fig. 3.4 Maximum anal canal pressure in response to rectal distension.

after a rectal distension of between 150–200 ml, the internal sphincter completely relaxes (Hancock, 1976; Lane and Parks, 1977); the balloon descends into the anal canal and only minimal straining is required to expel it. In patients with Hirschsprung's disease the reflex is absent and the internal sphincter fails to relax at all. In this condition the intrinsic neural plexus of the rectum is abnormal, which suggests that the receptor site is in the viscus itself.

The somatic component

The skeletal muscles of the pelvic floor have a dual role: they combat the force of intra-abdominal pressure, thus preventing a pelvic hernia, and the external sphincter group (which includes the puborectalis muscle) play the most important part in the maintenance of continence. Muscles which are actuated only by voluntary means would be useless for the task of maintaining continence or of combating gravitational forces, as the person's attention would need to be constantly drawn to them. An automatic mechanism is essential. If an electromyographic needle is inserted into most skeletal muscle no electrical activity at all is found at rest; it only develops as a result of voluntary or synergistic activity. The pelvic floor is quite different; the muscles are constantly contracting at rest and even during sleep. But this is not all as, by means of automatic reflex action, the muscles will either additionally contract or relax according to circumstance. Thus when intra-abdominal pressure rises (for example as a result of coughing, walking or

105

lifting) there is rapid reflex reinforcement of the tonic activity of the pelvic floor muscles to resist this pressure (Fig. 3.5). Voluntary contraction can be sustained for about 60 seconds but not much longer, after which activity fades.

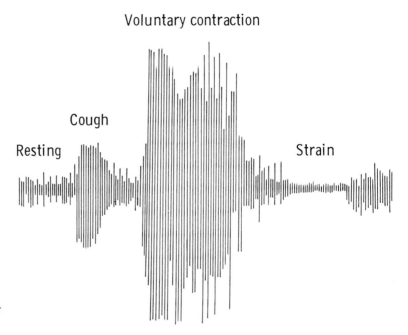

Fig. 3.5 External sphincter electromyography.

Distension of the rectum by a balloon first increases the activity of the skeletal muscles. This again will protect against involuntary evacuation. When inflated to a greater size, reflex relaxation of the entire sphincter mass occurs but rarely in normal circumstances. It is seen, however, when there is impaction of faeces, such as occurs in patients with idiopathic megacolon, in the elderly and in certain postoperative states. Here the rectum is grossly overloaded and the external sphincters are totally patulous. The main complaint of such a patient will be incontinence; he has no control at all. Liquid stool passing around the impacted mass leaks out without let or hindrance. This interesting physiological state also has clinical relevance, demanding vigilance on the part of the doctor, especially when looking after the elderly. Fortunately, it is readily corrected.

Normal defaecation straining also inhibits the activity of the pelvic floor reflex and allows a stool to be passed without difficulty (Fig. 3.5). However, if a person indulges in excessive defaecation straining over years, the pelvic floor is forced downwards at the same time as the muscles are relaxed and not counteracting this force. They are therefore passively stretched. Though recovery is almost certainly complete after a temporary episode of this nature, if the habit persists for years the pelvic floor will be gradually forced lower and the muscles become increasingly stretched. Not only may the muscles lengthen and become less efficient because of this, but the nerves supplying them are also stretched, in particular the branches supplying the external sphincter. This will be referred to in a later section.

The mechanical valve effect is maintained by the tonic contraction of the external sphincter and puborectalis muscles. The lower rectum makes a double right angle just before and on entering the upper anal canal (Fig. 3.2). As a result, the upper part of the canal is closed by the anterior wall of the lower rectum, which impinges upon it. Any increase in abdominal pressure will automatically force that part of the lower rectal wall even more firmly upon the closed upper anal canal and will block it provided the anal sphincters remain active. In this way a flap valve is formed between a zone of high and low pressure. Thus, any increase in abdominal pressure will automatically seal the upper anal canal and prevent stress incontinence occurring. The angulation between the anal canal and lower rectum is maintained by the puborectalis muscle.

Sensation

Assessment of any sensation, whether qualitative or quantative, is always difficult. However, there is no doubt that in the normal person rectal distension produces a sensation of fullness in the perineum associated with a feeling of impending evacuation. Distension above the ampulla produces only intestinal abdominal colic. It was originally thought that receptors responsible for 'rectal' sensation were present in the rectal wall. Recently, however, it has been shown that the sensory mechanism remains intact even after total excision of the rectum with anastomosis of the colon to the upper anal canal (Lane and Parks, 1977). It is therefore apparent that the rectum itself is not the site of sensory information. The rectal ampulla lies in a cradle formed by the levator ani muscles and it is probable that changes in volume stimulate stretch receptors in these muscles. Further evidence for this comes from patients who have had total excision of the colon and rectum for ulcerative colitis and have been given a pelvic pouch anastomosed to the anal canal. As the pouch distends, they get a sensation identical with that experienced in their previously normal state.

In summary, the internal sphincter keeps the anal canal closed and provides a pressure gradient acting against the rectum, the latter functioning as a reservoir for faeces and flatus. The tone of the levator ani and external sphincter is maintained by a reflex arc. Sensory impulses arises from receptors in the pelvic floor muscles and the squamous mucosa of the anal canal, providing information at both reflex and conscious levels. The tonic contractile activity of the pelvic floor muscles continually adjusts to changes in abdominal pressure. Contraction of the puborectalis muscle, situated at the anorectal junction, maintains the right angle between the axis of the rectal ampulla and the anal canal itself. This in turn establishes a flap valve mechanism which automatically occludes the upper anal canal. The seal of the valve is normally only broken by intra-luminal contents entering the lower part of the ampulla.

REFERENCES AND FURTHER READING

Hancock BD. Measurement of anal pressure and motility. *Gut* 1976; **17:** 645–51.

Ihre T. Studies on anal function in continent and incontinent patients. *Scandinavian Journal of Gastroenterology* 1974; **9:** Supplement 25.

Kerremans R. *Morphological and Physiological Aspects of Anal Continence and Defaecation.* Brussels: Arscia Vitgaven, 1969.

Lane RHS and Parks AG. Function of the anal sphincters following coloanal anastomosis. *British Journal of Surgery* 1977; **64:** 596–9.

DESCENDING PERINEUM SYNDROME

The normal position for the anal canal is above a line joining the ischial tuberosities and the ano-rectal junction lies immediately below a line joining the lower part of the pubic symphysis to the tip of the coccyx (Fig. 3.6). During the act of straining the anal canal should not drop more than 2 cm.

In patients with the descending perineum syndrome the anal canal will, in the resting, state, lie at a lower level and on straining the perineum may balloon well below the lowermost limits of the bony pelvis (Fig. 1.6). The incidence in the general population is unknown, although it is a quite frequent finding in patients attending a rectal clinic. It is more common in women and may occur at any age, although it is rare before the third decade.

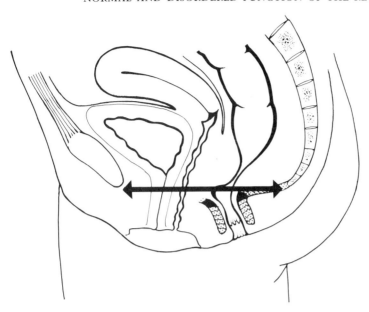

Fig. 3.6 The upper anal canal normally lies on the line joining the lower borders of the public symphysis and the coccyx.

AETIOLOGY

The majority of patients will admit to excessive straining efforts at the time of defaecation. It is probable that this is a major factor in the aetiology as prolonged periods of straining will weaken the pelvic musculature and in time reduce the normal anorectal angle. Furthermore the straining effort, by increasing intra-abdominal pressure, which is transmitted across the anterior rectal wall, will encourage prolapse of mucosa into the upper anal canal. This anterior mucosal prolapse (AMP) results in a feeling of incomplete evacuation of the bowel, to which the patient will respond by further straining efforts. Thus a vicious circle is set up (Fig. 3.7).

When pressure measurements are made in these patients, both the resting pressure in the anal canal and the normal increase in pressure during voluntary contraction are reduced. The pudendal nerve is tethered at two sites in the bony pelvis, where the nerve passes from the greater sciatic foramen over the ischial spine to gain access via the lesser sciatic foramen to the pudendal (Alcock's) canal. When the pelvic floor descends the pudendal nerve and its branches supplying the external anal sphincter (and levator ani) are stretched. Nerve function may be seriously affected by a stretching force and this may be the aetiology of both the external sphincter weakness and the perineal pain some of these patients experience (Parks, Swash and Urich, 1977).

109

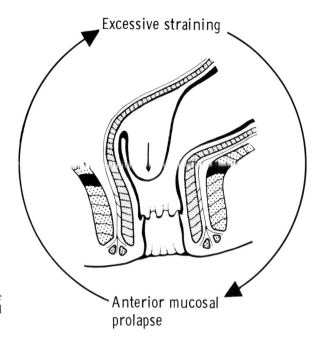

Excessive straining

Anterior mucosal
prolapse

Fig. 3.7 The vicious circle
of straining and mucosal
prolapse.

Parks, Porter and Hardcastle (1966) originally found that
electromyographic potentials recorded from the external
sphincter during a straining effort displayed rapid inhibition as
the pelvic floor descended. Further study has shown that this is
so where there is gross perineal descent. If, however, there is a
lesser degree of descent the converse may apply. That there is
failure of inhibition or even recruitment of activity in early cases
suggests this may be a significant source of some of the
defaecation difficulties.

CLINICAL FEATURES

Patients with the descending perineum syndrome usually
experience a sense of incomplete evacuation associated with a
constant desire to defaecate; there may also be the passage of
mucus and blood. Straining at defaecation is usually a major
feature and this may be accompanied by overt mucosal or
haemorrhoidal prolapse. There is frequently a past history of
haemorrhoidectomy.

Faecal incontinence of varying degrees and constant perineal
pain, characteristically precipitated or aggravated by sitting,
occur in the advanced case.

The perineum will often be observed to lie at least 1 cm
below the bony outlet of the pelvis at rest. Alternatively it may
lie in the normal position at rest, but descend more than 2 cm

when the patient is asked to strain, or 'bear down' as if to pass a stool. There may be prolapse of rectal mucosa or haemorrhoids at the anus. Digital examination usually reveals a reduced resting anal tone with a correspondingly poor 'squeeze' during voluntary contraction over the examining finger. Proctoscopy will demonstrate obvious anterior rectal mucosal prolapse. Occasionally a solitary ulcer of the rectum may be observed on sigmoidoscopy (see below).

MANAGEMENT

The fact that during prolonged straining the patient is effectively attempting to evacuate his own rectal mucosa should be very carefully explained to him. The steps necessary to avoid further straining need to be discussed and include: the correction of constipation, usually by means of a bulk laxative, the use of suppositories (glycerine or bisacodyl) and the administration of enemata. If the rectum is satisfactorily emptied each morning any further call to stool should be ignored, if at all possible.

Anterior mucosal prolapse or prolapsing haemorrhoids will require treatment. The former is best managed by injection sclerotherapy, but if this is not adequate then rubber band ligation, or even surgical excision will be necessary.

Where there is faecal incontinence, sphincter exercises accompanied by a course of pelvic Faradism may improve function. If conservative measures are not successful a post-anal repair should be considered.

REFERENCES AND FURTHER READING

Parks AG, Porter NH and Hardcastle JD. The syndrome of the descending perineum. *Proceedings of The Royal Society of Medicine* 1966; **59**: 477–82.
Parks AG, Swash M and Urich H. Sphincter denervation in anorectal incontinence and rectal prolapse. *Gut* 1977; **18**: 656–65.

SOLITARY ULCER SYNDROME

The solitary ulcer syndrome is a not uncommon condition but it is frequently misdiagnosed because of its protean manifestations. In the majority of cases a frank ulcer is present, usually situated on the anterior wall of the lower rectum. Occasionally the ulcer is situated higher in the rectum (usually from 7–10 cm). At this site there may be multiple ulcers which may involve the rectum circumferentially.

The ulcer is typically shallow, though it may be several centimetres in diameter, and is surrounded by clinically inflamed mucosa. Sometimes no frank ulceration is seen; there is only a localised area of inflamed mucosa which may even be polypoid. The characteristic histological features have been described by Madigan and Morson (1969) and consist of the replacement of the lamina propria by fibroblasts and smooth muscle cells which are arranged at right angles to the muscularis mucosae; that is, they pass towards the surface between the tubules of the mucosa.

CLINICAL FEATURES

Clinical and experimental evidence suggests that the changes are the response of the mucosa to trauma. This is usually the result of prolapse, either mucosal or complete, and is brought about by straining efforts (Rutter and Riddell, 1975). It is probable that the low anterior ulcers are associated with mucosal prolapse, the higher ones being due to an intussusception of the rectum. This latter situation can be demonstrated radiologically and can also be seen on sigmoidoscopy when the patient is straining. Frank ulceration of this type is seldom seen in true rectal prolapse in which the anal sphincters are weak and patulous. It is likely that mucosal trauma results from straining efforts in the presence of an actively contracting sphincter mechanism (physiological studies indicate that the puborectalis actually contracts when the patient strains down).

The commonest symptom is the passage of mucus, frequently associated with blood. Perineal pain may be experienced, particularly during and after defaecation. The patient often has a sense of anal obstruction (due to the mucosal prolapse), and this results in prolonged and excessive straining, perhaps the most important aetiological factor. Characteristically also there is a sense of incomplete evacuation which is present throughout the day, so that the person makes multiple, fruitless defaecation attempts. Such symptoms, together with the findings on examination, may be mistaken for carcinoma, and indeed rectal excision has been performed in error – a further reason for positive biopsy prior to cancer surgery. The second diagnostic difficulty is the confusion with non-specific inflammatory bowel disease. It is probable that diagnoses such as *mucous colitis* are in fact due to this syndrome.

MANAGEMENT

Treatment is nearly always conservative and in the first instance is aimed at explaining to the patient the exact nature of the condition. The prevention of straining is the all important factor in the relief of symptoms. However, the repetitive defaecation urge experienced by such people is often compulsive and in such cases the chance of success is small. They may learn to live with the condition, the symptoms being reduced to such a level that they are tolerable.

Operative intervention is seldom called for, though several authors have reported improvement following rectopexy in those patients who have marked internal intussusception. It is not yet possible to say whether this type of treatment will give permanent relief.

REFERENCES AND FURTHER READING

Madigan MR and Morson BC. Solitary ulcer of the rectum. *Gut* 1969; **10**: 871–81.
Rutter KRP and Riddell RH. The solitary ulcer syndrome of the rectum. *Clinics in Gastroenterology* 1975; **4**: 505–30.

RECTAL PROLAPSE

Rectal prolapse is defined as the protrusion of one or more layers of rectum through the anal sphincter. If mucosa alone is involved, the prolapse is called incomplete (Fig. 3.8); if all layers of the rectal wall protrude, it is termed complete (Fig. 3.9).

The terminology implies that incomplete rectal prolapse has the same causes and is merely an earlier stage of complete prolapse, but there are many reasons to doubt this assumption. Moschowitz (1912) stated that complete rectal prolapse is a true 'hernia-en-glissade' of rectum and distal colon through the pelvic diaphragm, and this clearly can occur without antecedent mucosal protrusion. Similarly, mucosal prolapse can result from a wide variety of causes of distortion of the tubular structure of the anal canal associated with laxity of the submucosa (such as third-degree haemorrhoids, pronounced rectocoele, perineal descent, anal sphincter weakness and after operations for fistula-in-ano) without any evidence of pelvic floor hernia and with little or no tendency to progress to a complete rectal prolapse. However, while there is considerable reason to doubt that the two types of rectal prolapse are of similar aetiology, they often co-exist and the terms complete and incomplete which have been hallowed by long clinical use serve to emphasise the major difference between them.

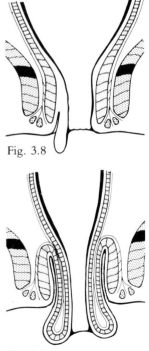

Fig. 3.8

Fig. 3.9

Mucosal (incomplete) prolapse can be treated by surgical manoeuvres directed at the mucosa (and its local supporting structures) but complete rectal prolapse can be cured only by operations which include retethering the rectum within the pelvic cavity.

Although complete rectal prolapse was described in the Ebers Papyrus of 1500 B.C., until recently it was regarded as untreatable since there was no practical method for permanently replacing the prolapsed rectum. Operations were devised in the 19th Century that amputated the excessive tissue protruding from the anus, but insofar as these did not affect the origin of the prolapse at the pelvic diaphragm they were usually unsuccessful and in the course of time further lengths of bowel inevitably descended through the weakened pelvic floor.

INCIDENCE AND AETIOLOGY

Rectal prolapse is commonest in children below the age of three, and in elderly women. In both age groups, straining at defaecation and pelvic floor weakness are common.

In children, an obsessional mother is often the cause of the straining, and pelvic weakness may be present as a result of malnutrition and absence of ischiorectal fat; whooping cough, measles and tuberculosis may also cause wasting and laxity of the levator muscles and may be associated with a chronic cough causing bursts of raised intra-abdominal pressure to stretch the tissues still further. Chronic urinary obstruction can also substitute for constipation as a cause for prolonged straining, and the shallow sacral curve of the infant has also been suspected as aggravating the tendency to pelvic floor deficiency. It is clear that most of these factors are reversible, and the great majority of childhood prolapses recover on conservative management; however, 10% of cases persist, and in these children some permanent abnormality of the pelvic floor or mental defectiveness is often present. In these instances careful search for spinal defects and paralysis of the pelvic diaphragm must be made by suitable radiographic studies, including myelography and electromyography. Cystic fibrosis is another cause.

In adults, females predominate in the proportion of 6:1 and most of them are thin, elderly women. In men the peak incidence falls off after the age of forty, whereas in women it climbs steadily to reach its maximum incidence in the seventh decade. The predominance of female patients might suggest that previous pregnancy and labour are important aetiological factors. Kupfer and Goligher (1970) investigated this and found that the incidence of complete prolapse was in fact higher in those female patients who were nulliparous. More than half the adult cases give a clear history of straining associated with intractable constipation and it is this which probably provides the abdominal squeeze that produces the prolapse.

Weakness of the pelvic floor is clearly an important aetiological factor. Neurological disorders affecting the cauda equina and the pelvic nerves (for example multiple sclerosis, tabes dorsalis, neoplasms or trauma) have a definite incidence of complete rectal prolapse, but overall only account for 1.5% of cases.

PATHOLOGICAL CHANGES

Defaecation is a delicately synchronised response in which relaxation and contraction of the large bowel, pelvic floor and

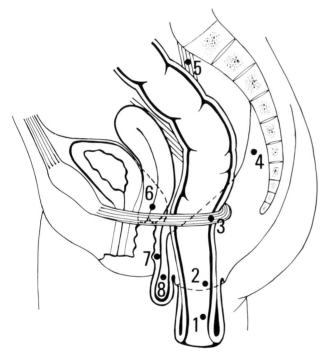

1   Prolapsed rectum

2   Gaping patulous anus

3   Stretched puborectalis

4   Increased presacral space

5   Attenuated lateral ligaments

6   Procidentia uteri

7   Atrophic rectovaginal septum

8   Large peritoneal pouch

Fig. 3.10 The patho-anatomy of complete rectal prolapse.

abdominal muscles are completely co-ordinated. Prolonged straining abolishes anal sphincter tone and if the puborectalis is weak or damaged by the factors already discussed, then the whole pelvic floor sags. With this downward descent there is a degree of invagination of the rectal wall which causes it to turn itself inside out as it emerges from the anal canal. Cineradiographic studies have shown that in many cases the prolapse starts as an internal intussusception of the rectum in the region of the middle to upper two-thirds (Broden and Snellman, 1968). Once the leading edge of the prolapse reaches the anal canal, it itself causes further reflex anal inhibition with the development of the typical gaping patulous anus which accompanies the condition. The prolapsed rectum becomes traumatised and the mucosa ulcerated with histological changes identical to those of the solitary ulcer syndrome. There is now considerable evidence that pelvic floor weakness may be associated with a traction neuropathy of the pudendal nerve as a result of downward displacement of the pelvic floor, for example during straining or child birth (Parks, Swash and Urich, 1977). This may be responsible in many cases not only for the prolapse, but also for the incontinence that frequently accompanies it. The patho-anatomical changes of complete rectal prolapse are diagrammatically shown in Fig. 3.10.

CLINICAL ASSESSMENT

Before embarking on treatment a thorough appraisal of each case is necessary. There are three equally important facets to this clinical assessment, viz: the degree of prolapse, the state of continence and the fitness of the patient.

In order to determine whether a prolapse is complete or not, it is essential that the full extent of the rectal protrusion should be produced to the examining surgeon. This can usually be brought about by asking an adult patient to strain, but can be almost impossible to achieve in children. In such cases of difficulty or doubt, the answer can often be obtaining by examining the patient immediately after an attempt at defaecation produced by a glycerine suppository. If the prolapse is small, visual examination may not be enough to decide if full rectal wall descent is present, but in complete prolapse while rolling the prolapse between the finger and thumb the surgeon will be able to feel the characteristic thickening present near the anal verge where the bowel wall doubles back on itself. Other aids to diagnosis include the observation that in complete prolapse concentric circular folds of mucosa are usually seen, and on sigmoidoscopy the mucosa of the rectum may be boggy, oedematous and friable, testifying that it has been prolapsing in the recent past. The upper limit of such mucosal changes provides a very accurate guide to the extent of prolapse that is present. Very rarely, the anterior hernial (rectovaginal) sac that is invariably found at operation in cases of complete prolapse may be seen or felt prior to surgery, and even when the prolapse cannot be extruded by the patient, small bowel in the sac may be felt with the finger between the rectum and the back of the vagina and uterus. Complete prolapse begins by descent of the anterior rectal wall and its accompanying peritoneal pouch, which causes the anterior wall to be characteristically more bulky than the posterior, and the lumen of the bowel to be directed posteriorly. If a markedly patulous anus is present, the case is likely to be one of complete prolapse.

The continence of the patient can be most accurately judged from the history when patients are prepared to divulge all the facts. If the anal sphincters are markedly patulous, this constitutes a subsidiary problem that may require treatment in addition to that aimed at the prolapse itself.

Differential diagnosis

In children complete rectal prolapse may have to be distinguished from an intussusception. This is usually very obvious from the history, but in any case of difficulty the finger should be inserted into the anal sulcus: if the finger passes freely into the rectal ampulla, the case is one of sigmoido-rectal intussusception and not rectal prolapse.

In both children and adults mucosal prolapse must be distinguished from a prolapsing anal polyp or third-degree haemorrhoids. The smooth glistening mucosa covering a juvenile polyp is easily differentiated from the rugose mucose of prolapse, and the presence of haemorrhoids is obvious once they are looked for.

In every case of prolapse the presence of other diseases of the colon or rectum must be excluded. Proctoscopy and sigmoidoscopy is mandatory in every case to exclude polyps or carcinoma of the rectum and lower sigmoid colon. In adults a radiographic appraisal of the whole colon should be made to exclude a carcinoma or severe diverticular disease, because in both instances treatment for the prolapse may have to be modified. Very occasionally a carcinoma presents as an ulcer on the prolapsing bowel, and any suspicious lesion should be biopsied.

MANAGEMENT

In adults the only way to control complete rectal prolapse is by operation. This is rarely the case in children where the condition usually resolves spontaneously on regulation of the bowel habit.

The general fitness of the patient to withstand an operation must be taken into account as many of them are elderly and enfeebled. However, in spite of this the operations are remarkably well tolerated, so that the clinician can afford to err generously on the side of giving the patient the chance of cure.

Bowel preparation is important and the operation should be covered by antibiotic prophylaxis. Pre-operative anticoagulation is not advisable since a pelvic haematoma might lead to the possibility of infection in an area which may contain unabsorbable foreign material (such as polyvinyl alcohol sponge – Ivalon).

There are two principal types of procedure, abdominal and perineal. The major abdominal repair operations provide excellent anatomical restoration with the fewest recurrences but may produce urinary or sexual dysfunction. The more minor perineal approaches, on the other hand, provide only a moderately good anatomical reconstruction with a considerable chance of recurrence, but a lower risk of pelvic nerve damage. In the elderly anatomical restoration is usually the overriding concern of the surgeon, and should be treated almost exclusively by major anatomical repair, whilst in the young adult a more conservative approach may be advisable.

Abdominal approach

There are many operations described aimed at fixing the rectum, removing redundant large intestine or repairing the pelvic floor from above. This is not the place for a detailed exposition of surgical technique. The rectopexy favoured by the author is based on that described by Wells in 1959. Ripstein's Teflon sling procedure is safe and gives good results (Ripstein, 1965), but serious complications have been reported. Anterior resection is a more major operation, and the risk to life is much greater than with those alternative abdominal operations which do not involve opening the bowel and performing an anastomosis. Excision of the rectum and a permanent colostomy is reserved for those cases whose rectal function is beyond salvage.

The technique of the extended Ivalon sponge rectopexy is summarised as follows. The rectum is mobilised posteriorly down to the level of the coccyx and the anterior peritoneal pouch is excised (this is the most difficult step). The lateral ligaments of the rectum are then mobilised and divided near the pelvic wall. The Ivalon sponge is not attached to the presacral fascia but instead is wrapped around the rectum to cover its posterior and lateral aspects: this avoids any danger of pricking the presacral veins, but nevertheless many surgeons do in fact attach the sponge to the presacral fascia. The edges of the sponge, which stiffens the rectal wall enough to prevent intussusception, while promoting adhesions between the rectum and surrounding tissues, are stitched to the rectal wall and the stumps of the lateral ligaments are sutured to the sacral promontary. A row of stitches is placed to obliterate the recto-uterovaginal space thus reforming the rectovaginal septum. The uterus is stitched to the anterior abdominal wall with stout unabsorbable sutures as a form of simple ventral suspension. Finally the peritoneum of the pelvic floor is closed at the level of the pelvic brim to cover completely the implant (Fig. 3.11).

This operation corrects all the major anatomical defects with

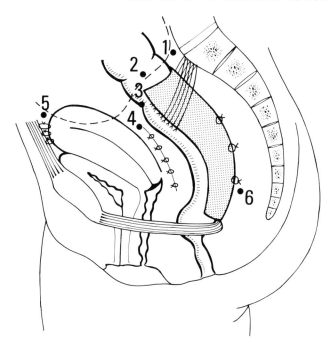

1. Lateral ligaments stitched to sacral promontory.

2. Peritoneum closed at higher level.

3. Ivalon sponge stitched to rectal wall.

4. Rectovaginal septum reformed

5. Ventrosuspension

[6. Stitches from sponge to fascia]

Fig. 3.11 Ivalon rectopexy.

the exception of the pelvic floor laxity. However, in approximately half the patients with pre-operative incontinence, satisfactory continence is restored.

Perineal approach

The perineal approach allows a repair of the puborectalis portion of the levator ani. The rectum itself cannot be fully mobilised or returned to its normal position, so that the operations necessarily have the aspect of 'plugging back' the descending tissues rather than a total correction of the situation. With these reservations, it is true to say that with a young patient who will co-operate in avoiding straining on defaecation postoperatively, a successful repair can be done through the perineum, with negligible risk to the pelvic nerves.

The operation of choice involves a posterior approach through the intersphincteric space. When the level of the puborectalis sling is reached, the rectum is pushed upwards into the pelvis and the puborectalis muscles are than drawn together behind the rectum using a darn of stout monofilament nylon. If the operation is carried out satisfactorily the gap in the pelvic floor is closed, the puborectalis sling made taut and the anorectal angle restored. At the same operation the patulous external anal sphincter muscle may be tightened. Recurrences with this technique seem more likely than with any of the abdominal operations.

119

The Thiersch operation is simple, but has very poor long-term results. It often increases the problem of constipation (by narrowing the anal orifice too much) or the wire fractures with immediate recurrence. The results are slightly better with new, more pliant, materials for the encircling stitch (nylon or Mersilene mesh). Rectosigmoidectomy has such a high recurrence rate that it has been virtually abandoned.

REFERENCES AND FURTHER READING

Broden B and Snellman B. Procidentia of the rectum studied with cine radiography: a contribution to the discussion of causative mechanisms. *Diseases of the Colon and Rectum* 1968; **11:** 330–47.

Kupfer CA and Goligher JC. One hundred consecutive cases of complete prolapse of the rectum treated by operation. *British Journal of Surgery* 1970; **57:** 481–7.

Moschowitz AV. The pathogenesis, anatomy and cure of prolapse of the rectum. *Surgery, Gynaecology and Obstetrics* 1912; **15:** 7–21.

Parks AG, Swash M and Urich H. Sphincter denervation in anorectal incontinence and rectal prolapse. *Gut* 1977; **18:** 656–65.

Ripstein CB. Surgical cure of massive rectal prolapse. *Diseases of the Colon and Rectum* 1965; **8:** 34–8.

Thomson JPS. Anorectal prolapse. In: Hadfield, J and Hobsley, M. eds. *Current surgical practice*, 2. London: Arnold, 1978; 66–86.

Wells C. New operation for rectal prolapse. *Proceedings of The Royal Society of Medicine* 1959; **52:** 602–3.

INCONTINENCE

The plight of the patient with anorectal incontinence is sad indeed. There is the obvious association with uncleanliness and the feeling of being a social outcast. It is thought to be a rare condition, but it is probably commoner than is generally believed; people conceal their symptoms from embarrassment and shame. Nothing can be done for them while they are social outcasts, as they pad themselves to prevent detection and become recluses. As they get older the problem becomes greater and, when the matter becomes known to the family, they are frequently rejected and institutionalised.

There are many causes of faecal incontinence. The following list gives the commoner ones:

Severe diarrhoea
Physiological disturbance (impaction of faeces)
Neurological disease
Deficiency of the muscle ring

SEVERE DIARRHOEA

Sudden, explosive diarrhoea may well cause an episode of incontinence even in a normal person. If, in addition, the subject has any pelvic floor defect, whether this be due to injury, neurological disease or the process of ageing, then he will be more susceptible to such relatively minor events. A frequent cause of this state of affairs is inflammatory bowel disease. A villous adenoma secreting considerable quantities of mucus can have the same effect, as indeed can a carcinoma. These possibilities must always be borne in mind when dealing with a patient who is partially or totally incontinent. Provided that no organic disease is present, a patient can often be rendered symptom-free by simply inducing a more solid stool. This can be done by dietary means or by the use of one of the well-known drugs having a delaying action on the intestine. It is important to avoid the converse situation as the straining efforts required to evacuate a constipated stool will weaken the pelvic floor muscles even more.

PHYSIOLOGICAL DISTURBANCE
(FAECAL IMPACTION)

Impaction of faeces is seen in the young with idiopathic megacolon, after operation and in the elderly. Psychological factors are often implicated in the young, but this is seldom the case and the child will almost always respond to corrective physical measures. The colon and rectum lack the necessary *vis-a-tergo* to propel faecal contents. A patient may be normal for years, but a temporary enfored bed rest due to illness may set a vicious cycle into action. The rectum becomes overloaded and it is impossible for such a mass to be evacuated normally. As we have seen, the sphincters lose their tone due to reflex inhibition. The child is incontinent, constantly soiling his clothing. This can go on for many years before treatment is instituted. Firstly the impacted mass must be removed and this may require a general anaesthetic. The distended colon is atonic and will require stimulation to restore its activity. Disposable enemas are therefore given daily for a week to ten days. Thereafter one or more glycerine suppositories are given each day after breakfast to induce rectal contraction. This regime may be required for several months. In the postoperative patient, evacuation followed by suppositories for a few days will usually suffice.

In the elderly the problem is more complex, as the sphincter activity may be partially lost before impaction occurs. Such people will often keep the stool hard to maintain normal continence. It is easy then for them to be tipped over into impaction. Incontinence is an even more marked feature than with the other groups. When examined the anal canal will be gaping and patulous. Once evacuated, however, sphincter tone returns. They may need a suppository routine almost indefinitely to prevent recurrence.

NEUROLOGICAL DISEASE

As reflex control of the pelvic floor is centred in the region of the cauda equina, lesions above this level, though capable of removing the conscious element, seldom cause grave impairment of function. Even in the case of a complete transection of the cord, reflex emptying of the rectum occurs once the stage of spinal shock has passed. Such patients learn how to induce reflex rectal contraction, usually by stimulating the lower anal canal. Without doubt, the most difficult neurological situation to manage is the cauda equina syndrome. If the lesion is complete, there is no muscle activity in the pelvic floor at all, nor is there sensation. These patients are totally incontinent. If they try to alleviate the situation by inducing a hard dehydrated stool, then they frequently become impacted. It is therefore usually necessary for them to keep the stool firm, but to induce defaecation with the aid of glycerine suppositories or even disposable enemata.

Another category of neurological incontinence used to be given the title of 'idiopathic'. The most obvious feature of this condition is that the sphincter muscles are lax and patulous on clinical examination. Careful assessment reveals an absent anal reflex, and no activity in the external sphincter itself. The puborectalis muscle usually contracts on voluntary effort and the activity in the levator muscles may be within normal limits. There is, however, loss of tone in the puborectalis muscle with the result that the normal anorectal angulation is lost and the efficiency of the flap valve mechanism is impaired.

Physiological testing of the sphincters usually shows that no power at all is developed at rest, either by the internal or external sphincter muscles. The pressures developed on voluntary contraction vary greatly but are usually considerably less than normal. Routine electromyography is not grossly abnormal. Biopsy of the various muscles constituting the pelvic floor has revealed changes characteristic of degeneration in the nerves supplying the muscles. These changes are very similar to those found in the carpal tunnel syndrome at the wrist and indicate a local neuropathy. This is believed to be due to stretching of the nerves supplying the pelvic floor either by straining efforts over many years, or in some cases the result of a difficult labour. A similar change is seen in association with rectal prolapse and here too the likely cause is pelvic floor descent resulting in lengthening and secondary degeneration of nerves supplying the sphincter muscles. It is this neuropathic change which can be detected by single fibre electromyography (Parks, Swash and Urich, 1977).

The muscle degeneration in these patients is most severe in the external sphincter with increasing function present as one ascends through the puborectalis muscle to the levator ani group. The tone in the puborectalis is grossly deficient so that the anorectal angulation is impaired. Nevertheless, some activity in this muscle remains and it can be used to restore almost normal function in these patients. Should the patient have a large rectal prolapse, then this is first dealt with by means of a rectopexy. After this operation about one-third of patients will still be incontinent and they will need an operative repair of their pelvic floor in exactly the same way as those patients previously categorised as having idiopathic incontinence.

Any operation designed to relieve this condition must take into account the fact that the muscles are manifestly weakened, and must aim at making the residual function maximally effective. An essential part of any procedure must be the reconstruction of the anorectal angulation, with restoration of the flap valve mechanism. This objective can be obtained by reconstructing the pelvic floor muscles from behind the rectum and anal canal. The principle of the operative technique is to lift the visceral component of the anal canal forwards, off the inner surface of the external sphincter, the puborectalis and levator ani muscles, and to place sutures from side to side across these muscles to shorten their effective length of action. At the same time the repair will restore the anorectal angle by approximating the two limbs of the pubococcygeus and puborectalis muscles. The technique may be difficult and it would be inappropriate to discuss it in detail. However, the mode of access to carry out this procedure is one of great anatomical interest. Advantage is taken of the previously mentioned inter-sphincteric plane of embryological fusion between the viscus and the somatic muscles surrounding it.

An incision is made behind the anal canal (Fig. 3.12) and the space between the internal and external sphincters is identified. This space is then opened up by a careful dissection and the internal sphincter is lifted off the skeletal muscles posteriorly and laterally (Fig. 3.13). In succession the external sphincter, the puborectalis and (after division of Waldeyer's fascia) the pubococcygeus and ileococcygeus muscles are identified. The plane is a bloodless one and no nerves cross it. Sutures are laid across from one limb of each exposed muscle to the other, starting with the ileococcygeus (Figs. 3.14 and 3.15).

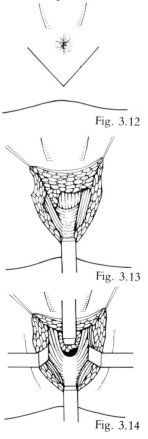

Postanal repair of pelvic floor muscles and external sphincter

Fig. 3.12

Fig. 3.13

Fig. 3.14

123

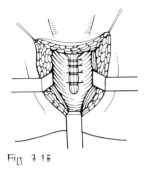

Fig 3.15

Postoperatively these patients either have a temporary colostomy to prevent disruption of the repair, or are given artificially induced diarrhoea for about ten to twelve days. Once this period has passed, the repair is sound. The need for careful management of these patients never ceases. If they return to their previous straining habits, the muscles will gradually lengthen again and they will revert to the same state as they were in pre-operatively. It is therefore essential that evacuation is induced each day with the aid of an evacuant suppository (such as glycerine). They are also encouraged to perform sphincter exercises routinely, though this is probably only effective in the long term. It is very important to explain to the patient precisely the nature of the original condition and the measures required to prevent its recurrence.

The operation has given satisfactory results in about 85% of 175 patients treated, which is not unreasonable, bearing in mind the degree of atrophy which exists in the muscles.

DEFICIENCY OF THE MUSCLE RING

Anorectal agenesis

This is a subject requiring specialised experience and skill. A general principle is that only pelvic floor muscle can be used in any restorative operation, as only this has the tonic activity previously described. Despite apparent difficulties, it is important to realise that children who are afflicted can often be helped and, if not restored to complete normality, at least to a manageable state.

Traumatic section

Trauma causing section of the muscle ring with retraction of muscle to 180° is found associated with childbirth, surgery for anal fistula and automobile accidents. The female pelvic floor is particularly susceptible to muscle damage; incontinence often follows a degree of damage which would not cause symptoms in the male. The anterior injury of childbirth is dealt with reasonably successfully by immediate reconstruction of the anterior perineum. A proportion fail, however, and these require formal reconstruction as a secondary procedure.

Sphincter injury may also be caused by automobile and other forms of trauma, including operative treatment for anal fistula. In the past pessimism has been expressed regarding the results of reconstructive surgery in such cases, particularly when the defect was lateral or posterior. However, provided there has been no neurological damage to the muscles, a satisfactory functional repair can almost always be achieved, no matter how bizarre the injury (Parks and McPartlin, 1977). It is essential to mobilise the ends of the divided muscle, freeing it from scar tissue binding it down to the fascia in the ischiorectal fossa. To achieve a satisfactory result, overlap of the muscle ends without tension is essential and the repair is usually protected by a temporary colostomy (Fig. 3.16).

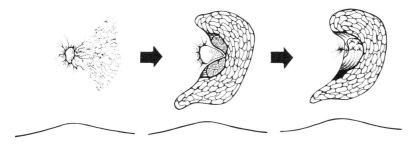

Fig. 3.16 Sphincter repair.

Our knowledge of the physiology and pathophysiology of the pelvic floor has greatly increased over the last twenty years. Most of the causes of incontinence can now be classified and their scientific basis is known. By one method or another most of them can be helped to overcome this very severe social disability. Equally important is the need for steps to be taken to prevent the causes of incontinence which set in with advancing age. The dietary habits of Western civilisation over the last hundred years have resulted in a high proportion of our people having to expel a hard stool with considerable difficulty. The straining efforts undoubtedly result in the neuropathic changes which have been described. It would be far better to prevent such changes occuring than to treat them once fully developed. It is therefore essential to educate the population to new dietary habits so that a more normal pattern of defaecation occurs spontaneously.

The influence of childbirth on the genesis of incontinence is at present unknown, though strongly suspected in certain cases. Correction of difficulties during labour may well be another important preventative measure we should be considering.

REFERENCES AND FURTHER READING

Parks AG. Anorectal incontinence. *Proceedings of The Royal Society of Medicine* 1975; **68:** 681–90.

Parks AG. Postanal pelvic floor repair. In: Tood IP, ed. *Colon, rectum and anus* (3rd ed. Operative surgery). London and Boston: Butterworths, 1977: 249–54.

Parks AG and McPartlin JF. Surgical repair of anal sphincters following injury. In: Todd IP, ed. *Colon, rectum and anus* (3rd ed. Operative surgery). London and Boston: Butterworths, 1977: 245–8.

Parks AG, Swash M and Urich H. Sphincter denervation in anorectal incontinence and rectal prolapse *Gut* 1977; **18:** 656–65.

PROCTALGIA FUGAX

Proctalgia fugax is a term used to describe intermittent attacks of severe, paroxysmal perineal pain, mostly occurring at night and lasting from ten to twenty minutes. The pain can be so severe as to be totally incapacitating. Another characteristic is that it usually only occurs three or four times a year often for many years. It is said to occur more frequently in neurotic individuals but this is very doubtful.

Little is known of the pathogenesis of the pain except that some have claimed to have examined a patient during an attack and found intense spasm of the puborectalis and pubococcygeus muscles which they have interpreted as being in the nature of a tetanic cramp. The patient may well learn methods of relieving the pain before its spontaneous cessation. The passage of wind, digital manipulation of the anal canal, or the insertion of a bland suppository may give rapid relief.

The condition disturbs the patient mostly because of fears as to its cause, rather than because of the actual pain itself, which is infrequent and transient. Once reassured, he may well not wish any active therapy. Two simple measures may be helpful in preventing attacks if they are severe enough to justify treatment; the first is the use of a small dose of a mild tranquilliser prior to going to bed. The second is quinine bisulphate (100–200 mg) which is usually successful in preventing attacks, probably because of its effect in preventing muscle cramps generally. Its mode of action in achieving this is quite unknown.

The diagnosis of proctalgia fugax should only be made when the story is characteristic, when the attacks are infrequent, and when they are relieved by simple measures. It is only too easy to make this diagnosis, which involves no further investigation or treatment, when in fact a definite abnormality is present. Conditions which tend to be given this label are fissure-in-ano, mucosal prolapse, fistula-in-ano and even more serious pathology such as carcinoma of the anorectal region or prostrate. Careful history taking and examination will avoid such errors.

4. Principles of Surgical Management

PRE-OPERATIVE BOWEL PREPARATION

Sepsis is the most important complication following surgery of the large bowel. It may present as septicaemia, peritonitis, a localised abscess or, most commonly, wound infection. Poor surgical technique may be responsible for anastomotic breakdown and other septic complications, but the source of infection is the endogenous bacteria of the faeces and bowel lumen. Pre-operative preparation of the bowel is directed at minimising bacterial contamination by removing faeces (mechanical preparation) and suppression of bacteria (antibacterial treatment).

MECHANICAL PREPARATION

The faeces contain $10^{10} - 10^{11}$ bacteria per gram, in addition to metabolites and particulate matter, which antagonise certain antibacterial agents and prevent phagocytosis. There is, therefore, no argument about the importance of successful mechanical cleansing of the large bowel. However, vigorous use of purges and enemas is not suitable for all patients, particularly the frail and elderly and those with intestinal obstruction. A preliminary defunctioning colostomy is necessary if there is complete obstruction. Where there is partial obstruction mechanical preparation may be difficult and may occasionally precipitate severe pain or even complete obstruction. A plain x-ray of the abdomen to show the contents of the colon may be helpful in these circumstances (Herter, 1972).

Methods

Dietary restriction

A low residue diet will reduce the amount of indigestible fibre and, therefore, decrease the faecal mass. It was suggested that a 'no residue' elemental diet, composed of amino acids, vitamins and glucose, reduced the numbers of bacteria isolated from the faeces. However, later studies have failed to confirm this reduction. The main effect of elemental diets has been to reduce the daily faecal output by an average of 70%.

Purgatives

Magnesium sulphate or castor oil are most frequently given. In some centres magnesium sulphate is preferred because it is easier to take and produces less colicky abdominal pain. However, its use requires more supervision because it produces a fluid stool which must be evacuated before an empty colon is achieved.

Enemas

Enemas are used to empty the left side of the colon the night before the operation. Simple saline washouts, contact laxatives, e.g. bisacodyl (Dulcolax) suppositories or oxyphenisatin (Veripaque) enemas, may be given. Enemas should not be given immediately before operation because of the risk of residual fluid within the colon.

Whole gut irrigation

In 1973, Hewitt and his colleagues instituted a method of continuous irrigation of the whole gut with an electrolyte solution introduced through a nasogastric tube. This technique can shorten the time spent preparing the bowel to between 2–6 hours and improves the success of preparation in certain circumstances. Neomycin was added to the fluid to suppress aerobic bacteria and the risk of systemic absorption of neomycin and overgrowth of resistant strains of bacteria was found to be reduced by the short exposure to this agent. Patients undergoing this form of preparation must be observed all the time and there is a particular risk of fluid overload in the elderly. Although the nasogastric tube and the resulting continuous 'diarrhoea' are tolerated well by most patients, a few find this method more exhausting than conventional preparations. A final important point is that this method is contraindicated in patients with obstructing tumours.

As a modification of the tube-saline irrigation technique, some centres have used the voluntary drinking of 3–4 litres of isotonic saline or 1–2 litres of 10% mannitol solution. There is a theoretical risk that mannitol (a sugar) may cause potentially explosive hydrogen formation by colonic bacteria.

A preliminary transverse colostomy may be undertaken for intestinal obstruction. Before definitive surgery the proximal colon is prepared in the same way as the whole bowel. The distal colon is washed through with saline introduced via the distal loop or, if that is not possible, from both above, and below through the rectum. There is no evidence that defunctioning, or even complete disconnection of the colon, reduces the number of bacteria.

Operations to defunction the large bowel

Mechanical preparation of the large bowel, with dietary restriction, purgatives, enemas and defunctioning when necessary, produces a good result, with a clean bowel in approximately 65%, a fair result in 20% and a poor result in 15% of patients undergoing elective resections of the colon; obstructing tumours are usually the cause of the poor results.

ANTIBACTERIAL TREATMENT

Most patients undergoing large bowel surgery are given antibacterial chemotherapy to reduce the incidence of infection. There is controversy about the effectiveness of such treatment because the development of postoperative sepsis is determined by many factors; in the absence of intestinal obstruction, faecal contamination or established infection (peritonitis or an abscess), good surgical technique is the most important, avoiding contamination of the wound and peritoneum by intestinal contents (Keighley, 1977). The bacteria released when the colon is opened are responsible for nearly all the infections after colonic surgery. New bacteriological techniques have shown that anaerobic bacteria, e.g. *Bacteroides fragilis*, are frequently isolated from infected wounds in addition to aerobic coliform bacteria, e.g. *Escherichia coli.*

Until recently the majority of regimes of pre-operative antibacterial treatment were ineffective against anaerobic bacteria but erythromycin, tetracycline and metronidazole (Goldring, Scott, McNaught *et al.*, 1975) have all been shown to suppress most components of the bacterial flora of faeces when given with neomycin or kanamycin. Metronidazole is now generally preferred to other antianaerobic agents, and especially to lincomycin and clindamycin because of their association with pseudomembranous colitis. If oral administration is not possible, metronidazole suppositories have been shown to be as effective as the intravenous form and considerably cheaper.

Choice of antibacterial agent

However, it must be emphasised that treatment with appropriate combinations of antibacterial agents will not eliminate bacteria from the gut. The term 'suppression' of the bacterial flora describes the effects of antibacterial treatment more accurately than the word 'sterilisation' commonly applied in this context.

Timing and route of antibacterial treatment

There are two main lines of approach: the first is to suppress the numbers of bacteria in the lumen of the gut by treatment with combinations of oral, poorly absorbed, antibacterial compounds (Marks, Hawley, Peach *et al.*, 1979).

The second is to enhance the clearance of bacteria from the peritoneal cavity and the tissues by having an adequate concentration of appropriate antibiotics *in the tissues at the time of contamination*. This is achieved by giving peroperative antibiotics 1–4 hours before or at the start of the operation but *not* afterwards.

A low incidence of postoperative infection has been reported following either pre-operative or peroperative treatment (Polk and Lopez-Mayor, 1969). Advocates of pre-operative treatment claim that these regimes suppress the numbers of bacteria to levels which can be cleared from the peritoneal cavity without additional peroperative antibiotic treatment. However, in a few patients appropriate pre-operative treatment may have no measurable effect on the numbers of faecal bacteria recovered from the colon at operation. Nonetheless oral medication regimes are preferred by many surgeons who reserve peroperative systemic antibiotics for surgery on the unprepared large bowel, e.g. in obstruction or inflammatory bowel disease. Commonly used antibacterial agents are indicated in Table 4a.

Table 4a. *Commonly used antibacterial treatment*

| Time | Route | Effective mainly against | |
		Aerobic bacteria	Anaerobic bacteria
Pre-operative	Oral	KANAMYCIN *Neomycin *Phthalylsulphathiazole	METRONIDAZOLE
Peroperative	Parenteral	GENTAMICIN CEPHRADINE *Ampicillin	METRONIDAZOLE

* Possible alternative treatment

Disadvantages of antibacterial treatment

In addition to hypersensitivity and other toxic reactions to individual drugs (e.g. ototoxicity after gentamicin) which are more likely with systemic antibiotics than the poorly absorbed oral agents, there are two major disadvantages; the balance between the antibiotic sensitive and resistant micro-organisms in the gut is altered and there may be enhancement of tumour implantation at the suture line. The risks of Staphylococcal superinfection and pseudomembranous colitis have discouraged some surgeons from the routine use of antibacterial treatment. There is a theoretical risk of tumour implantation at the suture line, but the majority of surgeons take precautions to reduce this by using tapes above and below tumours, irrigation of the bowel with cytotoxic agents and the use of iodised sutures. The shortage of prospective randomised clinical trials is another reason why surgeons have been reluctant to use these agents. There is a need for more trials before the role of prophylactic antibacterial treatment in large bowel surgery is established. Treatment may have to be modified with the changing antibiotic susceptibility of bacteria.

An example of a pre-operative preparation regimen is shown in Table 4b.

Table 4b. *Pre-operative preparation regimen for bowel surgery*

Pre-operative Day	Diet	Mechanical	Antibacterial
4 and 3	Low residue		
2 (admission)	Fluids only	Castor oil 30 ml	Metronidazole 200 mg/6 hourly to total six doses before operation
1	Clear fluids	Castor oil 30 ml in the evening Oxyphenisatin enema in the evening	
0	Nil		Gentamicin 1.8 mg/kg 1–4 hours before operation.

REFERENCES AND FURTHER READING

Goldring J, Scott A, McNaught W and Gillespie G. Prophylactic oral antimicrobial agents in elective colonic surgery. *Lancet* 1975; **2:** 997–9.

Herter FP. Preparation of the bowel for surgery. *Surgical Clinics of North America* 1972; **52:** 859–70.

Hewitt J, Rigby J, Reeve J and Cox AG. Whole gut irrigation in preparation for large bowel surgery. *Lancet* 1973; **3:** 337–340.

Keighley MRB. Prevention of wound sepsis in gastro-intestinal surgery. *British Journal of Surgery* 1977; **64:** 315–21.

Marks CG, Hawley PR, Peach SL, Drasar BS and Hill MJ. The effects of phthalylsulphathiazole on the bacteria of the colonic mucosa and intestinal contents as revealed by the examination of surgical samples. *Scandinavian Journal of Gastroenterology* 1979; **14:** 891–96.

Polk HC and Lopez-Mayor JF. Postoperative wound infection: a prospective study of determinant factors and prevention. *Surgery* 1969; **66:** 97–103.

ANAESTHESIA

This section is a summary of points of interest and importance in colorectal anaesthesia and can only be a supplement to the standard texts.

MAJOR ABDOMINAL PROCEDURES

The usual sequence of barbiturate, relaxant and nitrous oxide is appropriate; each anaesthetist will have his own preferences as regards relaxant and analgesic supplements. There is no contra-indication to the use of epidural anaesthesia, which might be expected to give a drier operating field for abdomino-perineal excision, but many anaesthetists (and surgeons) have been disappointed with the results and have abandoned its use. Major colorectal procedures, especially if radical for malignancy, will take more than two hours and, even in the absence of severe haemorrhage, will require intravenous fluid at a rate of at least one litre per hour.

A ventilator set to deliver a tidal volume of at least 650 ml with a correspondingly slow rate (12–14/min) will present a quiet operative field and minimise peripheral pulmonary atelectasis.

Mobilisation of the splenic flexure and the anchorage of an ileostomy to the under-surface of the abdominal wall are procedures demanding particularly profound relaxation; he is a fortunate anaesthetist (and patient) whose surgeon facilitates this by having the intestines outside the abdomen rather than packed up against the diaphragm. Paradoxically perhaps, the greater the experience of the surgeon the larger the incisions he allows himself for these operations and this in turn demands more relaxation for their closure—a demand readily met by a generous final dose of depolarising relaxant.

The use of the lithotomy-Trendelenburg position for most of these operations permits a change of operative strategy if indicated but calls for a slow return to the horizontal position postoperatively to avoid postural hypotension. Surgeons are occasionally apprehensive about the effect on a newly-fashioned intestinal anastomosis of the neostigmine required for relaxant reversal or the opiate used for postoperative analgesia; a soundly constructed anastomosis is jeopardised by neither, but it may sometimes be diplomatic for the anaesthetist to prescribe pethidine rather than papaveretum.

MINOR PROCEDURES

Anal operations call for relaxation of the sphincter muscles; low spinal blockade by either the intrathecal or epidural (caudal) approach is effective. Since most patients prefer to be asleep while in the lithotomy position, light general anaesthesia is more commonly used with the relaxation provided by infiltration of the ischiorectal fossae with 20–25 ml of 1% lignocaine and 1:200,000 adrenaline. Concern is sometimes expressed at the simultaneous use of such quantities of adrenaline and 0.5–1% halothane, or when as much as 0.5 mg of adrenaline in a 1:300,000 solution may be infiltrated subcutaneously (e.g. during the course of an extensive excision of perianal warts). In practice, cardiac arrhythmias have not been encountered in these circumstances nor when undiluted 1:1,000 adrenaline solution is applied topically to fistula wounds for haemostatis.

In operations for fistula, by contrast, the surgeon is better able to identify the skeletal muscle components of the sphincters (the puborectalis sling in particular) if they are not relaxed. On occasion, a cough, deliberately induced by giving a sudden brief inhalation of ether vapour, may be most helpful.

Most fistula wounds need to be reviewed under anaesthesia postoperatively at least once and sometimes at regular intervals. In this situation it is for each anaesthetist to make his own personal assessment of the hazards allegedly associated with the repeated administration of anaesthetic agents, such as halothane.

SURGICAL ANATOMY

The large intestine consists of the caecum (with the appendix), the ascending, transverse, descending and sigmoid colon, the rectum and anal canal. The terminal ileum joins the caecum in the right iliac fossa, and the colon then lies like a picture frame around the loops of the small intestine, although the actual position of any part of the large intestine varies with the build and the position of the subject.

COLON

The terminal ileum meets the large intestine at the ileocaecal valve. In general the mucosal lips of the valve stop regurgitation of the colonic contents into the small intestine, but the valve is frequently incompetent. This incompetence may result in barium filling the small intestine during a barium enema examination, or in small bowel distension in large intestinal obstruction. The appendix is attached to the lower pole of the caecum, and may lie within the true pelvis or in front of or behind the terminal ileum or caecum. The ascending colon is short and, having lost its peritoneal covering posteriorly, it is usually fixed. Beneath the right lobe of the liver the colon turns medially (the hepatic flexure) to become the transverse colon. The hepatic flexure is closely related to the gall bladder, duodenum and right kidney.

The first part of the transverse colon has no peritoneal covering posteriorly, and lies in front of the right kidney, the second part of the duodenum and pancreas. The main part of the transverse colon hangs in a loop on its mesentery (transverse mesocolon) below the greater curve of the stomach and attached to the posterior aspect of the greater omentum, which hangs like a curtain in front of the small bowel loops. Small parts of the omentum can undergo torsion giving rise to an

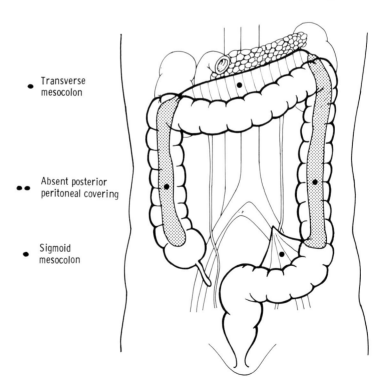

Transverse
mesocolon

Absent posterior
peritoneal covering

Sigmoid
mesocolon

Fig. 4.1 The peritoneal relationship to the colon.

acute abdomen. The distal part of the transverse colon is closely related to the lower pole of the spleen and the left kidney and makes an acute bend (the splenic flexure) to become the descending colon. The descending colon, like the ascending colon, usually has no posterior peritoneal covering and is consequently fixed. It becomes the sigmoid colon at the pelvic brim. The sigmoid colon is variable in length and also has a mesentery (sigmoid mesocolon) which has a comparatively short base making the sigmoid colon prone to volvulus, a problem which does not affect the transverse colon. As it is mobile, it often lies in the pelvis, but may lie in the left or right iliac fossa (Fig. 4.1).

The outer muscular coat of the colon is incomplete and appears as three bands called taeniae coli, which being shorter than the rest of the bowel give the colon its distinctive haustrated appearance. The fatty appendages are called appendices epiploicae.

RECTUM

The precise site where colon becomes rectum is debatable. Surgeons usually regard the sacral promontory as the junction, but anatomists favour the level of the third sacral vertebra. At one time it was thought that an anatomical sphincter existed at the junction but this is not the case, although there is some evidence of a physiological sphincter on pressure studies. The rectum is approximately 12 cm in length and follows the curve of the sacrum to the levator ani muscle where it angulates posteriorly to become the anal canal. At the junction of the middle and lower thirds of the rectum, the peritoneum sweeps forward on to the back of the bladder in the male (Fig. 4.2), and on to the upper vagina and uterus in the female (Fig. 4.3).

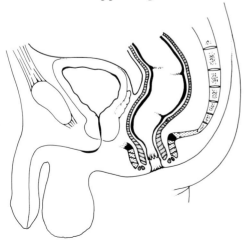

Fig. 4.2 Saggittal section of male pelvis.

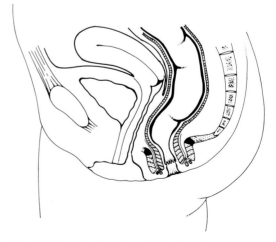

Fig. 4.3 Saggittal section of female pelvis.

Below the peritoneal reflection, lateral to the rectum, there are collections of fibro-fatty tissue containing the middle haemorrhoidal blood vessels which constitute the lateral ligaments and hold the rectum to the side wall of the pelvis. Anteriorly the extraperitoneal part of the rectum in the male is related to the bladder and ureters, seminal vesicles and the prostate, and in the female to the posterior vaginal wall, but is separated from all these structures by the fascia of Denonvilliers. Posteriorly the rectum is loosely attached to and separated from the sacrum, coccyx and the presacral vessels by the fascia of Waldeyer and a variable amount of fibro-fatty tissue. Each end of the rectum is in the midline, but the ampulla between deviates from side to side. This results in folds formed by the circular muscle layer and the mucosa which are best seen at sigmoidoscopy, usually two on the left side, with one on the right side between them – rectal valves of Houston. The longitudinal muscle coat of the rectum, unlike the colon, forms a complete covering. The mucosal lining of the colon and rectum is a glandular columnar epithelium.

BLOOD SUPPLY

The colon and rectum are primarily supplied by the superior and inferior mesenteric arteries (Fig. 4.4), the distribution of which may show considerable variation (Griffiths, 1956). As the vessels approach the bowel they bifurcate and form arcades so that a continuous chain of communicating vessels, the marginal artery, is formed that supplies terminal branches to the bowel wall. The inferior mesenteric artery becomes the superior haemorrhoidal artery as it crosses the left common iliac artery and enters the true pelvis. There is good communication between the inferior mesenteric and superior mesenteric arteries in the region of the distal transverse colon, and also between the last sigmoid artery and the superior haemorrhoidal artery. The middle haemorrhoidal artery, variable in size, is a branch of the internal iliac artery and reaches the rectum through the lateral ligament on each side. The inferior haemorrhoidal artery is a branch of the internal pudendal artery, which in turn arises from the internal iliac artery and reaches the anal canal by traversing the ischiorectal fossa. All three arteries to the rectum and their branches supply all layers of the rectum and colon, the contribution of each being very variable. Nevertheless the inferior haemorrhoidal arteries are always capable of supplying adequately a rectal stump to a point well above the peritoneal reflection, even after division of the middle haemorrhoidal arteries. The terminal branches of these vessels pierce the muscle of the bowel to reach the submucosal and mucosal

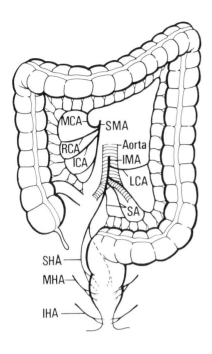

ICA	Ileocolic artery
RCA	Right colic artery
MCA	Middle colic artery
SMA	Superior mesenteric artery
IMA	Inferior mesenteric artery
LCA	Left colic artery
SA	Sigmoid arteries
SHA	Superior haemorrhoidal artery
MHA	Middle haemorrhoidal artery
IHA	Inferior haemorrhoidal artery

Fig. 4.4 Blood supply of colon.

layers. Blood vessels supplying the appendices epiploicae also pierce the muscle layer. It is at these sites of muscular perforation that herniation of mucosa occurs in diverticulosis.

The venous drainage closely follows the arterial supply. Veins from the right side of the colon form the superior mesenteric vein which joins the splenic vein to form the portal vein. The inferior mesenteric vein which is a continuation of the superior haemorrhoidal vein lies to the left of the inferior mesenteric artery and continues up beyond the origin of the artery for several centimetres to join the splenic vein.

LYMPHATIC DRAINAGE

Lymph drains from the lymphatic plexuses in the submucosal and subserosal layers of the colon to the extramural lymphatic vessels and nodes accompanying the blood vessels. Nodes may be found in close relationship to the bowel wall and along all the blood vessels to the pre-aortic nodes, which in turn drain to the cisterna chyli and the thoracic duct. In the rectum lymph drains from similar plexuses into channels which accompany all three sources of arterial supply, so that lymph may drain upwards to the pre-aortic nodes and laterally to the internal iliac nodes and thence to the para-aortic group. Lymph from the lower rectum only rarely joins that of the anal canal to drain to the inguinal nodes.

NERVE SUPPLY

The right side of the colon receives a sympathetic and a parasympathetic nerve supply. The former comes from the sympathetic chain on each side via the greater and lesser splanchnic nerves which join the plexus around the coeliac axis and origin of the superior mesenteric artery. The latter comes from the posterior vagus nerve via the same plexus. The nerves then accompany the blood vessels to the bowel.

The left side of the colon and the rectum receive a sympathetic supply from the sympathetic chain via the lumbar splanchnic nerves which join the pre-aortic plexus around the origin of the inferior mesenteric artery: from there they accompany that vessel and its branches to the bowel. This plexus also forms the presacral or hypogastric nerve which descends into the pelvis and divides to send a plexus of nerves to the side wall of the pelvis on each side. From here fibres pass to all the pelvic organs including the lower rectum. The parasympathetic supply comes from the sacral nerves via the pelic splanchnic nerves (nervi erigentes) which join the pelvic plexus of sympathetic fibres. Thence they supply the lower rectum and other pelvic organs, and passing up the presacral nerve are distributed to the left colon with the sympathetic fibres.

It is the hypogastric nerve which may have to be sacrificed in cancer operations of the lower large intestine – division of the sympathetic element leading to sterility in the male, there being normal erection and orgasm but failure of ejaculation. This nerve should therefore be very carefully preserved in less radical operations. Theoretically, division of the sympathetic supply to the bladder should cause incontinence of urine, but in practice only slight increase in frequency usually occurs. Division of nerves lower in the pelvis may theoretically cause retention of urine and failure of erection owing to division of the parasympathetic element. In practice there seems to be little permanent effect on the function of the bladder, on sexual function, or on anal reflex sphincter mechanisms, presumably because the nerve plexuses are largely spared.

REFERENCE AND FURTHER READING

Griffiths JD. Surgical anatomy of the blood supply of the distal colon. *Annals of the Royal College of Surgeons* 1956; **19**: 241–56.

PRINCIPAL OPERATIONS

The basic principles of colorectal operations are described below, but for complete technical detail the reader should refer to texts of operative surgery (Todd, 1977; Goligher, 1980; Maingot, 1980).

Position of the patient

Whilst operations on the right colon may be performed with the patient flat on the operating table, operations on the left colon and the rectum are best done with the patient in the lithotomy–Trendelenburg position (Fig. 4.5). This allows a second surgeon to operate synchronously to excise the anal canal and rectum or to operate through the anus (peranal approach). It also allows the rectum to be cleansed by irrigation for example during restorative resection.

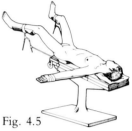

Fig. 4.5

Incisions

A variety of incisions may be used for large bowel operations. Personal preference is a major factor in the choice. Commonly used incisions are shown diagrammatically in Fig. 4.6. Some surgeons use a transverse or oblique lower abdominal incision, but this does not allow ready access to the splenic flexure and makes the siting of any subsequent stoma difficult.

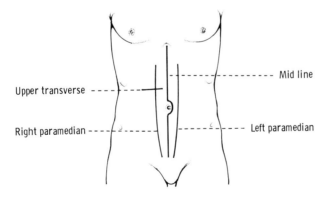

Fig. 4.6 Incisions.

LARGE BOWEL RESECTION AND EXCISION

Resection

The majority of resections are undertaken for the treatment of neoplasms, other indications being diverticular disease and inflammatory bowel disease. In all cases a careful laparotomy is carried out. In those patients with tumours, assessment is made of the degree of spread of the neoplasm, both locally and distally to the regional lymph nodes and to the liver.

The exact type of resection, a term which implies eventual restoration of bowel continuity, depends on the site and type of the pathology. Frequently used resections are listed and illustrated in Fig. 4.7.

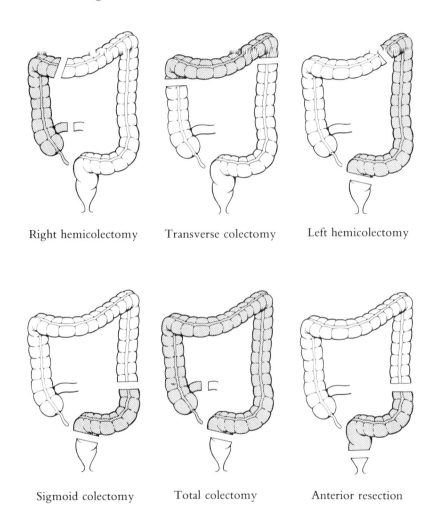

Right hemicolectomy   Transverse colectomy   Left hemicolectomy

Fig. 4.7 Resections.   Sigmoid colectomy   Total colectomy   Anterior resection

Such diagrams are clearly only a guide, as the amount of bowel removed in each case must depend on the pathology, and also on the variable anatomy of the arterial supply of the colon.

A restorative resection of the rectum is termed an 'anterior resection' because it is carried out from the front through the abdomen. Posterior approaches, for example by the trans-sphincteric or by the trans-sacral approach, have been described but are rarely used.

After resection the bowel ends are generally joined end to end. There are two principal techniques for doing this, either by hand suturing with single layer (Fig. 4.8) or double layer anastomosis (Fig. 4.9), or, more recently, by the use of a *Anastomoses*

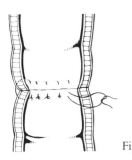

Fig. 4.8

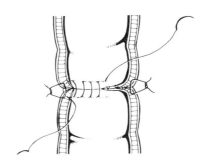

Fig. 4.9

stapling device (Fig. 4.10). The traditional method of anastomosis is the double layer technique. Some surgeons find the single layer method easier to perform, and more reliable, but for rectal anastomoses the staple method may prove to be superior to both.

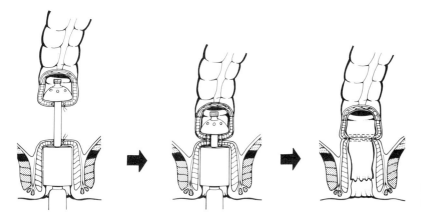

Fig. 4.10 The use of an automatic stapling device.

When an anastomosis is performed it is essential that the following points are observed. The suture line must be perfect (there must be no gaps and the mucosa must be inverted). There must be no tension on the anastomosis or on the blood vessels supplying it (in left-sided resections this will necessitate mobilisation of the splenic flexure). The bowel ends must have an adequate blood supply (this may necessitate resection of more

141

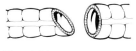

Fig. 4.11

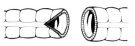

Fig. 4.12

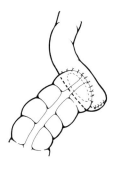

Fig. 4.13

bowel than the pathology itself calls for). Steps must be taken to avoid collections of serosanguinous fluid and so prevent potential infection (care is thus needed to achieve adequate haemostasis and, where necessary, to provide adequate postoperative drainage).

Should there be disparity in the size of the two bowel ends, one of the following manoeuvres may help in the construction of the anastomosis, namely oblique division of the bowel (Fig. 4.11), spatulation or antimesenteric slit (Fig. 4.12), or end-to-side anastomosis (Fig. 4.13). Occasionally side-to-side anastomosis is required, for example to relieve intestinal obstruction where resection is impossible.

In the case of a very low rectal anastomosis it is sometimes not technically possible to construct a conventional anastomosis using the anterior approach because of inadequate space, for example in an obese patient or if the pelvis is narrow. In these patients the staple method is now proving useful, but procedures for hand suturing are available including the Parks colo-anal (peranal) sleeve anastomosis (Fig. 4.14), or the Turnbull-Cutait pull-through technique, or by using the York-Mason trans-sphincteric approach or the Kraske trans-sacral approach (Todd, 1977).

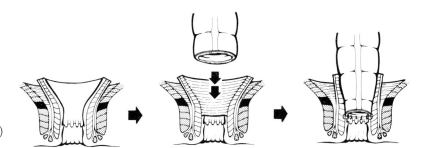

Fig. 4.14 Colo-anal (peranal) anastomosis.

Excision

For a variety of reasons part of the large bowel is excised, no restorative anastomosis is undertaken, and an end stoma is constructed. The chief indication is in those diseases which require the removal of the anal sphincter mechanism, or preclude restoration of intestinal continuity. The commonly used excisional operations are illustrated in Fig. 4.15.

When the rectum is excised there is also an incision in the perineum, and it is convenient for two surgeons to work together (synchronous combined abdomino-perineal excision of the rectum, unfortunately sometimes abbreviated to SCAPER).

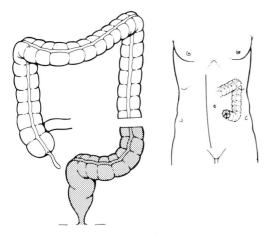

Excision of the rectum with terminal colostomy.

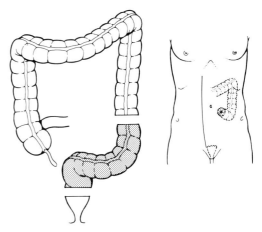

Hartmann's operation with oversewing of the rectal stump and terminal colostomy.

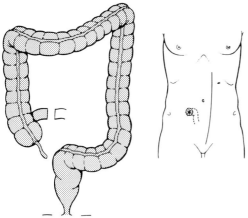

Proctocolectomy with terminal ileostomy.

Fig. 4.15 Excisions.

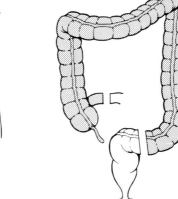

Subtotal colectomy with mucous fistula and terminal ileostomy.

Extent of operation

The extent of the operation will depend on the disease for which it is being performed. There is a need to be more radical when operating for malignant disease, removing at least five centimetres of bowel on either side of the limits of the tumour, with as much of the lymphatic drainage as possible. Since the lymphatics accompany the blood vessels this necessarily means that the length of bowel supplied by the artery in question may be devitalised, and in spite of the presence of the marginal artery, enough bowel must be removed to ensure that the subsequent anastomosis has an adequate blood supply. This accounts for the fact that a greater length of bowel is always removed than is necessary for the safe removal of the neoplasm. It is usual in patients with left-sided colonic or rectal tumours to divide the inferior mesenteric artery at its origin

143

from the aorta – the so-called 'high tie'. However, it is prudent to avoid this step in the very old, and in the very obese, thus sparing the left colic artery.

When excising the rectum for malignant disease a wide dissection is made and in the female the posterior vaginal wall is usually removed. For inflammatory bowel disease the perirectal fatty tissue is preserved, the perineal dissection takes place between the two anal sphincters, an intersphincteric dissection, and in the female the vaginal wall is left intact.

Drainage

Drains are inserted for two reasons. Firstly, to drain out serosanguinous fluid which may accumulate in body cavities such as the pelvis and secondly, to form a track from the site of an anastomosis to the surface so that should there be leakage of faecal matter it will be carried to the surface and away from the general peritoneal cavity. A variety of drains is available made of corrugated plastic or latex rubber, but tube drains attached to a closed vacuum or to a closed sump system are being used increasingly (especially to drain the pelvic cavity).

After excision of the rectum the perineal wound requires very careful drainage. In the male a latex rubber drain is used when the wound is partially closed, or a sump suction drain if the perineum is closed completely. In the female, if the posterior vaginal wall is removed the pelvis is drained through the vagina with or without suction.

STOMAS

Ileostomy

There are three types of ileostomy namely, terminal (spout), loop and continent (reservoir).

Terminal ileostomy. The stoma is sited just below the waistline well away from the umbilicus, the anterior superior iliac spine, any pre-existing scars and the incision through which the operation is being performed. Ideally the stoma site should be chosen pre-operatively with the patient in various positions to ensure that the appliance will adhere satisfactorily and that the patient can manage it. A trephine is made through the anterior abdominal wall, usually before making the main abdominal incision. The underlying muscle fibres are divided. The terminal ileum is prepared in such a way that a viable spout of bowel, approximately 2.5 cm in length, will protrude from the abdominal wall at the completion of the operation (Fig. 4.16). Care is needed to avoid possible sites of internal herniation of the small bowel, for instance by closing the 'lateral space' between the bowel and the abdominal wall.

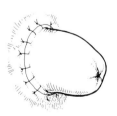

Fig. 4.16

Loop ileostomy. Occasionally a loop ileostomy is raised as a temporary measure to protect a distal ileorectal or colo-anal anastomosis (Fig. 4.17).

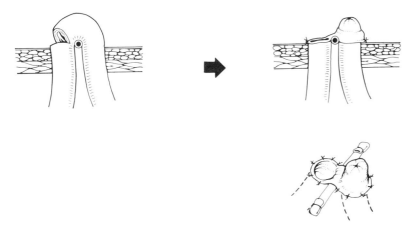

Fig. 4.17 Loop ileostomy.

Continent ileostomy. A recent development in the surgery of ileostomy construction has been described by Kock (1973). A reservoir is constructed from the terminal ileum just proximal to the stoma and this is emptied by the passage of a catheter through the stoma two or three times a day (Fig. 4.18). The

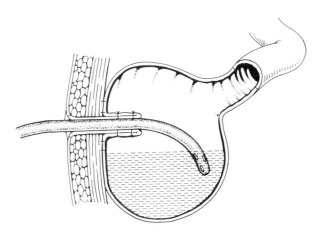

Fig. 4.18 Continent ileostomy.

stoma is flush with the skin and is sited lower than the standard ileostomy, which makes it cosmetically more acceptable.

An interesting new technique (Parks, Nicholls and Belliveau, 1980) is to site the reservoir in the pelvis and to suture the efferent spout of ileum to the dentate line in the anal canal so that the catheterisation is performed through the anus. In some of these patients voluntary evacuation is possible.

145

Caecostomy

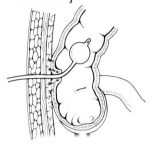

Fig. 4.19

Colostomy

Fig. 4.20

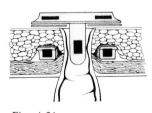

Fig. 4.21

A self-retaining catheter is inserted into the caecum (Fig. 4.19) to decompress the colon proximal to an anastomosis or occasionally to relieve large bowel obstruction. An appendicectomy is also performed.

Considerable nursing care is required to ensure that the catheter remains patent. A fistulous connection between the caecum and the abdominal wall is well established after a week. The catheter is then removed and the fistula closes spontaneously, provided there is no distal obstruction. Because caecostomy does not totally defunction the bowel its usefulness is limited.

There are four types of colostomy namely, terminal, loop, double-barrelled and divided.

Terminal colostomy. A terminal colostomy (Fig. 4.20) is almost invariably sited in the left iliac fossa in conjunction with excision of the rectum, or as part of Hartmann's operation. The siting and trephine are similar to those used for an ileostomy. When the bowel has been brought to the surface without tension, it is sutured to the skin with interrupted mucocutaneous sutures flush with the surface. A recent innovation has been the insertion of a magnetic ring in the subcutaneous layer of the anterior abdominal wall immediately superficial to the musculature. When healing is complete a magnetic stopper is inserted which allows some degree of continence. A cross-section is illustrated in Fig. 4.21.

Loop colostomy. A loop colostomy in the transverse or sigmoid colon is usually performed as a temporary measure. A transverse colostomy is used to relieve distal large bowel obstruction, or to cover a left-sided anastomosis. A sigmoid colostomy is used to defunction the rectum and anal canal as an adjunct to complex anal surgery such as for fistula or incontinence. A loop of bowel is brought to the surface through a small separate incision and held in place by a glass rod or rubber tube and mucocutaneous sutures (Fig. 4.22). A

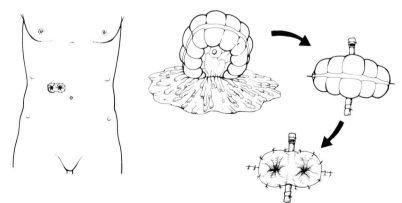

Fig. 4.22 Stages in construction of loop colostomy.

loop colostomy may be readily closed when no longer needed. The intact bowel may be returned to the abdominal cavity, or if the inevitable omental adhesions are not fully divided around the site of the stoma, it can remain outside the general peritoneal cavity, a so-called extra-peritoneal closure of colostomy.

Double-barrelled colostomy. For a double-barrelled colostomy the bowel is completely divided and a spur fashioned between the two ends of bowel. This was previously popular as part of the Paul-Mikulicz operation to avoid intraperitoneal anastomosis. The spur is subsequently crushed and the continuity of the bowel restored (Fig. 4.23). Although the opening should then spontaneously close, formal closure is often needed.

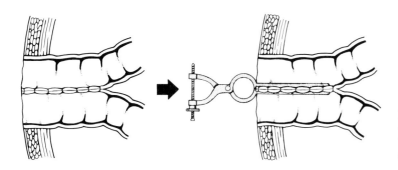

Fig. 4.23 Double-barrelled colostomy (left). Application of enterotome to crush spur (right).

Divided colostomy. The two ends of colon can be separated at the surface by a skin bridge of varying width. This achieves more effective defunctioning of the distal loop but is now rarely used.

REFERENCES AND FURTHER READING

Goligher JC. *Surgery of the anus, rectum and colon.* London: Ballière Tindall, 1980.

Kock NG. Continent ileostomy. *Progress in Surgery* 1973; **12**: 180–201.

Maingot R. *Abdominal operations.* New York: Appleton-Century-Crofts, 1980.

Parks AG, Nicholls RJ and Belliveau P. Proctocolectomy with ileal reservoir and anal anastomosis. *British Journal of Surgery* 1980; **67**: 533–38.

Todd IP. ed. *Colon, rectum and anus.* (3rd ed. Operative surgery). London and Boston: Butterworths, 1977.

POSTOPERATIVE CARE

The principles relating to the postoperative management of patients undergoing large bowel surgery are simple; the patient should be allowed to recover from the operation without undue interference but complications will require diagnosis and the correct management. Patients are liable to any of the standard complications that arise after all surgical procedures but these are well described in standard surgical textbooks and do not need to be repeated; there are, however, complications special to colorectal surgery.

When considering postoperative management it is important to remember that the rapidity with which an individual patient recovers matters little, providing that there are no complications. Normal colonic activity should, therefore, be allowed to return spontaneously without undue encouragement, for it is leakage from a colonic anastomosis that accounts for most of the significant morbidity and mortality (Chapter 5).

Careful observation by nursing and medical staff is mandatory. A patient with a normal temperature, pulse, blood pressure and respiration chart is probably running an uncomplicated course while any elevation of pulse rate or temperature will have an underlying pathological cause. If a cause cannot be found, this means a failure of diagnosis; there is no place for blind antibiotic treatment in a patient with an undiagnosed postoperative fever.

MANAGEMENT OF FLUID INTAKE

In many of the patients undergoing surgery to the colon and rectum, the operation is a planned procedure and the patient is in normal water and electrolyte balance. This may even be so in some emergency situations. Fluids by mouth should be restricted until the patient has established normal intestinal activity. This may be judged by the absence of abdominal distension, the presence of normal bowel sounds and the passage of flatus or a stool: flatus is more significant than a liquid stool. Once the patient tolerates fluids this may be followed by a return to normal diet after two or three days. Patients should normally have passed flatus by day three or four and have their bowels open by day four or five. In patients undergoing emergency surgery, such as for inflammatory bowel disease, particularly in the acute phase, the situation may be quite different and careful monitoring will be needed of the fluid requirements against urinary output and specific gravity, central venous pressure, packed cell volume, blood urea and electrolyte results. Patients may also require parenteral nutrition.

There is no need for routine nasogastric aspiration but should the patient complain of nausea or should vomiting occur, a tube will be required until the quantities aspirated are less than the small quantities being taken by mouth.

MANAGEMENT OF MICTURITION

All patients undergoing surgery of the left colon and rectum will require a catheter and continuous bladder drainage. The catheter should be removed early on day five; in the female patient, whose perineal dissection has included excision of the posterior vaginal wall, delay in removal of the catheter may make nursing care easier. Complications following removal of a catheter include acute and painful retention, retention with overflow, and incontinence. Pre-operative urological assessment which has included symptomatology, a mid-stream specimen of urine (MSU) and an intravenous urogram (IVU) may help to identify before surgery those patients who are at urological risk, although in the male it is sometimes difficult to be certain whether postoperative problems are due to bladder outflow obstruction or related to operative damage to autonomic nerves. Retention following catheter removal requires further catheterisation for a few days and a second attempt at catheter removal when the patient is more mobile. Micturition is often successful at this stage but a third catheter is sometimes required; if the third attempt at removal is unsuccessful carbachol 500 μg by subcutaneous injection is sometimes helpful in initiating micturition but the patient will almost certainly require specialist urological care.

Should the bladder be involved in the operation (e.g. partial cystectomy) then continuous drainage, sometimes encouraged by low pressure suction, may be needed for ten days. It is useful to perform a static cystogram before removal of the catheter to confirm healing of the bladder.

Incontinence with little evidence of retention is a more difficult problem, though with time, improvement may be spontaneous. Meanwhile, the patient should be fitted with an incontinence appliance and then reassessed with a further IVU and with bladder pressure studies, if available.

MANAGEMENT OF WOUNDS

The abdominal wound in most instances heals by first intention although infection may be a complication after large

Abdominal wound

149

bowel surgery: recent interest in pre-operative preparation should reduce this problem. It is usual to remove the sutures on the tenth day and to replace them with adhesive strips to give additional support while the scar is maturing and to prevent widening of the scar.

Drainage wound

Wounds created for drains usually heal when the drain is removed – at approximately the seventh postoperative day. Failure to heal may indicate anastomotic sepsis.

Stomas

Stoma construction is usually completed by suturing the bowel end to the margin of the cutaneous trephine with a muco-cutaneous suture. Inspection of the stoma in the early post-operative period is important to ensure complete viability of the stoma and to verify that it has not become detached.

Perineal wound

The main factor delaying the discharge of a patient from hospital, following successful excision of the rectum, is slow healing of the perineal wound. The practice of primary suture of the perineal wound has been introduced and this reduces this time. The pelvic space should be drained by means of a sump suction drain and left *in situ* until drainage is minimal, usually the fourth or fifth postoperative day. The drainage tube is brought out above the pubis or to one side of the perineal wound. Primary suture is contraindicated if there is any soiling of the wound at the time of surgery. The wound should be carefully observed in the postoperative period and if there is any clinical evidence of infection or a haematoma it should be opened widely and good drainage established; this usually means leaving a three finger defect. Evidence of a collection is provided by bulging of the wound, a discharge between the sutures and a fever. Further management of the perineal wound is the same as if there had been no primary closure.

If the perineal wound is not closed a corrugated drain is left in the centre of the wound with a large defect to provide good drainage. The drain is removed on day five.

Daily baths are probably all that is required to keep the perineal wound clean, but this may be helped by irrigation with dilute hypochlorite solution (e.g. 1 in 80 Milton solution). The perineal wound should be examined with a finger twice weekly and any fibrinous adhesions broken down. It should never be packed, but instead a flat dressing soaked in hypochlorite solution inserted to keep the skin edges apart and prevent healing at skin level before obliteration of the deep part of the cavity. In the long-term a perineal sinus with continuing perineal discharge always indicates the presence of a deep presacral cavity and the whole wound will need to be laid open and encouraged to heal from within outwards.

NUTRITIONAL CARE

Malnutrition is common among patients undergoing surgery (Hill, Pickford, Young *et al.*, 1977). It is caused by patients taking inadequate food pre-operatively because of the underlying disease and may be worsened in some with sepsis by abnormally high metabolic wastage of protein and energy (Kinney, Duke, Long *et al.*, 1970). Malnutrition causes reduced protein synthesis, poor tissue repair, immunological abnormalities and increased susceptibility to infection; awareness of it is, therefore, important. Its presence will sometimes be obvious from the general appearance of the patient, but even an obese patient, though he appears misleadingly rotund, may be losing lean body mass. The body weight is useful and should always be recorded when a patient is admitted to hospital so that comparison can be made later if necessary. If a patient has lost more than 10% of his usual weight and is likely to lose more, then particular attention must be paid to his food intake. Oedema may make body weight a poor guide; other means of simple nutritional assessment include measurement of skin folds and arm circumference, serum proteins and urinary creatinine.

Malnutrition is managed, preferably under the supervision of a dietician, by encouraging the patient to eat (his likes and dislikes are important), providing extra protein and energy by oral supplementation or by tube feeding through a fine nasogastric tube. It is only when these methods do not provide adequate nourishment that parenteral nutrition is indicated.

PARENTERAL NUTRITION

Nutrition is possible through either peripheral or central veins. It is easy to cannulate peripheral veins but they become inflamed and thrombose if strongly hypertonic solutions are infused through them or if the catheter is not changed regularly. The amino acid solutions most commonly available are hypertonic but can be infused in parallel with isotonic fluids, such as fat emulsion or saline, using a double giving set. For peripheral venous nutrition, fat provides the main source of energy and glucose is only used in 5% concentration. It is usually possible to provide about 6300 kJ (1500 kcal and 8–14 grams of nitrogen (gN) per day over one to two weeks by this method. Peripheral infusion of isotonic amino acid and electrolyte solutions, with or without any energy source, has been shown to improve nitrogen balance and might prove better than the conventional dextrose and saline solutions used postoperatively today. The use of such a system is, however, likely to be expensive and needs justification by controlled trial. Peripheral feeding is sometimes a convenient way of supplementing oral intake in patients in whom a nasogastric feed is inappropriate.

Most patients requiring parenteral nutrition need it for periods of longer than one to two weeks, and need larger inputs of energy and protein than can be provided peripherally. In them a catheter is inserted into the superior vena cava, using strict aseptic technique. A simple approach allows routine use of a skin-tunnelled silicone rubber catheter for this purpose (Fig. 4.24) (Powell-Tuck, 1978).

Central venous catheterisation is potentially dangerous; the risks include the catheter insertion, metabolic complications, and contamination of the infusate or catheter by bacteria or fungi. Metabolic complications can be minimised by keeping careful daily records of all the constituents of a feed. This includes not only calories, nitrogen and electrolytes, but also calcium, phosphate, trace elements and vitamins. The patient should be weighed daily and urine regularly tested for sugar. It is simple to measure urinary urea as a guide to the nitrogen requirements (urinary urea in mmol × 0.033 = gN catabolised), assuming losses of protein are not unusually high in stool or urine. Routine biochemical estimations suffice in most patients to provide further assessment.

The prevention of sepsis is crucial (Ryan, Abel, Assott, et al., 1974). The catheter entry site is sprayed, for example with povidone-iodine, and dressed occlusively. Bottle and infusion set changes are performed with obsessional care following strict nursing protocols. Any additions to the infusate containers, which are necessary for most patients, must be made with rigorous aseptic technique and preferably by a pharmacist using a laminar flow cabinet.

Parenteral nutrition should be organised by a team of interested medical, nursing and pharmacy staff, including bac-

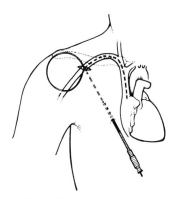

Fig. 4.24

teriologists and biochemists. If sufficient care is taken, it can be used to maintain or improve a patient's nutrition for weeks, months or even years; without such an approach it is dangerous.

REFERENCES AND FURTHER READING

Hill GL, Pickford I, Young GA, Schorah CJ, Blackett RL, Burkinshaw L, Warren JV and Morgan DB. Malnutrition in surgical patients. An unrecognised problem. *Lancet* 1977; **1:** 689–92.
Kinney JM, Duke JH, Long CL and Gump FE. Tissue fuel and weight loss after injury. *Journal of Clinical Pathology* 1970; **23:** Supplement **4,** 65–72.
Powell-Tuck J. Skin tunnel for central venous catheter. A non-operative technique. *British Medical Journal* 1978; **1:** 625.
Ryan JA, Abel RM, Abbott WM, Hopkins CC, Chesney TMcC, Colley R, Phillips K and Fischer JE. Catheter complications in total parenteral nutrition. A prospective study of 200 consecutive patients. *New England Journal Medicine* 1974; **290:** 757–61.

ANTIMICROBIAL THERAPY

Antimicrobial drugs including antibiotics, other chemotherapeutic agents and antiseptics are widely used in large bowel surgery as prophylaxis against infection and in the therapy of established infection and contamination. This widespread use needs careful review. The drugs are expensive and may easily lead to complacent surgery as a result of a false sense of security. Furthermore, their unbridled use may produce undesired side effects such as the emergence of resistant strains and toxic effects on the patient.

Wound infections, abscesses, peritonitis and septicaemia are common complications of large bowel surgery, so it is inevitable that antibiotics should have been used by colorectal surgeons to attempt to reduce this serious morbidity. However, the reports in the literature about the value of such therapy are very conflicting and any conclusions require careful study. This is because many of the so-called controlled trials of such treatment are open to criticism. Uncontrolled attempts to assess the value of any prophylactic procedure are useless, and many reports merely describe retrospective observations of infection following the use of various antibiotics. Since the definition of infection is difficult and varies in reports from simple inflammation to the actual drainage of pus from a wound, the significance of any retrospective studies must be viewed with caution. Thus for any clinical trial to be significant it must be prospective, well constructed and best carried out with the help of a nurse-epidemiologist who can inspect every wound.

For any therapy designed to reduce infection to be of value it must be appropriate to the bacterial flora encountered. There are two main sources of infection during large bowel surgery. The first is the exogenous flora of the environment and skin, which are aerobic. Antibiotic sensitivities of these are dependent upon the previous exposure of the organisms to these drugs. Infection with these organisms can be reduced by attention to air sterility in the operating room and adequate skin preparation with bacteriocidal agents at the time of surgery. The second and more important source of clinical infection is the faecal flora which is a mixture of aerobic and anaerobic organisms. The anaerobes outnumber the aerobes by ten thousand to one and consist mainly of *Clostridium welchii*, Peptostreptococcus species, Lactobacillus species and the most important *Bacteroides fragilis*. *Bacterioides fragilis* is sensitive to several antibiotics including lincomycin, clindamycin and metronidazole, and in some cases to tetracyclines, erythromycin and the more toxic chloramphenicol. The aerobic organisms include *Escherichia coli, Streptococcus faecalis and* Staphylococcus species; *Escherichia coli* is sensitive to the aminoglycocides and cephalosporins.

PROPHYLACTIC USE OF ANTIBIOTICS

Systemic

In elective large bowel surgery an attempt should be made to reduce the faecal flora by suitable mechanical and antimicrobial bowel preparation (see previous section). However, when this has not been carried out and in the emergency situation when time prevents it, the systemic use of a mixture of an aminoglycocide (e.g. gentamicin) with clindamycin or metronidazole peroperatively has been shown to reduce postoperative infective complications.

On balance it seems that the prophylactic systemic antibiotics are effective in reducing postoperative infection, especially in patients who have had no pre-operative bowel preparation (Keighley, 1977). However, it still remains to be proven conclusively that they are of value. If they are to be given, therapy should ideally be started pre-operatively or during the operation. They have no value at all if started later than four hours after contamination.

If prophylactic antibiotics and bowel preparations have not been used and peritoneal and wound contamination with gut contents occurs during surgery, local cleansing is needed and the above antibiotic combination should be started.

Local

The use of local antibiotics has always been controversial. For some years it has been stated that antibiotics used systemically should never be used locally in spray or powder form since the local high concentration is rapidly diluted by absorption and so only serves to stimulate the production of resistant organisms. It may also produce local tissue damage, toxic effects and hypersensitivity of the patient to the drug. However, these opinions may require review following results of a trial and subsequent clinical experience, in which it was shown that topical cephaloridine 1 g dissolved in 2 ml sterile water instilled into the wound before closure reduced the incidence of wound infection significantly (Pollock and Evans, 1975).

Other prophylactic measures

Plastic wound drapes are used by many surgeons to prevent wound contamination, especially from skin organisms introduced at operation. There is no conclusive evidence in the literature to support their value and since in rectal surgery the most likely source of infection is the gut flora, such a prophylactic measure cannot have even theoretical value.

Careful surgical technique during surgery is of great importance in reducing postoperative infection. Excessive trauma to tissues by rough handling, devascularisation by excessive dissection or tight suturing, haematoma formation and contamination of the wound by bowel contents all contribute to increased postoperative sepsis. Furthermore, any systemic therapy with steroids which patients suffering from inflammatory bowel disease may be receiving might predispose to infection by reducing the patient's defence mechanism.

Local instillation of antiseptics such as chlorhexidine or noxytiolin have not been shown to reduce wound infection, while the evidence for the value of local povidone iodine is controversial. Furthermore, irrigation of the peritoneal cavity with noxytiolin at the time of surgery has been shown to impair healing in experimental animals. The conclusion must be that at present there is no adequate evidence to support the use of these compounds in a prophylactic capacity.

THERAPY OF ESTABLISHED INFECTIONS

The incidence of wound infection following large bowel surgery varies in reports from 20% to 60%. The therapy of established abscess formation or wound infection following surgery of the large bowel is probably less controversial than prophylaxis. Treatment includes the establishment of free drainage of any pus and the use of antibiotics to which the cultured organisms are sensitive. It is necessary to ensure that anaerobic as well as aerobic cultures of any tissue fluids are carried out.

It is often difficult to recognise and treat septicaemia occurring after surgery because this may produce a very varied clinical picture. Any patient who becomes shocked or very unwell after large bowel surgery must be suspected of having septicaemia. Essential urgent investigations include blood culture, blood film and electrolyte estimation, urinalysis and culture, abdominal and chest x-rays and culture of any wound or stoma fluids. Careful clinical recording of pulse rate, blood pressure and in severe cases central venous pressure help in management. Fluid replacement and antimicrobial therapy, initially a combination of aminoglycocide with metronidazole in adequate doses, must be started immediately and therapy continued until the results of any microbiological studies are available.

REFERENCES AND FURTHER READING

Keighley MRB. Prevention of wound sepsis in gastrointestinal surgery. *British Journal of Surgery* 1977; **64:** 315–21.

Pollock AV, Evans M. Changing patterns of bacterial resistance in relation to prophylactic use of cephaloridine and the therapeutic use of ampicillin. *Lancet* 1975; **2:** 1251–4.

Strachen CJL, Wise R. *Surgical sepsis.* London: Academic Press, 1979.

STOMAS

The preparation of a patient who is to receive a stoma is most important. The exact nature of the operation must be explained and the patient must understand that a stoma is compatible with normal life and that with instruction the stoma can be managed without difficulty. This is often made easier by introducing the patient to someone who already has a similar stoma.

The correct siting of the stoma is also important. This must be the responsibility of the surgeon performing the operation. It should be sited on a part of the abdominal wall free from scars and well away from the umbilicus, the costal margin, the anterior superior iliac spine and the groin crease, so that an appliance may be fitted without difficulty. The selected position should be checked with the patient in several different postures. Incorrect siting is responsible for many of the problems which may occur in the long term. Details of stoma construction should be obtained from operative textbooks (Todd, 1977).

PHYSIOLOGY

The way a particular stoma functions depends entirely on the part of the intestine used for the stoma: the more proximal the stoma, the more liquid will be the effluent. Thus an ileostomy will have a liquid effluent, which averages between 500–700 ml/day (Hill, 1976), and a colostomy constructed with the sigmoid colon will very often result in the passage of solid faeces. Stomas sited between these two points will have an intermediate type of effluent. The liquid intestinal fluid contains proteolytic enzymes, which are traumatic to the skin; for this reason an ileostomy is constructed as a spout so that the effluent may be readily collected in the appliance, rather than leak under the flange on to the skin. This is not necessary with a colostomy since the formed effluent is much less irritant to the skin, as well as being less in contact with it.

APPLIANCES

There are many different types of stoma appliance available. They fall into two groups – those which are totally disposable after each action, suitable only for patients with a colostomy, and those which can be drained. The latter may only need changing once or twice a week. The most satisfactory appliances have a skin protective, together with an adhesive backplate, and often a supporting belt is worn in addition (Fig. 4.25). It is very important to fit an appliance of the

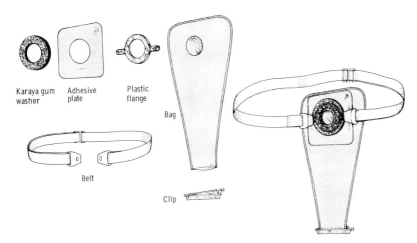

Karaya gum washer   Adhesive plate   Plastic flange   Bag   Belt   Clip

Fig. 4.25 An example of a drainable ileostomy appliance.

correct size so that the skin protective fits closely to the edge of the stoma, but does not cause pressure on it with consequent ulceration. The size of the stoma varies and it is usually much bigger in the immediate postoperative period, when it may be oedematous, than it is a month later. It may at this time be necessary to change to a different size of appliance.

Appliances are usually made of transparent material, permitting the vascularity of the stoma to be readily checked in the immediate postoperative period. However, some patients find transparent bags unacceptable and patterned opaque covers are available to conceal both the stoma and the contents. Excess gas production may be a problem, resulting in ballooning of the bag, and a small pinhole in the top of the bag covered with a charcoal filter will allow gases to escape without leakage.

COMPLICATIONS

Structural problems

Necrosis. During the construction of a terminal stoma the bowel may become ischaemic. This causes first discoloration and then necrosis of the stoma. For this reason, it is very important that a stoma be regularly examined in the postoperative period.

Detachment. It is now customary to suture the margin of the stoma to the skin at the conclusion of the operation (mucocutaneous suture). Although it is very unlikely for the stoma to become detached, this does sometimes happen, and is another reason for regular examination of the stoma in the early postoperative period.

Recession. The spout of an ileostomy may retract and the stoma may flatten. This may cause leakage under the appliance.

Stenosis. Stenosis seldom occurs when a mucocutaneous suture is performed at the time of the operation. It may be a problem when healing of skin and skin mucosa is allowed to occur by second intention.

Prolapse. Prolapse is really a form of intussusception of the bowel, and can be exceedingly difficult to treat. The appliance can be filled with intestine, which may become congested and ulcerate.

Ulceration. Ulceration is most commonly caused by the stoma rubbing on the appliance or because the flange is too tight. It is usually satisfactorily treated by attention to stoma care.

Hernia. Peristomal hernia is more common after colostomy than ileostomy. It is usually caused by the opening through the abdominal wall being too large, and occurs into the plane of the abdominal wall between the external oblique muscle and the fibrous layer of the superficial fascia. The appliance may then be difficult to keep in place and an unsightly bulge results, which bothers the patient.

Fistula. Fistulation may occur in ileostomy patients between the two layers of the spout. Local necrosis caused by the sutures used to hold the spout everted is usually the reason.

Skin soreness. Peristomal skin soreness is usually caused by the contact of effluent with skin for prolonged periods and is mainly the result of leakage. Many factors predispose to leakage; these include incorrect siting of the stoma, irregularities of the surrounding skin, lack of manual dexterity on the part of the patient, and such problems as recession, stenosis and fistula formation. Other causes of skin soreness include hypersensitivity to the materials of the appliance, too vigorous cleansing of the skin, and peristomal fungus infection.

The recently-formed nursing speciality of stomatherapy has greatly advanced stoma care. Stomatherapists offer considerable expertise in advising patients about appliances and the use of skin protectives. Often this is all that is necessary to solve a particular problem.

Functional problems

Excessive action will occur with those conditions which produce diarrhoea in the normal person, such as acute infective episodes, transit disorders, malabsorption syndromes including lactase deficiency, and sensitivity to antibiotics. More specific causes occurring in patients with stomas include intestinal obstruction, para-intestinal sepsis and recurrent inflammatory bowel disease (Crohn's disease). However, in some patients no obvious cause is found. The management of ileostomy over-action must if possible be directed towards the cause. If no cause is found, various medications may be used to reduce the volume of effluent. These include codeine phosphate, loperamide (Imodium) or diphenoxylate (Lomotil).

Reduced action in the absence of abdominal colic is probably of no significance provided it is temporary. However, a complete cessation of stoma function may indicate the presence of intestinal obstruction, especially when associated with abdominal pain. With an ileostomy this is most likely to be due to a bolus obstruction at the site where the small bowel passes through the anterior abdominal wall, which is especially likely to occur after the ingestion of excessive amounts of vegetable matter.

Excessive smell and noise may embarrass the patient. Smell is not such a problem with the newer types of appliances, which are odour-proof, but excessive smell may indicate the presence of abnormal bacterial colonisation, such as may occur with a partial small bowel obstruction. Bismuth subgallate (400 mg before meals) is said to help. Excessive noise is difficult to cope with, but may be associated with air swallowing.

General problems

Metabolic problems do not usually occur with a colostomy unless there is excessive action, but with an ileostomy there is a risk of fluid depletion and hyponatraemia. Any increase in the volume of effluent should, therefore, be investigated and vigorously treated. There is an increased incidence of biliary and renal stones in ileostomy patients.

Psychosocial problems affect patients to a varying degree, depending upon their age, sex and personality (Thomson and Lennard-Jones, 1977.) Patients are naturally concerned by the alteration of their structure and function. They often wish to restrict knowledge of the fact that they have a stoma to a limited circle of relatives and friends; this desire for privacy makes the stoma patient selfconscious about factors such as a bulky appliance, noise and odour, which could draw attention to the fact that he or she is different from other people. Young women are especially conscious of the appearance of a stoma. Disguise of the stoma and appliance, as far as possible, is thus important. An ileostomy is no bar to marriage or to pregnancy. In men the stoma itself does not affect sexual function, but rectal excision, especially for malignant disease, may result in impotence by damage to the pelvic nerves. Stomas present special problems in children and teenagers, in the elderly and those who are mentally and physically handicapped.

Considerable help may be obtain from stomatherapists and also through the various stoma clubs, such as the Ileostomy Association of Great Britain and Ireland, and the Colostomy Welfare Group (Todd, 1978).

REFERENCES AND FURTHER READING

Hill GL. *Illeostomy – surgery, physiology and management*. New York: Grune and Stratton, 1976.

Thomson JPS and Lennard-Jones JE. Life with an ileostomy. *Clinics in Gastroenterology* 1977 **6**: 699–708.

Todd IP, ed. Colon, rectum and anus. (3rd ed. Operative surgery). London and Boston: Butterworths, 1977.

Todd IP. *Intestinal stomas*. London: Heinemann, 1978.

5. The Management of Complications

LARGE BOWEL OBSTRUCTION

Many diseases of the colon cause some degree of obstruction. This section, however, deals only with management of patients with *total* obstruction to the onward passage of gas and faeces.

AETIOLOGY

Apart from congenital abnormalities (Chapter 10) there are two common causes of complete colonic obstruction, and others that are less common. The common ones are cancer and diverticular disease; the others include Crohn's disease, volvulus of the sigmoid colon or caecum, toxic megacolon of ulcerative colitis, and colonic ileus (also known as pseudo-obstruction or Ogilvie's syndrome). The detailed treatment of each of these diseases is different, but the fundamental principles are the same – to relieve the obstruction and to cure the underlying condition.

DIAGNOSIS

The patient with total obstruction always presents with abdominal distension and constipation, usually with pain and frequently with vomiting. Unless perforation has caused peritonitis, fluid and electrolyte disturbances are later features.

The diagnosis depends on the history and physical examination and is confirmed by plain abdominal x-rays in the erect and supine positions. These, in addition to confirming the distension of the colon, may indicate the site of the obstruction and (a very important measurement) the size of the caecum. Sigmoidoscopy should be done, partly because at least a third of all obstructing lesions occur in the sigmoid colon, and partly because it may allow non-operative relief of an obstruction due to a sigmoid volvulus. If this examination is negative, and the caecum is less than nine centimetres in diameter on the plain abdominal x-ray, then the time spent on doing an emergency gastrografin enema is justified as an aid to planning treatment.

MANAGEMENT

Pre-operative management

All patients with colonic obstruction must have a period of pre-operative assessment and treatment. The first essentials of treatment should be the passage of a nasogastric tube and the setting up of an intravenous infusion. If the caecum is not grossly distended an enema should be given.

Assessment of cardiovascular and respiratory function should include electrocardiography and estimation of the central venous pressure, of ventilatory function, and of arterial blood gases where indicated. Gross abnormality may indicate the danger of respiratory failure postoperatively which would call for assisted respiration. Blood estimations should include the concentration of haemoglobin (does the patient need a blood transfusion?) and of urea and electrolytes (is he fluid and/or electrolyte deplete?). Fluid intake and output must be monitored, urine volume and specific gravity being especially useful in the control of fluid balance.

Obstructions due to sigmoid volvulus and colonic ileus are best managed conservatively, but it must be stressed that if the caecum exceeds nine centimetres in diameter on x-ray, laparotomy should not be delayed. Many other patients benefit from the initial resuscitative measures, and spontaneous relief of obstruction may occur. They can then be prepared for elective surgery.

Operations

Laparotomy should not be delayed for more than six hours if no flatus is passed.

'Blind' decompression

A small incision (under local anaesthesia if necessary) to perform a caecostomy or a tranverse colostomy has attractions if the patient is very ill, but the possibility of misdiagnosis (including failure to discover a simultaneous perforation) makes this course undesirable.

Laparotomy

Abdominal x-rays, sometimes supplemented by sigmoidoscopic findings or an emergency gastrografin enema, enable the surgeon to plan his incision. The choice of vertical or tranverse incision may be left to individual judgement but if a staged operation is envisaged, the incision must be placed so as not to interfere with the subsequent resection. It should not be less than 10 cm long so that the whole hand can be introduced to feel the liver and the site of obstruction. The precise pathology of a stenosing lesion is usually not obvious, but if a staged procedure is planned it is unwise to do any dissection at the site of obstruction.

A loop of transverse colon denuded of omentum is brought out (preferably through a separate short incision) and held by a rod until after abdominal closure. The colostomy should be opened immediately and a glass Paul's tube tied in, or the colostomy and rod enclosed in an appliance which can be attached to the skin preventing faecal leakage. Bacteriological study of the colonic contents or mucosa at the time of operation gives valuable guidance if an antibiotic should subsequently be needed.

Tranverse colostomy

A caecostomy should always be done if the muscle and peritoneum over the distended caecum are found to be split, or it there is a frank caecal perforation. It should also be considered if the caecal gas shadow on x-ray is more than nine centimetres wide. Satisfactory results are obtained with a tube caecostomy with a large bore catheter brought out through a stab incision in the right iliac fossa (Fig. 4.19). Exteriorisation of the caecum is advocated by others; it has the merit of allowing freer drainage of faeces but the disadvantage of causing greater contamination of the abdominal wall. Apart from the indications above, there is no place for caecostomy.

Caecostomy

Obstructing carcinomas of the caecum or ascending colon are usually treated by primary right hemicolectomy with ileocolic anastomosis. In patients with more distal malignant obstructions the advantages of primary resection are, first, the possibility of a better long-term prognosis than after staged resection and, secondly, that primary resection deals more efficiently with a lesion which is also perforating. The proximal distended colon is brought out as a terminal colostomy and the distal colon either delivered as a mucous fistula or sutured and replaced in the peritoneal cavity (Hartmann's operation). Colonic anastomosis should never be done in the presence of obstruction, infection or faecal loading.

Primary resection

There is a technique for overcoming these adverse factors and allowing primary anastomosis after resection of an obstructing lesion of the colon. After isolating the lesion between clamps, a length of stiff corrugated polyvinyl tubing with a bore of 2.5 cm (anaesthetic gas scavenger tubing is suitable) is introduced into the dilated colon proximal to the lesion. The upper clamp is then released and faecal effluent allowed to flow into a bucket. A Foley catheter is inserted into the terminal ileum and thence through the ileocaecal valve into the caecum. It is connected to a bladder-irrigation reservoir containing saline. The entire obstructed colon can now be irrigated until the effluent is clear; 6 to 10 litres are required. The empty bowel may safely be anastomosed (Dudley, Radcliffe and McGeehan, 1980).

Postoperative management

Sepsis prophylaxis, starting before the operation, is recommended (Chapter 4). In patients in whom gross contamination of the abdominal wall has occurred skin suture should be delayed for five days. There is no place for long term prophylactic antibiotics, but existing peritonitis requires treatment; the combination of parenteral gentamicin and rectal suppositories of metronidazole is logical.

Until the colon obstruction is manifestly overcome it is wise to rest the intestine by regular aspiration of the nasogastric tube and to continue with intravenous fluid and electrolyte replacement.

The colostomy should be inspected frequently, and therefore the stoma appliance must be transparent. The two complications of a terminal colostomy are necrosis and retraction. Either of these may require surgical revision of the colostomy. The main complication of a loop colostomy is prolapse, and if this happens the bowel must be pushed back. Sepsis around a colostomy is common but usually requires no active treatment.

Chest complications are common, and their prevention demands effective pain relief and encouragement to breathe deeply and cough. Intermittent positive pressure ventilation is needed if the pO_2 while breathing oxygen-enriched air is below 60 mm Hg. Occasionally serious pulmonary insufficiency may arise from inhalation of gastric contents or complicate severe sepsis. If sepsis occurs, a valuable guide to the choice of therapeutic antibiotic will be given by the results of cultures taken from the colonic contents during operation.

PROGNOSIS

Operations for colonic obstruction entail a higher morbidity and mortality than the same operations done electively. Why should this be so?

If the first place, patients with obstruction are usually old, their reserves are low, they come to operation acutely ill and cardiac and respiratory complications are common and lethal.

Many obstructing cancers are incurable because of local spread or distant metastases.

The incidence of septic complications is also high, partly due to the lack of antibiotic preparation of the bowel but even more to the colon being loaded with faeces so that contamination during operation is likely. In addition, an anastomosis of obstructed bowel (as in right hemicolectomy) is far more prone to break down than one in a fully-prepared bowel.

For these reasons the mortality within 30 days in patients with complete colonic obstruction is between 20 and 40%. The presence of a perforation either at the site of a lesion or of the caecum increases the mortality to 50–80%.

The late mortality also is much higher in patients operated on for obstruction, partly because of the advanced state of the cancer, partly because of the higher average age of these patients, and partly – it has been suggested – because staged resections are less curative than primary resections. Out of every 100 patients presenting with complete colonic obstruction due to cancer, only 15 are likely to live five years.

REFERENCES AND FURTHER READING

Dudley HAF, Radcliffe, AG and McGeehan D. Intra-operative irrigation of the colon to permit primary anastomosis. *British Journal of Surgery* 1980; **67**: 80–81.

Fielding LP and Wells BW. Survival after primary and after staged resection for large bowel obstruction caused by cancer. *British Journal of Surgery* 1974; **61**: 16–18.

Goligher JC and Smiddy FG. The treatment of acute obstruction or perforation with carcinoma of the colon and rectum. *British Journal of Surgery* 1957; **45**: 270–4.

Hughes ESR. Mortality of acute large bowel obstruction. *British Journal of Surgery* 1966; **53**: 593–4.

Lowman RM and Davis L. An evaluation of cecal size in impending perforation of the cecum *Surgery, Gynecology and Obstetrics*, 1956; **103**: 711–18.

Welch JP and Donaldson GA. Management of severe obstruction of the large bowel due to malignant disease. *American Journal of Surgery* 1974; **127**: 492–9.

COLONIC PERFORATION

Perforation of the colon may occur in diseased or in healthy bowel. In this section discussion is confined to perforation complicating pathological processes affecting the colon. Perforation of normal bowel as a result of trauma is discussed in Chapter 6.

A breach in the wall of the colon may occur as a result of increased intraluminal pressure consequent to occlusion of the bowel lumen. The perforation may be at a site which is remote from the obstruction. For example, perforation of the anterior wall of the caecum is sometimes associated with obstruction of the left colon by carcinoma or diverticular disease. In such a case the raised intraluminal pressure interferes with the blood flow through the wall of the organ which predisposes to the development of an area of localised necrosis. This devitalised area gives way readily under the stress of pressure within the obstructed bowel.

Perforation of a segment of diseased colon may be the result of mechanical weakness, inflammation, ischaemia or malignant change. In these circumstances rupture of bowel may occur without any rise in intraluminal pressure.

The management of patients with perforation of the colon depends upon the pathological condition responsible. A wide variety of operations is available but the choice as to the most appropriate procedure depends upon the general condition of the patient, the degree of localisation of infection subsequent to perforation and the underlying pathology as well as the experience of the surgeon.

PERFORATION WITH LOCALISED ABSCESS

This is a not uncommon complication of diverticular disease. A small paracolic abscess may settle on a conservative regime. On occasion a well walled-off pericolic abscess in the left lower quadrant which is not associated with obstruction of the colonic lumen may be treated by incision and drainage. Larger abscesses require drainage and usually a proximal defunctioning colostomy, a loop colostomy formed in the right transverse colon being generally satisfactory. Division of the loop is seldom warranted.

In patients with 'sealed perforations' due to acute ulcerative colitis, Turnbull and his colleagues (1970) have recommended decompressing transverse and sigmoid colostomies, together with a diverting loop ileostomy, as an alternative to excisional surgery in the emergency situation. These authors contend that if proctocolectomy is carried out in the acute case of ulcerative colitis in which small perforations have become sealed by adherence of the colon to the parietal peritoneum, mobilisation of the colon may lead to leakage of intestinal content into the peritoneal cavity.

PERFORATION WITH GENERALISED PERITONITIS

Suture of the perforation with drainage, but without a defunctioning colostomy, is mentioned to be condemned. When perforation occurs in diseased bowel the tissue around the defect tends to be oedematous, inflamed and friable. Simple closure of the perforation and the insertion of a drain is, therefore, an unsafe procedure.

Suture of the perforation with drainage together with a proximal defunctioning colostomy gives added protection following the closure of a perforated colon. However, it must be realised that this supplementary procedure may be limited in its effectiveness. There are two reasons for this: firstly, the actual closure of the inflamed or necrotic bowel may be unsatisfactory because of the nature of the tissue being sutured. Secondly, if the segment of colon between the colostomy and the site of the closed perforation is loaded with faeces, then further leakage is still liable to occur should the suture line break down.

In some cases of generalised peritonitis secondary to diverticular disease of the colon, no obvious perforation may be identifiable at the time of laparotomy. If a decision is made to drain the peritoneal cavity and establish a tranverse colostomy rather than resect the diseased segment then an over-enthusiastic search for a sealed perforation should be avoided since disturbance of the area might lead to further leakage.

Where the perforation occurs in the thinned-out wall of the caecum in cases of distal obstruction of the colon, it may be feasible to close the caecum around a large caesotomy tube which is brought out through the anterior abdominal wall in the right iliac fossa; the anterior caecal wall being tacked to the parietal peritoneum. While this procedure helps in dealing with the defect in the caecum it does not allow very satisfactory decompression of the obstructed colon. It is, therefore, advisable to form a transverse loop colostomy in addition.

Operations in which the perforated segment is left *in situ*

Diversion of the faecal stream by a transverse colostomy, as previously stated, does not remove the potential source of further contamination by the contents already within the left colon. This hazard may be avoided either by exteriorisation of the perforated segment or by primary resection with or without anastomosis.

Clearly, patients with faecal peritonitis due to a breach in the colonic wall should have the segment excluded from the peritoneal cavity. Adoption of this policy in cases of purulent peritonitis is more controversial but it also has a place in the management of selected cases from this group.

Operations in which the perforated segment is removed from the peritoneal cavity

167

When rupture of the colon follows necrosis due to volvulus or ischaemia, it is essential to excise the gangrenous segment. Perforation of a colonic carcinoma at or near a growth is best treated by excision rather than attempting to close the defect, which is generally a rather unsatisfactory procedure. There are several available techniques and these are described.

Exteriorisation

On occasions when the perforation is situated, for example, at the apex of the sigmoid loop, it is easy to exteriorise it. Further leakage into the peritoneal cavity is thus eliminated but this procedure does not stop the toxic products from the septic focus entering the blood stream. If the diseased segment is easily exteriorised it is easily excised. It seems best therefore to remove this portion of the colon as this adds relatively little to the time required for the operation and makes for more rapid progress and easier management postoperatively.

Excision of segment with end colostomy and mucous fistula

When perforation occurs in a mobile part of the bowel or in a segment which can be easily mobilised it may be feasible to excise the diseased portion at the initial operation and bring out the proximal bowel as an end colostomy and the distal end as a mucous fistula, thus removing the septic focus at this stage in the management.

Excision of segment with end colostomy and closure of distal stump

In those cases where the perforation is low in the sigmoid colon and where the mesentery is short, the formation of a mucous fistula may be impossible and it may be necessary to close the distal stump (Hartmann's operation).

Paul-Mickulicz operation

If sufficient length of intestine is available and if the operation is for a benign condition, some surgeons prefer to excise the diseased bowel and construct a double-barrelled colostomy. While this policy may be feasible in the management of patients with sigmoid volvulus where there is much redundant bowel, it is not often possible in perforated diverticular disease where the bowel tends to be shortened. In this operation only a limited segment of bowel is removed and the procedure does not allow for a very adequate excision of the field of lymphatic drainage in malignant disease.

Primary resection and anastomosis with or without proximal colostomy

In the various procedures just described, the primary aim is to save the patient's life, and the ultimate aim is to re-establish continuity of the colon after a suitable interval. However, there have been numerous reports in the literature of good results obtained by one-stage resection with anastomosis for perforated diverticular disease. Most of these series come from experienced surgeons who have used wise judgement in the selection of cases. The inexperienced surgeon should be aware of the risk of anastomotic leakage where this procedure is undertaken in the presence of frank peritoneal sepsis on an unprepared colon. The consequences of leakage may be reduced but not abolished by the formation of a simultaneous proximal colostomy.

Free perforation due to ulcerative colitis or amoebic dysentery or necrotising colitis is a highly lethal condition. Under these circumstances, especially when operating on patients with ulcerative colitis, surgeons generally feel it desirable to leave the rectum *in situ*. A decision as to further management can be made subsequently.

Subtotal colectomy with ileostomy and mucous fistula

REFERENCES AND FURTHER READING

Turnbull RB, Weakley FL, Hawk WA and Schofield P. Choice of operation for the toxic megacolon phase of non-specific ulcerative colitis. *Surgical Clinics of North America* 1970; **50**: 1151.
Jones PF. *Emergency abdominal surgery*. Oxford: Blackwell, 1974.

COLOVESICAL FISTULA

The commonest cause of colovesical fistula is diverticular disease of the colon, but it may also occur in Crohn's disease and other benign inflammatory conditions. Carcinoma of either the colon or the bladder may also lead to fistulation between these two organs. The segment involved is almost invariably the sigmoid colon, but on occasion the communication is with the caecum. The management, therefore, depends on the underlying cause, but in general a colovesical fistula should be treated surgically as it is unlikely to heal spontaneously and usually leads to ascending urinary tract infection and prolonged ill health. However, in advanced malignancy surgical excision is not always feasible.

In the definitive surgical management of colovesical fistula arising as a complication of diverticular disease, a three-stage procedure has generally been more widely practised than the one-stage operation. There are many factors, local and general, which influence the surgeon in his decision as to the procedure of choice.

Primary resection with anastomosis is justifiable, if the colovesical fistula is small, the inflammatory reaction is well localised, there is no pericolic abscess, the colon available on either side of the resected portion is healthy so that a sound anastomosis is feasible, and the patient's general health is good. Often the operation is more straightforward than anticipated.

A preliminary proximal colostomy is indicated in those cases in whom the inflammatory reaction is extensive, or in whom a pericolic abscess has formed. If it is clear that the fistula is due to benign disease, then a period of approximately 2–3 months is allowed for the inflammation to settle, at which stage resection is undertaken. Again, if a significant degree of obstruction is present, then preliminary diversion is obligatory.

Surgical management involves excision not only of the fistulous tract but also the diseased segment of bowel. The defect in the bladder should be closed directly and, if feasible, omentum is placed between the colon and bladder to prevent the two suture lines adhering. An indwelling catheter is left *in situ* for 10 days. In patients unfit for major surgery long term antibiotics may help control urinary infection, but it is unusual for the fistula to heal spontaneously.

ANASTOMOTIC BREAKDOWN

The overall mortality for large bowel resection and anastomosis is approximately 5%. One third of these deaths are due to sepsis (generalised peritonitis, abscesses, or fistulas) which follows leakage at the anastomosis. On many occasions restorative surgery has to be undertaken when there is a high risk of leakage from factors over which the surgeon has no control. However, if the increased risk is recognised it may be possible either to improve the general condition of the patient before definitive surgery, or to limit the surgery to that required immediately, e.g. colostomy in intestinal obstruction.

AETIOLOGICAL FACTORS

The situation of the anastomosis

Emergency procedures are often followed by anastomotic leakage, particularly those involving left sided colocolic and colorectal anastomoses for inflammatory complications of diverticular disease (Schrock, Deveney and Dunphy, 1973). A similar incidence of breakdown (10.5%) was found following elective surgery for diverticular disease in the presence of infection. With this exception the leakage rates of all types of elective intraperitoneal anastomoses are similar whether they involve the right or left colon. When extraperitoneal anastomoses are examined thoroughly a 69% incidence of breakdown has been reported (Goligher, Graham, and de Dombal, 1970). In this situation a poor blood supply to the bowel, accumulation of fluid after mobilisation of the rectum, and the absence of a serosal peritoneal layer on the rectum may be contributory factors. It may also be important that an anastomosis in this position is often excluded from the normal decontaminating mechanisms of the peritoneal cavity.

Poor surgical technique is the most important determinant of anastomotic leakage. Good pre-operative mechanical preparation of the colon will reduce the faecal bulk but spillage of any residual faeces must be avoided when the bowel is opened. Topical antiseptics, e.g. chlorhexidine, are helpful in minimising the effects of contamination with bacteria. The crucial point is that the segments of bowel to be anastomosed must have a good blood supply and must not be joined under tension. Before the bowel is anastomosed the segments enclosed within the clamps should be excised and the viability of the remaining bowel confirmed by its colour, the presence of pulsating vessels and bleeding from the cut ends. It should be noted that previous irradiation may predispose to ischaemia of the bowel by damaging small blood vessels.

Surgical technique

An inverting suture should be used for all large bowel anastomoses. Although a narrowed lumen is a theoretical possibility, a stricture is usually the sequel of peri-anastomotic infection after leakage. Goligher, Graham and de Dombal, (1970) have shown that there is an unacceptable incidence of infection, anastomotic leakage, and stricture after everting anastomoses in the colon.

Type of suture

When a colonic anastomosis is particularly at risk there is controversy about the advantages of an anastomosis constructed with one or two layers of sutures. When two layers are used it is possible that more reliable mucosal inversion is achieved than with a single layer of interrupted stitches. However, the inverted bowel inside the continuous inner layer stitch will slough eventually due to the loss of its blood supply in contrast to that enclosed by the interrupted sutures, most of which will be preserved. When the anastomosis is very low and difficult to construct it may only be possible to insert one layer of interrupted sutures. In these circumstances the anastomosis should be covered by a transverse colostomy to reduce the consequences of anastomotic leakage. The introduction of stapling devices has enabled some surgeons to carry out these low colorectal anastomoses more readily.

Drainage

It is customary, although probably not necessary, to drain most intraperitoneal colonic anastomoses. Bacteria and debris deposited during surgery will be rapidly diffused throughout the peritoneal cavity and removed through the lymphatics. The accumulation of fluid or haematoma in the pelvis may be an important cause of anastomotic leakage and it may be possible to prevent this accumulation by a technique of continuous irrigation using sump drains.

General factors

Old age, cardiovascular disorders, metabolic disorders such as diabetes mellitus, and advanced malignancy, may all prejudice anastomotic healing. Steroid and cytotoxic drugs have also been incriminated.

THE CRITERIA FOR ANASTOMOTIC BREAKDOWN

There is a high incidence of anastomotic breakdown after colorectal anastomoses, particularly low anterior resections. The means of detection of leakage from anastomoses in this position have been studied extensively. The failure of a colorectal anastomosis to heal may lead to specific postoperative complications, or be demonstrated by clinical and radiological examinations. There are three important postoperative manifestations.

Generalised peritonitis

Generalised peritonitis is the most serious complication with a high mortality. It is uncommon and usually follows leakage from intraperitoneal, rather than extraperitoneal anastomoses.

Localised peritonitis

Localised peritonitis leads to pyrexia, pain and localised tenderness suggesting the presence of an abscess (paracolic or pelvic). A pelvic abscess is the common manifestation of local sepsis after a colorectal anastomosis. It usually follows anastomotic leakage, but may occasionally occur without the demonstration of a defect in the suture line.

Faecal fistula

A faecal fistula is an accepted criterion for anastomotic breakdown, but its absence does not imply anastomotic healing

172

without complications. Everett (1975) found radiological evidence of anastomotic leakage (without one faecal fistula) in 15% of patients after colorectal anastomoses. The incidence of this complication may also depend on the adequacy of mechanical bowel preparations and whether or not the anastomosis is defunctioned by a colostomy.

INVESTIGATIONS

Abnormalities are seen on sigmoidoscopy in all patients with anastomotic dehiscence below the peritoneal reflection (Goligher, Graham and de Dombal, 1970). Defects in the suture line are usually large and barium enema studies, although useful in delineating the size of the defects are not necessary for their detection in contrast to those unsuspected defects revealed in patients with intraperitoneal anastomoses.

Sigmoidoscopy

It is well known that routine postoperative contrast studies will demonstrate leakage from a colonic or particularly a colorectal anastomosis in the absence of any other evidence (Fig. 1.25). Any series of patients examined in this way will have a higher incidence of anastomotic dehiscence than a comparable series without this examination. There may be little correlation between the size of a leak and symptoms and signs. When large leaks are demonstrated on x-ray, there is often no pain, rise in temperature, or drainage of pus or faecal fluid, and conversely all these may occur with a very small leak.

Contrast radiology

MANAGEMENT

In most cases there is no need for further surgery in patients with anastomotic breakdown. It is usual to cover an anastomosis at particular risk of breakdown with a colostomy. The colostomy will not prevent anastomotic breakdown, but it will divert faeces away from the anastomosis. It is more effective than a caecostomy, which in addition requires careful irrigation to avoid blockage with faeces.

If there are signs of spreading peritonitis in the absence of a colostomy, laparotomy with construction of a colostomy must be carried out urgently, together with drainage of the anastomosis. If there is severe contamination with either pus or faeces, the peritoneum should be washed out with an antiseptic solution and the patient started on treatment with a combination of parenteral antimicrobial drugs (e.g. gentamicin and

General peritonitis

metronidazole). After the patient has recovered satisfactorily a barium enema must be carried out before the colostomy is closed to determine that healing has occurred. If there is a tight stricture at the site of the anastomosis it may be necessary to excise it and re-anastomose the bowel.

Local peritonitis

The most frequent manifestation of anastomotic leakage is an abscess around the anastomosis, for example a pelvic abscess. The abscess usually discharges spontaneously, but it sometimes requires operative drainage. Many of these patients will already have a colostomy, although occasionally this problem can be managed without one. If there is evidence of a major leak the patency of the anastomosis must be confirmed before the colostomy is closed.

Faecal fistula

A faecal fistula may occur several days after operation without any signs of peritonitis. The faecal discharge will often resolve over a few days, or at the most a few weeks, provided there is no obstruction distal to the anastomosis. It is very seldom necessary to resect the fistula.

REFERENCES AND FURTHER READING

Everett WG. A comparison of one layer and two layer techniques for colorectal anastomosis. *British Journal of Surgery* 1975; **62:** 135–40.

Fielding LP, Stewart–Brown S, Blesovsky L and Kearney G. Anastomotic integrity after operations for large-bowel cancer: a multicentre study. *British Medical Journal* 1980; **2:** 411–14.

Goligher JC, Graham NG and de Dombal FT. Anastomotic dehiscence after anterior resection of rectum and sigmoid. *British Journal of Surgery* 1970; **57:** 109–18.

Goligher JC, Morris C, McAdam WAF, de Dombal FT and Johnston D. A controlled trial of inverting versus everting intestinal suture in clinical large bowel surgery. *British Journal of Surgery* 1970; **57:** 817–22.

Schrock TR, Deveny CW and Dunphy JE. Factors contributing to leakage of clonic anastomoses. *Annals of Surgery* 1973; **177:** 513–18.

6. Injuries to the Large Intestine

Abdominal trauma may damage the large intestine, its vascular supply and its mesenteric supports; the injury may be nonpenetrating or penetrating (Table 6a). Injuries can occur in isolation but are frequently associated with damage to other organs either intra-abdominal or elsewhere.

Table 6a. *Classification of colonic injuries*

Nonpenetrating	Crush
	Blast
Penetrating	Stab
	Gunshot
Intraluminal	Endoscopic
	Hydrostatic
	Pneumatic

INJURIES TO THE COLON

Causes of injury

Nonpenetrating abdominal trauma is most commonly due to road traffic accidents but may also be caused by a fall or blow on the abdomen at work or during participation in sport. The various mechanisms responsible for colonic injury are: a shearing force causing tearing of the colon near to its point of fixation, crushing of the colon, especially the tranverse colon against the vertebral column and bursting due to increase in intraluminal pressure (McKenzie and Bell, 1972).

Blunt trauma sometimes causes a superficial muscular tear of the colonic wall. It may produce a complete laceration of the entire thickness, resulting in faecal contamination of the peritoneal cavity. Occasionally an intramural haematoma may develop. The mesentery of the colon may be damaged. Rupture of a major vessel can lead to acute haemorrhage and if a segment of the bowel is devascularised, necrosis may lead to perforation. If ischaemia is less acute stenosis may develop subsequently.

Seat-belt injuries of the colon are of two types: discrete perforations which may be multiple, usually on the antimesenteric border of the bowel and complete or almost complete transections. The caecum and splenic flexures are the areas of the colon most likely to rupture.

The large bowel may be penetrated by sharp objects such as metal spikes or knives, by low or high velocity bullets and by fragments of shrapnel, mortar, glass or wood propelled at various velocities in bomb blasts. The prognosis depends on the severity of the injury and the nature of the agent causing it.

A high velocity bullet gives up a large amount of kinetic energy in passing through tissues. This may result in massive destruction of the colonic or rectal wall and disruption of the surrounding tissues. It usually causes a small entrance wound, a rather larger exit wound and a trail of destruction and cavitation in its path. Adjacent tissues may subsequently undergo necrosis because of cellular injury by the shock wave.

A low velocity bullet, gives up less kinetic energy. It often lodges in the tissues and whether it makes an exit or not, it is much less destructive.

Shotguns which discharge large numbers of pellets cause extensive damage to tissues if fired at close range. Bomb blast injuries can have devastating effects on the abdominal wall and the colon. Injury to the anorectum is usually associated with extensive trauma to the buttock region and shrapnel may be deeply embedded in these and in the pelvic organs. The bursting effect of bomb explosions may cause avulsion of the rectum from the anal and peri-anal tissues.

Large bowel trauma occurs much more often in association with injuries to other organs than it does in isolation. Often there are multiple lesions in the large and small bowel. The prognosis is worse when several abdominal organs are involved, for example the pancreas, duodenum, liver and major blood vessels.

Initial management

In the initial management of patients with large bowel injuries it is important to make as rapid and accurate a general assessment as possible. The co-existence of injuries at other sites should be borne in mind. It is important to ensure that urgent resuscitation is instituted, in particular that ventilation is adequate, and the blood volume restored.

Penetration of abdominal organs may occur not only via the

abdomen or flank but also from the back or perineum. Missiles entering the chest or even the neck may pass into or through the abdomen.

If the patient fails to respond to urgent resuscitative measures and it is apparent that considerable blood loss is occurring, then immediate laparotomy should be undertaken. While the patient's condition permits, x-rays of the abdomen may reveal free gas in the peritoneal cavity or gas trapped in the retroperitoneal region. There may be displacement of loops of bowel by retroperitoneal haematoma. X-rays taken in two planes help in the localisation of foreign bodies. Normal x-ray findings do not, however, exclude serious injury to the bowel wall, its supporting mesentery or its blood supply.

Nonpenetrating injury

In nonpenetrating abdominal trauma the decision to undertake laparotomy depends on the physical signs, although special investigations may be of some help. Careful initial assessment and subsequent re-appraisal are necessary.

Peritoneal aspiration with a fine bore needle in the four abdominal quadrants has been commonly used in an attempt to detect haemorrhage or perforations. The test may be negative unless there is a considerable amount of blood or intestinal content in the peritoneal cavity. On the other hand, a false positive result may occur if the needle used during aspiration inadvertently pierces an intact colon.

Peritoneal lavage via a peritoneal dialysis catheter is now accepted as a relatively safe diagnostic procedure yielding a much higher degree of accuracy than the four quadrant tap. The presence of blood or intestinal content in the lavage fluid should lead to urgent laparotomy. However, it should be remembered that with retroperitoneal colonic injury, peritoneal lavage may be negative.

Penetrating injury

While there is controversy as to whether selected cases of stabbing of the abdomen should be managed initially by observation rather than by laparotomy, there is no doubt that all abdominal gunshot wounds should be explored unless death is imminent from another cause, (for example, concomitant severe brain damage). Although injury to the large bowel may be anticipated prior to laparotomy, it is only at the time of surgery that a full assessment can be made. The size of the external wound bears little relationship to the depth of the penetration or to the severity of the intra-abdominal injury.

Operative management

Control of infection is vital if morbidity is to be kept at the lowest possible level. Potential sources of continuing contamination should be eliminated where possible. It is most important to excise all dead or dying tissue. Direct control of bleeding and the provision of drainage to prevent haematoma formation are most important. Antibiotics are important but should not be expected to solve all the problems if basic surgical principles are not followed. A broad spectrum antibiotic with metronidazole to meet the challenge of both aerobic and anaerobic organisms should be started before laparotomy. Tetanus toxoid is given if the patient has not been immunised.

The entrance and exit wounds should be thoroughly excised and drained. Skin is closed by delayed primary suture. It should be remembered that following stabbing the weapon may have been heavily contaminated by large bowel organisms which are deposited in the abdominal wall during withdrawal of the weapon.

A long paramedian or midline incision is essential to allow adequate access. Examination of all the contents of the abdominal cavity must be meticulous.

If there has been no significant vascular injury, a rent in the mesentery can be easily closed. When injury to a sizeable vessel has occurred the viability of the segment of bowel must be assessed and if necessary the segment excised.

Lacerations may be concealed in areas of retroperitoneal colon at the flexures or where the colon is hidden by omentum. It may be necessary to mobilise a segment of bowel or a flexure to make sure that it is intact. In gunshot injuries it is important to count the number of holes in the bowel and apply the 'rule of two'. If an uneven number of holes is found then a missed exit wound in the retroperitoneal area of the colon must be most carefully sought.

A tangential injury can lead to the count being uneven but this explanation may only be accepted after a thorough and detailed search.

When perforations are found in the gastro-intestinal tract these are temporarily isolated with non-crushing clamps to prevent further spillage of intestinal content. Specimens are sent for culture and particulate matter or foreign bodies are removed from the peritoneal cavity. If significant contamination has occurred it will be advisable to irrigate the peritoneal cavity with saline at a later stage in the operation.

Surgical options

There is no single policy of management which is applicable to all cases of colorectal injury. Table 6b outlines the commoner surgical options in the management of perforating injuries of

Table 6b. *Surgical options in the management of perforating injuries of the colon*

Primary suture

Primary suture with proximal decompression

Exteriorisation of perforation

Exteriorisation of sutured perforation

Resection with anastomosis
    with colostomy and mucous fistula
    with colostomy and closure of stump

---

colon. The procedure adopted should not be sterotyped but should depend upon the site of the colonic injury, the extent of the damage, the nature of the wounding agent, the general state of the patient and the expertise of the surgeon. There is a vast difference between the patient with a single small stab wound in the anterior wall of the caecum and the patient who has extensive devitalisation of tissue due to a high velocity bullet or bomb blast which has not only damaged the colon and other intra-abdominal organs but also caused widespread peritoneal faecal contamination and massive blood loss.

Nevertheless, there are surgical principles which may influence the procedure to be adopted. The consistency of the faecal stream in the right and left colon is different; an ileocolic anastomosis is safer therefore than a colocolic anastomosis. Some segments of the colon lend themselves more readily to exteriorisation than others and extensively injured colon should always be excised.

Primary closure is reasonable if there is a limited colonic wound of less than four hours duration with minimal peritoneal soiling, blood loss and associated injuries. Absolute contra-indications to primary closure are: delay in operation associated with frank peritonitis, massive contamination, high-velocity bullet wounds, explosive and shotgun injuries causing shattering of the tissues, blunt trauma, severe tissue destruction with extensive intramural haematoma or mesenteric vascular change, massive whole body trauma, extreme shock, severe pancreatic and duodenal injuries. In these circumstances, exteriorisation or resection should be the basis of management of the damaged colon.

In most penetrating wounds of the right colon, the treatment is either primary closure or resection with anastomosis. In stab injuries the edges of the colonic wound are trimmed and closure is effected in two layers using interrupted non-absorbable suture for the outer seromuscular coat. Under satisfactory conditions small low-velocity bullet wounds may be primarily

179

repaired. For more extensive trauma a right hemicolectomy is advised.

Wounds of the transverse colon are generally suitable for exteriorisation, the perforated area being converted into a colostomy. The colostomy can subsequently be closed or, if necessary, a segment resected and an end-to-end anastomosis performed.

When injury to the tranverse colon is so great that resection is obligatory, it is best to bring out the proximal end as a colostomy and the distal end as a mucous fistula, rather than to attempt an anastomosis at the initial operation.

In the descending colon primary suture or primary resection and anastomosis should be protected with a right transverse loop colostomy. This can be closed at a later date when the colon has soundly healed. Good results from primary closure have been achieved in selected cases of left colon injury, in which there was a clean, fresh, localised wound, with little contamination (Walt, 1976). In cases of extensive injury to the left colon, in which resection is required, it is sometimes better to delay the anastomosis until a subsequent operation, the proximal end being brought out as a colostomy and the distal end as a mucous fistula initially.

As in the case of the transverse colon, the sigmoid colon is suitable for exteriorisation, particularly if the rent is near to the apex of the loop. Lesions that are low in the sigmoid should be closed by direct suture if this is feasible, and generally proximal colostomy is advisable.

INJURIES TO THE RECTUM AND ANAL CANAL

There are various ways in which the rectum and anal canal can be injured. The causes are listed in Table 6c. If injury is suspected then careful examination of the pelvic area, both anteriorly and posteriorly, should be undertaken. The buttocks and anus are inspected and the anal canal and the lower rectum carefully palpated. If the patient has a gunshot wound, rectal injury should be suspected if the path of the missile is in the proximity of the rectum, if the sacrum is fractured, or if there is blood in the lumen of the bowel. The wound in the rectum may be beyond the reach of the palpating finger and even a small lesion within reach can be easily missed if the defect is plugged by mucosa.

Other organs in the pelvis are commonly damaged, particularly the bladder and urethra. The pelvis itself may be fractured, an injury which is often associated with extensive haematoma formation. Injury to the major blood vessels in the pelvis, particularly the veins, may lead to considerable blood loss.

Table 6c. *Causes of rectal injuries*

Swallowed foreign bodies
   chicken or fish bone, nail, needle

Objects inserted per anum
   enema tube
   sigmoidoscope
   thermometer

Impalement

Gunshot

Bomb blast

Pneumatic injury

Associated with pelvic fractures

Associated with surgical procedures
   gynaecological
   urological
   anorectal

Associated with childbirth

Radiation injury

Initial management

The general principles are the same as for colonic trauma. Sigmoidoscopy should be carried out with great care and with the insufflation of as little air as possible in order to avoid forcing any faecal material out through a rupture in the bowel should this have occurred.

Impalement injuries can be serious, the damage being much more extensive than is apparent initially. A spike may have passed deeply into the body injuring many organs. If the patient arrives at hospital with the foreign body still *in situ*, no attempt should be made to withdraw it until he is on the operating table, anaesthetised and the abdomen has been opened. If this policy is followed then it is easier to assess the exact track of the foreign body and the damage it is likely to have caused. When the foreign body is withdrawn severe haemorrhage is liable to occur. Clearly it is preferable for the patient to be in the operating theatre in these circumstances.

Operative management

The general principles in managing colonic injury also apply to the rectum.

Intraperitoneal rectal injury

After initial resuscitation, laparotomy is undertaken so that perforation or laceration may be repaired. For most intraperitoneal lesions it is advisable to have the safeguard of a proximal colostomy. This is obligatory if the rectal defect is large or difficult to close, or if there is bladder or urethral injury.

181

Extraperitoneal rectal injury

The primary surgical treatment depends to a large extent upon the nature and the extent of the injury. Laparotomy should be undertaken and adequate débridement carried out. Repair of the defect should be carried out *per abdomen*, where this is feasible. If this involves extensive dissection, however, there may be an increased chance of complications. Unless easy to repair it is better avoided therefore. It is vitally important that the region is adequately drained as there is a tendency for infected fluid and necrotic débris to pool in the retrorectal space. It may furthermore be advisable to insert a perineal drain through an incision just anterior to the coccyx into the retrorectal space. In the past coccygectomy was often advised to allow better drainage but because of the potential risk of oesteomyelitis, removal of the coccyx is better avoided.

In extraperitoneal penetrating rectal injury a diverting colostomy should be made. This is generally formed in the left iliac fossa using the sigmoid colon. It is also helpful at the time of initial operation to irrigate the distal sigmoid and rectum to clear it of faeces, thus reducing the likelihood of subsequent contamination of the perirectal tissue.

Anal canal injury

When the anal sphincters are damaged, every effort should be made to preserve as much sphincteric tissue as possible. Primary repair of the sphincters is recommended as this gives the best functional results. The skin is not approximated initially but can usually be closed later by delayed primary suture. If there has been extensive skin loss, as may occur in bomb explosions, then skin grafting is required later.

If there has been superficial damage to the buttock and perineal regions with only minor injury to the sphincters, then a diverting colostomy may be omitted. Otherwise, it is essential to provide proximal faecal diversion.

IATROGENIC INJURY OF THE LARGE BOWEL

Iatrogenic injury of the large bowel is occasionally associated with nursing or medical diagnostic procedures, e.g. rectal temperature measurement in infants, barium enema, sigmoidoscopy or colonoscopy. Ischaemic colitis may occur due to inferior mesenteric artery occlusion or spasm following selective angiography. The large bowel may be damaged during operations on adjacent organs.

The rectum and colon may be damaged by ionising rays in treatment of uterine and vesical cancer. Irradiation may cause a proctitis, ulceration or stricture formation in the rectum and fistulation into the vagina or bladder. Some of these complications can come on years after the therapy.

Patients with radiation proctitis have a very friable musoca which can bleed profusely; it is aggravated by constipation which should be avoided by using lubricant laxatives. Anaemia should be corrected, if necessary, by transfusion.

Surgery may be required for severe or intractable symptoms. Patients with severe proctitis or ulceration sometimes benefit from a prolonged period of faecal diversion by proximal colostomy. Where a rectovaginal or rectovesical fistula has developed it is essential to establish that this is not due to a recurrence of the neoplasm. A preliminary colostomy is essential before any attempt at repair. The surgical options include procedures in which the rectum is separated from the vagina and omentum or gracilis muscle is interposed. Alternatively, some form of sphincter-saving resection involving a colo-anal anastomosis may be undertaken. (Parks, Allen, Frank *et al.*, 1978).

Abdomino-perineal excision of the rectum may be required for severe continuing proctitis with marked tenesmus, for life-threatening haemorrhage and in some cases with fistula or marked stenosis.

FOREIGN BODIES IN THE RECTUM

Most sizeable objects that are found in the rectum have been inserted *per anum*, although smaller objects may have been ingested. Rarely they may erode through from adjacent organs. Care and at times not a little ingenuity are required for their removal. This may be made easier by suction apparatus, obstetric forceps, snares and even corkscrews for soft objects. Withdrawal of a large globular foreign body may induce a negative pressure above the object, hindering its extraction. It is often helpful to pass a catheter alongside the foreign body to allow air to enter the upper rectum.

A foreign body lodged high in the rectum may not be accessible. It is then reasonable to wait 24 hours or more in the hope that the object will descend into the lower rectum spontaneously. Enemas are best avoided as they will tend to push the object to a higher level. Ocassionally it is necessary to undertake laparotomy to remove the foreign body through an incision in the anterior wall of the intraperitoneal part of the rectum or to facilitate its removal through the anus.

REFERENCES AND FURTHER READING

Kirkpatrick JR and Rajpal SG. The injured colon: therapeutic considerations. *American Journal of Surgery* 1975; **129**: 187–91.
McKenzie AD and Bell GA. Nonpenetrating injuries of the colon and rectum. *The Surgical Clinics of North America* 1972; **52**: 735–46.

Towne JB and Coe JD. Seat belt trauma of the colon. *American Journal of Surgery* 1971; **122:** 683–5.

Walt AJ. Injuries and iatrogenic disorders of the colon and rectum. In: Bockus HL, ed. *Gastroenterology, 3rd ed. Volume 2.* Philadelphia: W.B. Saunders, 1976: 1120–7.

Parks AG, Allen CLO, Frank JD and McPartlin JF. A method of treating postirradiation fistulas. *British Journal of Surgery* 1978; **65:** 417–21.

7. *Inflammatory Bowel Disease*

PATHOLOGY

Two tasks face the Western pathologist, firstly to separate Crohn's disease and ulcerative colitis from other causes of colitis (Fig. 7.1) and, secondly, to separate them from each other. In

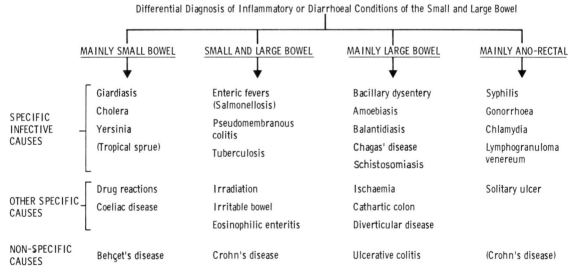

Differential Diagnosis of Inflammatory or Diarrhoeal Conditions of the Small and Large Bowel

	MAINLY SMALL BOWEL	SMALL AND LARGE BOWEL	MAINLY LARGE BOWEL	MAINLY ANO-RECTAL
SPECIFIC INFECTIVE CAUSES	Giardiasis Cholera Yersinia (Tropical sprue)	Enteric fevers (Salmonellosis) Pseudomembranous colitis Tuberculosis	Bacillary dysentery Amoebiasis Balantidiasis Chagas' disease Schistosomiasis	Syphilis Gonorrhoea Chlamydia Lymphogranuloma venereum
OTHER SPECIFIC CAUSES	Drug reactions Coeliac disease	Irradiation Irritable bowel Eosinophilic enteritis	Ischaemia Cathartic colon Diverticular disease	Solitary ulcer
NON-SPECIFIC CAUSES	Behçet's disease	Crohn's disease	Ulcerative colitis	(Crohn's disease)

Fig. 7.1

general this is possible on rectal or colonic biopsies, but a percentage of patients undergo colectomy before a tissue diagnosis is made; even after examination of the surgical specimen some 10–15% of cases cause difficulty in final classification. The colon has a limited pattern of response to inflammatory events and consequently there are only a few absolute distinguishing morphological criteria by which to separate many of these conditions. This is especially true for Crohn's disease and ulcerative colitis where considerable overlap exists. The final diagnosis in inflammatory bowel disease must, therefore, be a cumulative one made in conjunction with clinical, radiological and histopathological data. Every opportunity to obtain biopsy material should be taken so that a dynamic picture of the disease processes can be established. It is important for the laboratory to handle these biopsy specimens correctly, a subject considered in Chapter 1, and for the clinician to remember that normal sigmoidoscopic or colonoscopic appearances do not necessarily mean normal histology. Whenever inflammatory bowel disease enters the differential diagnosis, the pathologist must be given the opportunity to examine a biopsy.

Though the list of differential diagnoses is long, in practice the commonest problem is to separate out ischaemic colitis, pseudomembranous colitis, tuberculosis, the bacillary dysenteries, amoebiasis and the solitary ulcer syndrome.

Ischaemic disease

In ischaemic bowel disease (Chapter 9) infarction of the mucosa or fibrous obliteration of the lamina propria with attenuated glands are the main histological patterns. In the operative specimen submucosal granulation tissue, fibrosis and iron deposition are seen in chronic cases while haemorrhagic infarction characterises acute-onset disease. Biopsies taken after recovery from a mild episode may be normal or show only regenerative changes often with residual haemosiderin within macrophages.

Pseudomembranous colitis

In pseudomembranous colitis, provided a plaque is examined, focal 'explosive' disruption of groups of crypts with an overlaying layer of polymorphs, mucin and fibrin is seen. Adjacent mucosa is often relatively normal. When the plaques coalesce distinction from acute ischaemic colitis with mucosal necrosis is difficult. In antibiotic-associated colitis the biopsy may simply show non-specific inflammation.

Tuberculosis

Tuberculosis must always be considered when granulomas are seen. In operative specimens the granulomas are confluent, strictures when present are short and frequently multiple and the muscularis propria is obliterated by inflammation and fibrosis: all findings that are in contrast to those of Crohn's disease. When granulomas are found in biopsy material, especially in anal lesions, tuberculosis should be excluded prior to embarking on therapy for Crohn's disease.

The biopsy appearance of the bacillary dysenteries may be indistinguishable from ulcerative colitis but classically shows the initial stages of crypt abscess formation with a marked polymorphonuclear cell infiltrate in the absence of chronic inflammatory cells or significant glandular alteration. In amoebiasis the amoebae can be demonstrated by the periodic-acid Schiff stain, taking care to look at the mucosal surface and any amorphous debris on the slide.

Dysentery

The solitary ulcer syndrome (Chapter 3) shows typical histological features, some resembling ischaemia but including telangiectasia of superficial capillaries, and muscle fibres from the muscularis mucosae extending upwards from their usual position to lie between the dilated crypts in the lamina propria.

Solitary ulcer syndrome

The pathology of Crohn's disease and ulcerative colitis is described later in this chapter.

REFERENCE AND FURTHER READING

Morson BC and Dawson IMP. *Gastrointestinal pathology 2nd ed.* Oxford: Blackwell, 1979.

SPECIFIC INFECTIVE CONDITIONS – including diseases of the tropics

Although reported incidence rates are often strikingly different, most diseases of the large intestine which are common in the western world also exist in the developing countries. Ulcerative colitis is uncommon in tropical Africa, and Crohn's disease is rare; colonic and rectal carcinoma are unusual in most developing countries. Although altered bowel function associated with blood in the stool in an African or Arab undergoing investigations in the West will probably be associated with bacillary or amoebic dysentery or schistosomiasis, other lesions such as ulcerative colitis and colonic carcinoma must also be considered in the differential diagnosis. Tuberculosis of the ileocaecal region, which (like most other forms of the disease) is now unusual in white patients in the West, is still a major problem in third-world countries and must be seriously considered in Africans and Asians undergoing investigation.

The reverse situation is however equally, if not more, important; western patients, especially those who have travelled in tropical areas at some stage in their lives, must be adequately investigated for amoebiasis, giardiasis and other forms of parasitic or infective colitis before a confident diagnosis of non-specific inflammatory bowel disease is made. A number of cases of amoebic colitis have been misdiagnosed as ulcerative colitis in England; treatment consisted of colectomy and/or corticosteroids with resultant death of the patients. A course of metronidazole would doubtless have resulted in permanent cure.

Instead of classifying diseases under the headings of causative organisms this account will first outline the major diseases – the dysenteries, schistosomiasis and intestinal tuberculosis – and then the diseases of lesser practical importance which involve the caecum, colon and anorectal region.

AMOEBIC DYSENTERY (AMOEBIASIS)

Although common in all parts of the tropics, numerous cases of amoebiasis are on record in Westerners who have never left their own country.

The disease is caused by the protozoon *Entamoeba histolytica*, which, in its cystic stage, infects man via the gastro-intestinal tract in food or drink (usually water). Enzymes in the gastro-intestinal tract destroy the cyst-wall and the trophozoites released invade the large intestinal tissues, producing colonies in the intestinal wall and subsequently ulceration.

Initially, lysis of the epithelium produces superficial erosions. Extension then occurs to the submucosa, forming deeper lesions. Although there is virtually no leucocyte response and little oedema, secondary bacterial infection rapidly occurs with associated bacteria such as *Escherichia coli* and other Enterobacteria which play an important role in the survival of the trophozoites. Rarely, extreme and rapid invasion may produce severe haemorrhage from the large intestine.

Entry of the trophozoites into the portal vein radicles leads to liver lesions (see below). Some trophozoites pass to the rectum, cyst formation takes place and the life-cycle of the parasite is completed by defaecation and further infection of man. The cysts are destroyed by drying and are rapidly killed at 55°C, but will survive for as long as a month at 10°C.

Clinical features and management

Intestinal amoebiasis may result in severe, often bloody, diarrhoea, which can alternate with normal bowel function or even constipation, or may be entirely asymptomatic (cyst-carriers). Men are affected more often than women.

In acute amoebic dysentery, the incubation period may be as short as eight to ten days and in about 50% of patients the onset is sudden. Headache, nausea, chills, fever and colic may accompany the diarrhoea but between bouts the patient may be entirely free of symptoms. Without treatment chronic dysentery can result, associated with intermittent attacks of fever and bloody diarrhoea which cause progressive scarring and deformity of the colon. Amoebic appendicitis and amoeboma are other sequelae; rectal amoebomata may closely mimic carcinoma as irregular friable tissue masses.

The commonest clinical type, however, is the cyst-carrier, only a minority of whom experience symptoms. A carrier may either have acquired an infection but not have suffered the active disease or may be convalescent from an acute attack and continue to excrete cysts in the stools.

Diagnosis depends on finding amoebae (either cysts or trophozoites) in pus or stool specimens, pus being preferable. The specimen must be fresh and warm since it is impossible to detect the motile trophozoites after more than a few minutes; it should also be cultured if facilities are available. If the stools are formed, only cysts are likely to be found.

Proctosigmoidoscopic examination and biopsy of the mucosa are also important in diagnosis, but less so than fresh stool microscopy.

The white blood count may show a mild or moderate polymorphonuclear leucocytosis. Serology is of value in the invasive stage; it is more likely to be positive if there is hepatic involvement. The fluorescent antibody-titre (FAT) remains positive long after successful treatment and is of no value in assessing a cure.

Treatment has been revolutionised by the discovery that metronidazole (Flagyl) is an effective and safe antiamoebic agent. An acute attack of amoebic dysentery will respond to 800 mg given three times daily for five days. Mild side effects such as nausea and lethargy are common. The patient should be warned that the drug may cause unpleasant interreactions with alcohol. Tinidazole (2 g daily for 3 days) is an alternative agent.

In a particularly severe attack of dysentery (e.g. in a child, a debilitated adult, or a patient on immunosuppressive therapy) the metronidazole regime can be combined with tetracycline (250 mg orally six-hourly) for ten days together with a course of diloxanide furoate (Furamide). For the cyst-carrier state, diloxanide furoate is given alone (500 mg three times daily for ten days).

Older therapeutic regimes involving emetine hydrochloride combined with chloroquine and other anti-amoebic agents are now rarely used.

Hepatic amoebiasis is the commonest extra-intestinal complication. In most cases intestinal symptoms are not present and presentation is with a large tender liver in a sick patient. Pyrexia is usual but jaundice uncommon. The right diaphragm is usually raised and signs are often present in the right lower lung. Serological tests for invasive amoebiasis are usually strongly positive and a leucocytosis and raised serum alkaline phosphatase are likely. Liver scan and ultrasound will frequently demonstrate any abscess formation.

Treatment of hepatic amoebiasis also requires metronidazole or tinidazole, or alternatively one of the older regimes including emetine, chloroquine and tetracycline. If the abscess is large and the patient severely ill, needle aspiration is indicated; small abscesses will resolve with drug treatment alone. A space-occupying defect on the liver scan often persists for many months after successful treatment.

BACILLARY DYSENTERY (SHIGELLOSIS)

Bacillary dysentery is caused by organisms of the Shigella genus, confined to the intestinal tract and excreted in high concentration in the faeces but causing complications by absorption of toxin. Human carriers constitute the main reservoir of infection. The disease is highly contagious and is spread by food handlers and contaminated objects including bed-linen; the organism is readily destroyed by direct sunlight. There are many species of the causative organism. Those of major importance are: *Shigella dysenteriae (shigae), Sh. flexneri, Sh. boydii* and *Sh. sonnei. Sh. shigae* produces a powerful exotoxin and is usually responsible for the most severe disease; *Sh. sonnei* produces a mild disease and is often seen in temperate climates.

The disease affects the whole colon, especially the distal portion, but the ileum can also be involved. The organisms after being swallowed multiply in the colon with great speed, where they largely take the place of the normal bacterial flora. A rapidly developing hyperaemia of the mucosa is followed by oedema and haemorrhage. Infiltration with leucocytes and macrophages extends down to the submucosa. Necrosis and desquamation of the epithelium with formation of a 'membrane' are followed by the appearance of ulcers – a few millimeters in diameter – which may extend deeply into the muscularis mucosae. In fatal cases there is extensive necrosis of the intestine.

Clinical features and management

The incubation period is from one to seven days; usually one or two days. It is followed by an abrupt onset of fever (up to 40°C) and tachycardia. Within 24 hours, diarrhoea and colic follow: the stools (often 20 or more in 24 hours) are watery and contain blood and mucus; later pieces of necrotic mucosa and pus may be passed. Vomiting may occur with tenderness, mimicking an acute abdomen. If the diarrhoea is severe, dehydration and vascular collapse dominate the picture and can lead eventually to renal and circulatory failure. Untreated, the condition is usually self-limiting after a period lasting up to 3 weeks, but occasionally a chronic state results, associated with severe emaciation and postinfective malabsorption. There can be a high mortality rate, especially in children.

Local complications are perforation, which is unusual, and haemorrhage. Prolapsed haemorrhoids sometimes prove troublesome. Portal pyaemia with multiple liver abscesses occur rarely. Inflammatory lesions of the eyes (conjuctivitis and iridocyclitis), joints (polyarthopathy) and peripheral nerves may complicate an otherwise straightforward attack. Reiter's syndrome (non-specific urethritis, conjunctivitis and arthritis) is an occasional sequel. In severe shigellosis circulating endotoxin from the colon can produce a coagulopathy, thrombocytopenia, renal micro-angiopathy and haemolytic anaemia (haemolytic–uraemic syndrome). Convulsions may occur in children.

Diagnosis is assisted by finding a contact history; the disease is often epidemic. Proctoscopy or sigmoidoscopy shows a diffusely reddened mucosa, usually with a purulent and bloody exudate. Stool microscopy shows a polymorphonuclear leucocytosis with red blood cells and macrophages. Diagnosis is dependent on isolation of the causative shigella from the stools and several fresh stool specimens or rectal swabs should be examined for the organism and its sensitivities determined. Shigellae survive for only a short time in faeces. Serology is of very limited value in diagnosis.

Treatment of an attack includes: replacement of fluid loss, which may be considerable, symptomatic treatment and eradication of the infecting organism.

Fluid replacement can frequently be accomplished orally with dilute normal saline (saline diluted ×4) mixed with fruit juice, with added potassium chloride (2 g four-hourly). Alternatively, an oral solution such as that used in cholera may be given:

glucose	20.0 g
sodium chloride	3.5 g
sodium bicarbonate	2.5 g
potassium chloride	1.5 g
made up to 1 litre with water	

It is virtually impossible by the oral route to overload the circulation in an otherwise fit person. When vomiting is severe, intravenous therapy is often necessary, and especially in children fluid replacement by that route is sometimes of great urgency.

Symptomatic treatment such as propantheline bromide (Pro-Banthine) or diphenoxylate (Lomotil) may be of value.

In most cases specific treatment should be reserved until a clear diagnosis has been made. Indiscriminate use of antibiotics can be responsible for resistant strains of Shigellae and in a case of average severity caused by *Sh. Sonnei* specific treatment is not required. In a severely ill patient on the other hand, treatment may have to be started before bacteriological proof of diagnosis, the regime being changed if necessary when the antibiotic sensitivities become available. For many years, sulphonamides have been the main standby; they are still of great value, especially in the developing countries where their low cost is a great advantage. Their main risk is due to crystalluria in a dehydrated patient, especially in a hot climate. However, non-absorbable compounds – e.g. sulphaguanidine (3 g four-hourly for 5–7 days) and phthalylsulphathiazole (2 g four-hourly for 5–7 days) are relatively safe. Mixtures of sulphonamides (e.g. sulphadiazine, sulphathiazole and sulphamerazine), some of which are absorbed, are advocated by some physicians on the basis that an attack on bacteria via the blood-stream, in addition to that via the lumen of the intestinal tract, produces a more rapid cure. Antibiotics may be used as an alternative especially where there is sulphonamide resistance. Oral tetracycline (500 mg four times daily for 5–7 days), streptomycin (2 g daily for 5–7 days), ampicillin or chloramphenicol (500 mg four times daily for 5 days) are also effective. Neomycin, and combinations of antibiotics and sulphonamides are also of value.

Prophylaxis depends on prevention of faecal contamination of food, water and bed linen, avoidance of foodstuffs likely to be contaminated, and sterilisation of water. Flies are a source of much infection.

Fig. 7.2

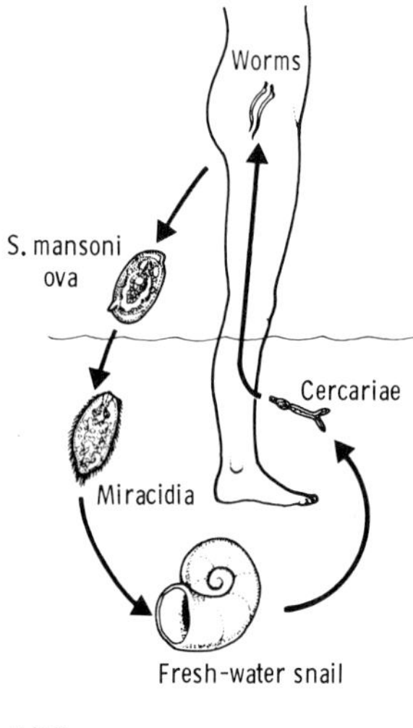

SCHISTOSOMIASIS

Three species of schistosomes (blood–flukes) commonly produce intestinal disease: *Schistosoma mansoni, S. intercalatum* and *S. japonicum*, although other species occasionally affect man. The various species can be distinguished by their characteristic ova.

Schistosomiasis affects many millions of people in the tropics – especially in Africa. The world incidence is at present increasing, because the habitat of the intermediate host – various species of fresh water snail – is increasing as new dams and irrigation schemes are constructed.

Man acquires infection (Fig. 7.2) when fresh water containing cercariae comes into contact with his skin. Whenever he is exposed, even briefly, by paddling, swimming, fishing, sailing etc., in contaminated water there is danger of infection. The cercariae penetrate intact skin and reach the liver via the circulation; from there they enter the portal system and develop into adult worms which can live there for up to 20 years. The females, after fertilisation, migrate to the terminal tributaries of the portal venous system against the blood flow; eggs are deposited, extruded into the intestine and excreted in the faeces. If the ova reach fresh water, a larva (miracidium) emerges and swims around until a suitable species of snail is found. Within the snail the life cycle is completed with the production and liberation of many new cercariae.

Intestinal schistosomiasis (S. mansoni and S. intercalatum)

Africa, the Middle-east, South America and the Caribbean are the main areas affected. Lesions develop in the walls of the large intestine, granulomatous reactions giving rise to ulceration, bleeding polyps and fibrosis; carcinomatous change is rare. Embolisation of ova to the liver gives rise to periportal fibrosis and eventually portal hypertension results with an enlarged spleen, ascites and bleeding oesophageal varices. Ova sometimes embolise to the lungs causing pulmonary hypertension; or to the spinal cord and occasionally to the brain, giving rise to space-occupying lesions.

Clinically the disease may begin with a short-lived local erythematous reaction of the skin following penetration by the cercariae. After 4–6 weeks a general allergic reaction occurs (with fever, malaise, muscle pains and urticaria accompanied by an eosinophilia) and lasts for several weeks. After months or years, intestinal symptoms appear including diarrhoea with blood and mucus, and tenesmus. Exacerbations occur every few weeks and may resemble amoebic colitis. The colon becomes thickened and tender. The mucosal ulcers become secondarily infected and polyp formation and colonic fibrosis may occur. Hepatic involvement and portal hypertension appear late in the course of the disease. Pulmonary involvement is heralded by haemoptysis and signs of cor pulmonale. A spinal cord lesion may result, usually a transverse myelitis.

Far eastern schistosomiasis (S. japonicum)

South-eastern China and the Philippines are the main areas involved. As with *S. mansoni* infection, the disease is primarily an intestinal one. The superior as well as inferior mesenteric vein, and thus the small intestine and proximal colon, are involved; liver pathology and portal hypertension are similar to those in *S. mansoni* infection but pulmonary involvement is less common, and central nervous system involvement (mainly the brain) much more common.

Clinically the allergic phase (Katayama syndrome) occurring 2–3 weeks after infection, is severe and is followed more rapidly by symptoms of intestinal involvement than with *S. mansoni*. The clinical manifestations are more severe than with the other schistosomal infections.

Diagnosis and management

Diagnosis depends on finding ova in the stool: lateral-spine = *S. mansoni*; terminal spine = *S. intercalatum*; spine-less *S. japonicum*. Numerous stools may have to be examined before a positive diagnosis can be made. Sigmoidoscopy may show ulceration. Rectal biopsy and aspiration liver-biopsy are of great value in diagnosis. Barium enema shows an immobile colon with irregular constrictions. As liver involvement occurs, liver function tests, portal venography and liver scans will give additional information. Chest radiography, if pulmonary involvement is present, shows right ventricular hypertrophy, an increased pulmonary artery component to the cardiac outline, and mottling of the lung parenchyma.

In all forms of schistosomiasis serology is of value approximately 4 weeks after infection but is no substitute for finding the ova. Complement fixation, fluorescent antibody and precipitin techniques may be used; the antigens are prepared from adult schistosomes or from viable ova. Intradermal tests are also used in diagnosis although there are some false positive reactions. None of the reactions is group specific.

Treatment is most commonly with niridazole (Ambilhar) in a dose of 25 mg per kg daily for 7 days. The least successful results are in *S. japonicum* infections. Toxic effects occur in the presence of portosystemic anastomoses when the unmetabolised compound has a direct effect on cerebral metabolism resulting in confusion, hallucinations and convulsions. Niridazole is, therefore, contra-indicated in the presence of severe hepatocellular disease and known portal-systemic shunting and also in psychotic patients. Recently, oxamniquine (Vansil) (20 mg per kg daily for 5 days), and praziquantel (Biltricide) (single dose of 20–40 mg per kg) have proved successful, and furthermore have few side-effects. Hycanthone (Etrenol) given as a single intramuscular dose has given promising results; however, hepatocellular toxicity can be severe.

Assessment of cure in schistosomiasis is difficult; survival of a few adult worms can give rise to the recurrent output of ova. Continued absence of viable ova 3 months after treatment suggests cure. Dead ova in urine, stool or biopsies after treatment are of no pathological significance.

Treatment of liver disease and portal hypertension may require portocaval anastomosis and other measures for arresting bleeding from oesophageal varices. Urinary tract infection and carcinoma of the bladder are treated on their merits. Brain and spinal cord involvement may require surgery, and respiratory and cardiac complications need appropriate treatment.

TUBERCULOSIS

Throughout tropical countries, tuberculosis of the ileocaecal region is an important and under diagnosed cause of intestinal disease including malabsorption (Anand, 1956). Colonic or anal tuberculosis alone is very rare. It is probable that tuberculosis has contributed to many of the cases designated as tropical sprue since Sir Patrick Manson's description of sprue in 1880.

Tuberculosis should be suspected in all immigrants from Africa and Asia with symptoms suggesting malabsorption, even after several years residence in the United Kingdom and also in the indigenous people of tropical countries.

Clinical features and management

The clinical picture is of diarrhoea and weight loss, often with symptoms suggesting malabsorption. A low grade pyrexia and anaemia are common. Lymphadenopathy is sometimes present and a tender mass is occasionally felt in the right iliac fossa. Barium meal and follow-through or barium enema will often show multiple ileal strictures; there may also by shortening of the ascending colon and caecum with loss of the normal ileocaecal angle. Chest radiography is normal. Acid-fast bacilli are rarely identified in the stool. The diagnosis is difficult however and, in spite of colonoscopy, diagnostic laparotomy is frequently necessary. Treatment is with antituberculosis agents with resection of any caecal mass or ileal strictures (Logan, 1969).

OTHER INFECTIONS INVOLVING THE LARGE BOWEL

Yersinia enterocolitis

Yersinia enterocolitis is an infection caused by small gram-positive coccobacilli (*Yersinia enterocolitica*) which are common in birds, hares, pigs and dogs (Winblad, Niléhn and Sternby, 1966). The commonest presentation is with acute ileitis. Over the past two decades it has become clear that the disease is by no means uncommon in man and presents with acute disease in the ileocaecal region; the distal colon is rarely involved.

Pathologically the infection produces white nodules closely resembling tubercles in the ileocaecal region, with regional lymph node involvement. Serology is of value in diagnosis and has given positive results in patients with symptoms suggesting acute appendicitis. Treatment is with parenteral streptomycin or oral sulphonamides.

Balantidiasis

Balantidiasis is a relatively uncommon condition which produces a severe chronic form of dysentery. It is caused by a large ciliated protozoon (*Balantidium coli*) which is a common parasite of pigs, guinea-pigs and monkeys. It is seen mainly in areas where pigs are kept in poor hygienic surroundings.

The disease is contracted by swallowing the cysts of *Balantidium coli* which have the same life cycle as *E. histolytica*. The trophozoite can exist in the colon without symptoms for long periods but when invasion occurs irregularly rounded ulcers are produced; they tend to be larger than those in amoebic dysentery.

Clinically like amoebiasis, the condition may be asymptomatic but in most cases there is dysentery with blood and mucus in the stool. There may be tenderness over the caecum or colon. During attacks of diarrhoea the trophozoites are present in the stool but between attacks only the cysts of the organism are found. Extra-intestinal infection does not occur.

Treatment is with tetracycline or one of its derivatives (500 mg twice daily for 10 days). Ampicillin may also be used.

Trichuriasis

Trichuriasis is a common, world-wide infection due to *Trichuris trichiura* (the whipworm). The disease is acquired by ingestion of ova; the worms hatch out in the caecum and colon anchoring themselves to the mucosa.

Clinically the disease is usually asymptomatic and ova are discovered on routine stool examination. Heavy infections in children occasionally produce rectal bleeding and prolapse, and anaemia. A mild eosinophilia is occasionally found in the peripheral blood.

If it is decided to attempt eradication of the organism, mebendazole (100 mg three times daily for three days) should be given.

Trypanosomiasis

South American Trypanosomiasis (Chagas' disease) is an infection caused by *Trypanosoma cruzi* which is transmitted to man in the faeces of a reduviid bug in which it has a cycle of development (Fig. 2.8). Dogs, cats, and many wild animals (including the armadillo and opossum) can harbour the infection and act as reservoirs.

The importance of the infection in the colon is that in the chronic state Auerbach's plexus is destroyed with resulting dilatation (megacolon) of the colon (Chapter 2).

Diagnosis is largely based on a geographical history. Exposure in a rural area of South America or Southern USA and West Indies is a prerequisite for diagnosis. There may be a history of an acute illness (acute Chagas' disease) in the past, especially in infancy and childhood.

Trypanosomes are present in low concentration in the peripheral blood. The complement-fixation test is of very limited value in diagnosis in chronic cases. No effective treatment is available. Prophylaxis is of paramount importance.

Oxyuriasis

Oxyuriasis, caused by *Enterobius vermicularis,* otherwise known as the threadworm or pinworm, is a very common infection especially in children and can involve whole families. Infection occurs when ova are ingested in contaminated food or drink, or from hands contaminated with faeces. Larvae are liberated in the upper small intestine and pass to the ileal region. The females migrate to the caecum or colon and as their ova develop they pass through the anus showering sticky eggs over the peri-anal skin.

Clinically there is intense pruritus ani resulting in scratching which leads to auto-infection. Loss of sleep and irritability are common. Local dermatitis, eczema, secondary bacterial infections and vulvovaginitis (with vaginal discharge) may be produced and the infection is a rare cause of appendicitis. There may be an eosinophilia.

Diagnosis is by identifying ova in peri-anal skin, in faeces or under the finger-nails. The ova can often be obtained for identification by placing a piece of transparent adhesive tape across the anus and then sticking it to a microscope slide. This may have to be repeated on several occasions.

Treatment is with piperazine (repeated after 2 g daily for 7 days) or mebendazole (200 mg as a single dose, repeated after one week). Children's nails should be cut short to prevent auto-infection. It is often advisable to treat all members of the family simultaneously.

Actinomycosis

Actinomycosis is an uncommon disease of the colon, the rectum being slightly more commonly involved. Induration without mucosal ulceration is seen and fistulae may occur. The disease should be considered if smooth submucous strictures of the rectum are seen. It seems likely that the organism is frequently a secondary invader following primary ulcerating lesions. Diagnosis is by biopsy when characteristic colonies of actinomyces can be identified. Treatment is with high doses of penicillin.

Giardiasis

The protozoon *Giardia lamblia* is a worldwide parasite, endemic in certain areas and an important cause of diarrhoea and abdominal symptoms to be considered in the differential diagnosis of inflammatory or functional bowel disease. Although the main site of infection is the duodenum and small intestine (often resulting in steatorrhoea and features resembling coeliac disease) there may be colonic involvement with reddened mucosa on proctosigmoidoscopy.

The organism may be seen on microscopy of diarrhoea stool but in some cases diagnosis will only be established (or excluded) by examination of duodenal aspirate, conveniently taken at the same time as a small intestinal biopsy. Treatment is with metronidazole (Flagyl) 2 g as a single dose each day for 3 days.

Campylobacter enterocolitis

Campylobacter enterocolitis results from infection with Campylobacters, tiny curved-rod bacteria, different from the classical cholera vibrios and related organisms. These are now recognised as a world-wide cause of a severe short-lived enterocolitis characterised by diarrhoea and abdominal pain, sometimes with other systemic features. Human and animal carriers occur and transmission is usually by food (particularly poultry) or water. The clinical picture is usually suggestive of an infective cause with a short period of fever and malaise followed by severe abdominal pain and then profuse diarrhoea. The small intestine is probably predominantly affected but there may be bleeding with sigmoidoscopic inflammatory changes, the rectal biopsy showing appearances of infective colitis.

Stool culture with selective media is simple. Treatment, when indicated, is with erythromycin 500 mg four times a day and is rapidly effective.

Pseudo-membranous colitis

Pseudomembranous colitis is the severest form of antibiotic induced diarrhoea and now shown to be due to *Clostridium difficile* toxin. It may follow the use of a wide range of antibiotics, especially clindamycin and lincomycin and less commonly ampicillin, tetracycline and others. The normal bacterial flora of the colon are disturbed and colstridial overgrowth occurs. The clinical picture ranges from simple diarrhoea to the severe forms of pseudomembranous colitis in which epithelial necrosis, usually visible sigmoidoscopically as characteristic white membranous plaques, may lead to colonic dilatation, systemic features or even death. Treatment is with vancomycin or possibly metronidazole, with supportive or resuscitatory measures as necessary.

Sexually transmitted diseases

Venereal infections involving the anorectal region, for example syphilis, gonorrhoea, lymphogranuloma venereum and granuloma inguinale (Donovanosis), occur commonly, especially in the tropics. They are discussed in Chapter 12.

REFERENCES AND FURTHER READING

Anand SS. Hypertrophic ileocaecal tuberculosis in India with a record of fifty hemicolectomies. *Annals of the Royal College of Surgeons* 1956; **19:** 205–22.

Cook GC. *Tropical gastroenterology*. Oxford: Oxford University Press, 1980

Editorial. Antibiotic associated colitis – a bacterial disease. *British Medical Journal* 1979; **2:** 349–50.

Hunter GW, Swartzwelder JC and Clyde DF. *Tropical Medicine*, 5th ed. Philadelphia: Saunders, 1976.

Logan V StCD. Anorectal tuberculosis. *Proceedings of the Royal Society of Medicine* 1969; **62:** 1227–30.

Vantrappen G, Agg HO, Ponette E, Geboes K and Bertrand P. Yersinia enteritis and enterocolitis: gastroenterological aspects. *Gastroenterology* 1977; **72:** 220–27.

Winblad S, Niléhn B and Sternby NH. *Yersinia enterocolitica* (pasteurella X) in human enteric infections. *British Medical Journal* 1966; **2:** 1363–6.

SPECIFIC NON-INFECTIVE CONDITIONS

RADIATION ENTEROCOLITIS

About 10% of patients receiving 5000 rads or more of abdominal or pelvic irradiation can be expected to develop gastro-intestinal symptoms. These may be due to damage to either small or large intestine, particularly if a loop is tethered by adhesions.

Acute symptoms after 1–2 weeks include diarrhoea, tenesmus etc., (resembling those of acute ulcerative colitis), or cramping small intestinal pains, and result from damage to the rapidly-dividing epithelial cells. Visible mucosal changes at this stage may be slight unless very large doses of irradiation have been used.

Delayed symptoms some weeks later may be similar or worse but are mainly due to the ischaemic effects resulting from damage to small vessels in the submucosa. The mucosa may be ulcerated or necrotic.

Late symptoms, six months or several years after the end of irradiation, result both from the continued thickening and obliteration of small vessels and from secondary ischaemic fibrosis. Ulcers, abscesses, fistulae or strictures may occur; the mucosa looks pale with telangiectases and bleeds easily.

There is no specific treatment, and although prostaglandin inhibitors (aspirin, indomethacin) may help in the acute stage, symptomatic management of the bowel disturbance and maintenance of iron stores is all that is usually possible. Corticosteroids are not proven to help. Surgery is avoided unless essential because of the poor healing and high complication rate of operating on the ischaemic bowel (Chapter 6).

OTHER SPECIFIC CONDITIONS

Other specific causes of inflammatory disease or mimicking conditions (referred to in Fig. 7.1 and described elsewhere) include irritable bowel syndrome, diverticular disease and cathartic colon (Chapter 2), ischaemic disorders (Chapter 9) and solitary ulcer syndrome (Chapter 3).

Eosinophilic gastro-enteritis is an uncommon condition of unknown aetiology which may affect any part of the gastro-intestinal tract. It presents with diarrhoea, abdominal pain or rectal bleeding. An eosinophilia is present both in biopsies and the peripheral blood (Johnstone and Morson, 1978). Steroid therapy is usually effective.

REFERENCES AND FURTHER READING

DeCosse JJ, Rhodes RS, Wertz WB, Reagan JW and Holden WD. The natural history and management of radiation induced injury of the gastro-intestinal tract. *Annals of Surgery* 1969; **170**: 369.

Duncan W and Nias AHW. *Clinical Radiobiology*. Edinburgh: Churchill Livingstone, 1977.

Johnstone JM and Morson BC. Eosinophilic gastro-enteritis. *Histopathology* 1978; **2**: 335–48.

PATHOLOGY OF NON-SPECIFIC INFLAMMATORY BOWEL DISEASE

The presence of significant small bowel disease or the finding of a giant-cell granuloma eliminates a diagnosis of ulcerative colitis; these are the only two absolute distinguishing pathological features between this condition and Crohn's disease. However, there is a small additional group of reliable, but not absolute criteria, and a host of lesser features that influence an opinion towards one or other disease (Morson and Dawson, 1979).

Ulcerative colitis (Fig. 7.3), unlike Crohn's disease (Fig. 7.4), is a mucosal disease that almost invariably involves the rectum, but then may spread proximally. There are morphologically recognisable periods of activity and remission, during which the extent of disease may increase and then decrease again as it becomes quiescent. Inflammation is limited to the mucosa except in acute and severe colitis. On gross inspection little may be visible from the serosal aspect of the bowel. The mucosa

Ulcerative colitis

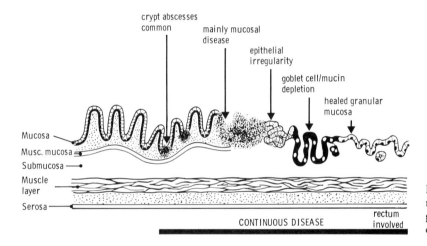

Fig. 7.3 Diagrammatic representation of histopathological changes in ulcerative colitis.

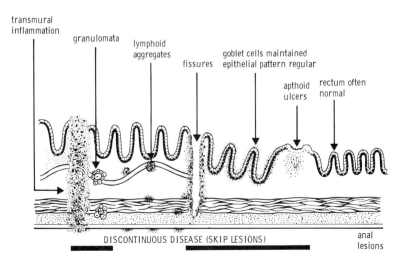

Fig. 7.4 Diagrammatic representation of histopathological chages in Crohn's disease.

201

most often appears congested and has a friable velvet-like texture. The degree of ulceration is variable. The left side of the colon is predominantly involved though improvement due to steroid enemas may produce an artificial sparing of this side of the bowel, and very rarely true rectal-sparing or right-sided disease may occur.

Microscopical examination in the active case shows a diffuse infiltrate of acute and chronic inflammatory cells limited to the mucosa. The glandular pattern is distorted, the goblet cell population depleted (mucin depletion) and crypt abscesses are numerous. As activity subsides the goblet cells return but the glandular pattern remains irregular often becoming atrophic – (widened spaces between and below the shortened glands). In remission the shortened disorganised glands are a diagnostic feature. In long-standing cases dysplasia of the epithelium may occur and can be graded as mild, moderate or severe. Severe dyplasia (precancer) is frequently associated with carcinoma somewhere in the colon, and when detected in rectal or colonoscopic biopsies, proctocolectomy has to be carefully considered (see below). Crohn's disease is also now accepted to carry a slightly increased risk of carcinoma but precancerous features have not been described.

Crohn's disease

Crohn's disease restricted to the colon occurs in some 20% of cases with another 60% having ileocolonic involvement. Generally the disease is right-sided but limited left-sided disease can occur, particularly in the elderly. In its classical form colonic Crohn's disease is a chronic discontinuous granulomatous condition with transmural aggregates of inflammatory cells and penetrating fissuring ulceration. The operative specimen shows a thickened bowel wall with an opaque serosa. Strictures and fistulae between bowel segments may be evident while large fleshy lymph nodes occur in the mesentery or pericolic fat. The mucosa is oedematous and characteristically traversed by linear serpiginous ulceration imparting an overall 'cobble-stone' appearance to the surface. Areas of non-involved bowel (skip-lesions) separate diseased segments although cases with diffuse disease are not rare. Inspection of normal-looking mucosa may show tiny 'aphthoid ulcers' which start as ulcerating lymphoid follicles and may be the initial lesion in the disease. Care should be taken to inspect the resected margins of an operative specimen for such changes. In proctocolectomies rectal sparing and anal disease are frequent features.

The key distinguishing attributes on microscopy are granulomas (aggregated foci of inflammatory cells) scattered throughout the bowel wall and like beads along the surface of the serosa, fissuring, ulceration and a regular glandular pattern with a maintained goblet cell population despite marked mucosal inflammation. Granulomas however are only found in some 60% of cases and fissures in 30%. Fibrosis in the submucosa is common and responsible for strictures but other features such as neural proliferation, pyloric gland metaplasia and a vasculitis are rare and less specific (Cook and Dixon, 1973). In contrast to Crohn's disease of the small bowel, colonic Crohn's disease rarely shows the full range of features.

Rectal biopsy is usually more helpful in ulcerative colitis than in Crohn's disease because there is no sampling error. The advent of multiple colonoscopic biopsies however, to some extent overcomes this drawback. The distinguishing criteria between the two diseases are much like those for the surgical specimens – granulomas, disproportionate inflammation in the submucosa, uneven mucosal inflammation with scanty crypt abscesses, and a preserved epithelial architecture favouring Crohn's disease; whereas goblet cell depletion, diffuse inflammation with prominent crypt abscesses, epithelial destruction, and degrees of glandular atrophy favour ulcerative colitis.

The place of biopsy

A normal rectal biopsy is strong evidence against a diagnosis of ulcerative colitis. Again it must be stressed that normal appearances on protoscopy or sigmoidoscopy do not necessarily imply normal histology. In Crohn's disease the chances of finding an abnormal biopsy increase the closer the diseased segment is to the anal canal, but even with disease restricted to the ileum diagnostic rectal biopsies are obtained in up to 12% of cases. Rectal biopsy can be used to monitor activity, treatment and the onset of dysplasia (precancer) in ulcerative colitis.

From colonoscopic biopsy one can now obtain an even more precise knowledge of the extent of involvement than that provided radiologically. In ulcerative colitis this improves the pick-up rate of mild total colitis and those with the greatest cancer risk. In Crohn's disease colonoscopic biopsy is particularly helpful in the milder cases with equivocal gross findings or doubtful recurrence. However, because of the small size of colonoscopic biopsies the incidence of granulomas is below that detected in most series of rectal biopsies.

Fulminating severe relapses happen in both ulcerative colitis and Crohn's disease, though more commonly in the former. Histopathological distinction between the two is most difficult in this phase and most of the unclassified cases in the literature fall into this category. In the severe phase the inflammation in ulcerative colitis becomes transmural, multiple groups of acute

Fulminating colitis

fissures may be seen and glandular irregularity with goblet cell depletion is less obvious. Thus the picture in fulminating ulcerative colitis presents a confusingly close resemblance to Crohn's disease and to interpret correctly it helps the pathologist to know the clinical state of the patient at the time of surgery. Occasionally the dilemma is not even settled after study of the operative specimen but has to await more characteristic follow-up biopsies taken subsequently from unresected bowel (Price, 1978).

REFERENCES AND FURTHER READING

Cook MG and Dixon MF. An analysis of the reliability of detection and diagnostic value of various pathological features in Crohn's disease and ulcerative colitis. *Gut* 1973; **14:** 255–61.

Morson BC and Dawson IMP. *Gastrointestinal pathology* 2nd ed. Oxford: Blackwell, 1979.

Price AB. Overlap in the spectrum of non-specific inflammatory bowel disease – colitis indeterminate. *Journal of Clinical Pathology* 1978; **31:** 567–77.

Price AB and Morson BC. Inflammatory bowel disease – the surgical pathology of Crohn's disease and ulcerative colitis. *Human Pathology* 1975; **6:** 7–29.

EPIDEMIOLOGY OF NON-SPECIFIC INFLAMMATORY BOWEL DISEASE

Non-specific inflammatory bowel disease has now been reported from most countries and many races. There have always been difficulties in differential diagnosis from endemic diseases in tropical and subtropical areas. It seems probable that the highest incidence is found in temperate climates and in Caucasian races with the population of Europe, Australasia and North America being most affected.

Epidemiological studies of inflammatory bowel disease aim to define the pattern of these diseases in a community but there are special difficulties over and above those of most other epidemiological work. Both ulcerative colitis and Crohn's disease are uncommon; diagnosis and differential diagnosis may not be easy. Rarity results in these studies dealing with small numbers and conclusions may then be based on disturbingly few patients.

Diagnosis and differential diagnosis rely on clinical, radiological and histological criteria which vary between studies; the extent to which histology is used will depend on the availability of biopsy material and the surgical composition of the series. Reasons for exclusion of cases are rarely given.

There is no uniform approach in dealing with clinical variants. A transient idiopathic proctitis unsubstantiated by histology leads to difficulties. Epidemiological studies of Crohn's disease may include or exclude patients with a clinical diagnosis of acute ileitis. The question of inclusion or exclusion of asymptomatic patients with Crohn's disease or surgically-treated patients with ulcerative colitis in prevalence data remains undecided and frequently unmentioned.

Many studies are incomplete through failing to include outpatients, patients under the care of private practitioners, or all age groups. There is wide variation in the definition of residential qualifications.

All these difficulties are augmented by the retrospective nature of much of the published work. Prospective studies using internationally-agreed criteria of inclusion are needed before substantial further progress can be made in this subject.

Incidence

Epidemiological studies are confined mainly to Europe and the United States of America. Annual incidence rates are defined as the number of new cases diagnosed (occasionally symptomatic onset is used) per 10^5 population per year and are set out in Tables 7a and 7b. Ulcerative colitis appears to be

Table 7a. *Ulcerative colitis: average annual incidence rates per 10^5 population*

Location	Rate	Years of study
Oxford	6.5	1951–60
Malmo	6.4	1958–70
Uppsala	6.0	1955–64
Copenhagen	7.3	1961–66
Tel Aviv	3.7	1961–70
⋆ Baltimore	4.6	1960–63
† Rochester	9.7	1935–64
Norway	3.3	1964–69

⋆ Hospital admission rates, whites only, 20 years and older.
† Includes patients with a transient proctitis.

Table 7b. *Crohn's disease: average annual incidence rates per 10^5 population*

Location	Rate	Years of study
Copenhagen	1.3	1960–70
Northern Ireland	1.3	1966–73
Gloucester	1.5	1966–70
Basle	1.6	1960–69
Aberdeen	2.2	1955–68
Uppsala	3.3	1956–73
Malmo	4.8	1958–73
★ Baltimore	1.8	1960–63
Norway	1.1	1964–69

★ Hospital admission rates, whites only, 20 years and older.

about two to three times more common than Crohn's disease.

There is little evidence to show that ulcerative colitis is increasing whereas most studies from Great Britain and Europe show a rising incidence of Crohn's disease. More recent awareness of the disease and its delineation from ulcerative colitis are generally considered to be insufficient to account for this increase. Two series (Kyle, 1971; Bergman and Kranse, 1975) show this rise to be due to more women developing the disease.

Age distribution

All authors agree that both diseases are most commonly diagnosed in patients in the age groups from 15 to 40 years. The actual peak incidence varies with the series and the way the material is subdivided. Most workers have found a secondary incidence peak in later years.

Sex

Ulcerative colitis is more common in men in about half the published series; figures from the Hospital In-Patient Enquiry show that more women than men are discharged with this diagnosis in England and Wales.

Crohn's disease has been found to have a higher incidence in women in over half of the epidemiological series, significantly so against the background population in one series.

Jewish population

North American series based on selected populations or specialised groups suggest that both diseases have a higher incidence among Jewish people. One epidemiological study in ulcerative colitis (Evans and Acheson, 1965) and one in Crohn's disease (Brahme, Lindstrom and Wenckert, 1975) also arrive at this conclusion, but the relatively low incidence and prevalence figures in an entirely Jewish population in the Tel Aviv study of ulcerative colitis (Gilat, Ribak, Benaroya *et al.*, 1974) should be noted.

Prevalence

An estimate of the number of affected persons in a community is usually assessed as a point prevalence rate, i.e. the number with the disease per 10^5 population at risk at a given date, usually the end-point of the study. The figures from some of the main studies are shown in Tables 7c and 7d.

Table 7c. *Prevalence rates per 10^5 population at a given date – ulcerative colitis*

Study	Rate	Year
Oxford (Evans)	79.9	1960
Malmo (Brahme)	89.0	1968
Copenhagen (Bonnevie)	44.1	1967
Tel Aviv (Gilat)	37.4	1970

Table 7d. *Prevalence rates per 10^5 population at a given date – Crohn's disease*

Study	Rate	Year
Aberdeen (Kyle)	32.5	1969
Nottingham (Miller)	26.5	1971
Uppsala (Bergman)	50.0	1973
Malmo (Brahme)	75.2	1973

Mortality

Annual mortality rates for ulcerative colitis from various countries are in the range 0.4–0.7 per 10^5 population. Recent figures for Crohn's disease are 0.15 and 0.14 per 10^5 population.

In England and Wales in 1975 ulcerative colitis was the stated cause of death in 327 patients and Crohn's disease in 233.

In ulcerative colitis, the highest mortality is found in the acute attack usually after surgical treatment: in Crohn's disease the mortality tends to occur late in the illness after multiple resections.

REFERENCES AND FURTHER READING

Bergman L and Krause U. The incidence of Crohn's disease in Central Sweden. *Scandinavian Journal of Gastroenterology* 1975; **10**: 725–9.

Bonnevie O, Riis P and Anthonisen P. An epidemiological study of ulcerative colitis in Copenhagen County. *Scandinavian Journal of Gastroenterology* 1968; **3**: 432–8.

Brahme F, Lindstrom C and Wenckert A. Crohn's disease in a defined population. *Gastroenterology* 1975; **69:** 342–51.

Evans JG and Acheson ED. An epidemiological study of ulcerative colitis and regional enteritis in the Oxford area. *Gut* 1965; **6:** 311–24.

Gilat T, Ribak J, Benaroya Y, Zemishlany Z and Weissman I. Ulcerative colitis in the Jewish population of Tel-Aviv Jafo. I Epidemiology. *Gastroenterology* 1974; **66:** 335–42.

Humphreys WG and Parks TG. Crohn's disease in Northern Ireland – a retrospective survey of 159 cases. *Irish Journal of Medical Science* 1975; **144:** 437–46.

Kyle J. An epidemiological study of Crohn's disease in Northeast Scotland. *Gastroenterology* 1971; **61:** 826–33.

Miller DS, Keighley AC and Langman MJS. Changing patterns in epidemiology of Crohn's disease. *Lancet* 1974; **2:** 691–3.

AETIOLOGY OF NON-SPECIFIC INFLAMMATORY BOWEL DISEASE

Genetic factors

There is an increased incidence of inflammatory bowel disease among the close relatives of patients with ulcerative colitis and Crohn's disease; the fact that both disorders can occur in the same families suggests that there is a similar genetic predisposition. There is also evidence that ankylosing spondylitis can occur in the same families with or without inflammatory bowel disease. Tissue antigen type HLA W27 is found in most patients with colitis or Crohn's disease in association with ankylosing spondylitis but no tissue antigen is clearly associated with inflammatory bowel disease occurring alone.

It has been argued that the increased incidence of inflammatory bowel disease in some families is due to the similar childhood environment rather than to inherited factors; however, the rarity of either disorder in spouses and the occurrence of disease in different generations and widely separated branches of a family, makes this unlikely.

Immune mechanisms

Circulating humoral antibodies to an antigen present in colonic epithelial cells and certain bacteria can be demonstrated in the blood of some patients with inflammatory bowel disease. An antibody-dependent cytotoxicity against colonic epithelial

208

cells can be demonstrated in tissue culture. Normal lymphocytes become cytotoxic after incubation with the serum of a
patient with colitis; conversely the lymphocytes of a patient
with colitis lose their cytotoxic effect after colectomy.

The role of immune complexes in these reactions is uncertain. They can be demonstrated both in the circulation and
within the mucosa. It is possible that the complexes within the
lamina propria cause activation of the complement pathway
with attraction of leucocytes and local tissue damage.

A characteristic feature of Crohn's disease is the epithelioid
cell granuloma. It is known that epithelioid cells are derived
from macrophages. There is no evidence that macrophages
have a phagocytic function in the granuloma but they are
metabolically very active. The granuloma may develop either
because an unusual antigen is present which resists destruction,
or because the macrophages of a patient with Crohn's disease do
not have the normal ability to destroy antigens.

Sensitivity to one or more food antigens has been suggested
as a factor in inflammatory bowel disease. The frequency of
antibodies to milk proteins has been extensively studied but the
presence or absence of such antibodies, or their titre, does not
appear to be correlated with the duration or severity of the
disease. It is probable that the normal permeability of the intestinal wall to antigens from the lumen is increased when the
mucosa is inflamed. The presence of circulating antibodies to
food or bacterial antigens may thus be a secondary effect.

Microbiological aspects

The faecal or intraluminal bacterial flora in ulcerative colitis
or Crohn's disease shows no striking departure from normal.
Similarly, the intimate mucosal flora is similar to normal.

No specific pathogen has been isolated as a cause of inflammatory bowel disease. Animal transmission experiments
have suggested that a transmissible agent may be present
capable of passing a filter small enough to remove normal
bacteria. Viruses have been proposed as specific causes of both
ulcerative colitis and Crohn's disease but the evidence is conflicting. Similarly, cell wall deficient bacteria have been studied
as possible causes of Crohn's disease but reproducible results
have not been obtained.

If no specific organism can be isolated, the possibility remains
that the normal bacterial flora may play a role in pathogenesis of
ulcerative colitis, Crohn's disease or both. Cross-reactivity
between a bacterial antigen and a mucopolysaccharide present
in colonic epithelial cells led to the suggestion that a self-
perpetuating auto-immune mechanism could result from sensitivity to the bacterial antigen. Local mucosal antibodies to
anaerobic organisms can also be demonstrated. The fact that the

first attack of ulcerative colitis often seems to follow a bowel infection gives support to the idea that contact with bacterial antigens due to damage of the normal mucosal defence mechanisms, could play a role in colitis and Crohn's disease.

Environmental factors

The rarity of non-specific inflammatory bowel disease in Africa and the Far East, and the fact that the disorders are relatively common throughout the western world, suggests that an environment factor may be important. Controlled studies have shown that patients with Crohn's disease tended to eat more refined sugar and unrefined fruit and vegetables than matched control subjects before the onset of their illness. It is possible that diet plays an important role in the liability to inflammatory bowel disease perhaps by an effect on the intestinal bacterial flora.

DIAGNOSIS AND MANAGEMENT OF NON-SPECIFIC INFLAMMATORY BOWEL DISEASE

Two types of non-specific inflammatory bowel disease may be distinguished from each other and from infective, ischaemic or irradiation colitis. The absence of a single defining feature which in other disorders is usually related to aetiology, renders the classification of non-specific colitis difficult and that of the individual case sometimes impossible. Thus infective colitis can be recognised by the presence of the infecting organism, or by evidence of its past involvement by serological or other methods, but ulcerative colitis is recognisable only by a pattern of histopathological changes in the colon. A recognisable group of symptoms and signs making up the clinical picture of ulcerative colitis usually corresponds with the characteristic pathological changes. Crohn's disease can be similarly recognised in overall terms but it is important to realise that both these disorders are classified primarily on an anatomical basis; at present no laboratory test is helpful. Since there is no single defining feature present in all cases of one and absent in all cases of the other, overlap is bound to occur. In most cases the weight of evidence favours ulcerative colitis or Crohn's disease, but in some the balance of evidence is such that the disorder must be described as 'indeterminate'. It must also be recognised that further subdivision of non-specific inflammatory bowel disease may become possible in the future as new tests are developed. The interaction between one or more environmental factors and various inherited or constitutional factors may then become apparent.

CLINICAL DIFFERENTIATION BETWEEN ULCERATIVE COLITIS AND CROHN'S DISEASE

At present it is convenient to recognize a relatively homogeneous disorder, ulcerative colitis, and a more heterogeneous disorder, Crohn's disease. Broadly, these two differ in several important respects as shown in Table 7e.

Table 7e *Differentiation between ulcerative colitis and Crohn's disease.*

Ulcerative colitis	Crohn's disease
Idiopathic proctocolitis	Granulomatous enteritis or colitis
Confined to the large intestine	Affects all parts of the gut
Confined to the mucosa (except in very severe cases).	Affects all layers of the gut wall
Continuous	Discontinuous
Can be cured by surgical removal of the colon and rectum	May recur after excisional surgery

Anatomical site

As a consequence of the anatomical differences, discriminant clinical features result. Ulcerative colitis is mucosal and almost always involves the rectum with a variable proportion of the colon in continuity with the rectum. Rectal symptoms are therefore common, namely: urgent defaecation, frequent defaecation and rectal bleeding.

Crohn's disease shows a predilection for the terminal ileum and the anal region. Terminal ileal disease leads to: obstructive symptoms; a mass or tenderness in the right iliac fossa; fistulation. Anal Crohn's disease can be suspected by the finding of oedematous skin tags, a bluish-pink colouration of involved skin, ulceration of the anal canal or perianal skin, fissures, recurrent abscesses, complex fistulae and nodularity of the anorectal junction, sometimes with stenosis.

Type of ulceration In ulcerative colitis, despite its name, there may be no ulceration. When ulceration develops it is usually restricted to the mucosa or submucosa and is a late feature in a generally inflamed mucosal surface. Deeper ulceration with penetration into the external muscle layers is associated with loss of large areas of mucosa. Destruction of, and damage to, muscle may lead to dilatation of the colon with incipient perforation and reduced tensile strength of the bowel wall at operation.

Crohn's disease is sometimes associated with deep cleft-like fissuring ulcers. These ulcers may penetrate to the serosa with a tender, thickened, persistently painful segment of bowel; possibly localised perforation with a pericolic abscess; internal or external fistulae; or occasionally acute perforation. At an earlier stage the ulcers are small and superficial but set in a background of apparently normal mucosa.

Continuity or discontinuity The mucosal lesion of ulcerative colitis extends continuously from the anus to its proximal junction with normal mucosa, as judged by endoscopy or x-ray.

Table 7f. *Clinical differences between Ulcerative colitis and Crohn's Disease*

	Ulcerative colitis	Crohn's disease
Symptoms		
Bleeding	very common	sometimes
Abdominal pain	sometimes	common
Urgent defaecation	very common	sometimes
Abdomen		
Abdominal mass	rare	sometimes
Spontaneous fistulae	never	sometimes
Anal region		
Ulceration	rare	common
Infection	occurs	common and complex
Lesions preceding bowel symptoms	never	sometimes
Endoscopy		
Rectum involved	95%	50%
Appearance	uniform, continuous hyperaemia, granularity, friability	oedema, ulcers, normal patches
Prognosis		
Medicine	adequate in 80%	inadequate in 80%
Surgery	'cure' possible	liability to recurrence
Cancer risk	definite	slight

The discontinuity of Crohn's disease may be observed on endoscopy or x-ray as the presence of discrete ulceration or discrete areas of inflammation with normal intervening mucosa.

Fibrosis is not a feature of ulcerative colitis and fibrous strictures do not, therefore, occur, though smooth concentric narrowing of the colon may result from muscular thickening. In Crohn's disease, fibrosis is a feature and fibrotic strictures occur with possible obstructive symptoms.

Presence or absence of fibrosis

Ulcerative colitis is usually associated with epithelial damage and regeneration. Precancerous and cancerous change may occur. Such changes are very uncommon in Crohn's disease.

Nature of the epithelial change

These clinical differences between ulcerative colitis and Crohn's disease are summarised in Table 7f. Other radiological and pathological features are illustrated in Figures 1.34, 1.35, 7.3 and 7.4.

ASSOCIATED DISORDERS

Ulcerative colitis by causing severe diarrhoea may result in secondary anal problems such as acute fissures, excoriation and prolapse or thrombosis of haemorrhoids. Another more worrying complication is the increased incidence of carcinoma of the large intestine among patients who have had symptoms for ten or more years and inflammation affecting most or all of the large intestine (see below).

Local complications

Crohn's disease, by its nature, tends to involve adjacent structures. Thus the anorectal lesion of Crohn's disease may spread to involve the external genitalia or give rise to a rectovaginal fistula. Colonic Crohn's disease may involve the bladder (with a possible colovesical fistula), the fallopian tube, the ureter, or other intra-abdominal structures. A chronic retroperitoneal abscess may spread to the psoas sheath. Incision of a chronic abscess tends to lead to an enterocutaneous fistula as the abscess is caused by local perforation of diseased intestine.

All types of non-specific inflammatory bowel disease may be associated with changes in other systems of the body. Some of these manifestations tend to accompany exacerbations of inflammation in the gut, others tend to follow an apparently independent course – Tables 7g and 7h.

Systemic complications

Table 7g. *Transient disorders occuring at the same time as activity of the intestinal disorder*

Skin	Erythema nodosum or, less commonly, spreading areas of ulceration (pyoderma gangrenosum).
Mucous membranes	Aphthous ulceration of the mouth or vagina
Eyes	Iritis or episcleritis
Joints	An arthritis tending to affect large joints, and involving first one joint and then another

Table 7h. *Persistent or slowly progressive disorders without obvious relation to the activity of the intestinal disorder*

Joints	Sacro-iliitis or ankylosing spondylitis, sero-negative polyarthritis
Liver	Chronic active hepatitis, cirrhosis
Biliary system	Pericholangitis, sclerosing cholangitis, bile duct carcinoma
Renal	Amyloidosis (only in Crohn's disease)

DIETARY AND NUTRITIONAL TREATMENT

Diet as a specific treatment

Bowel rest

It has been suggested that removing food from the intestinal lumen may reduce inflammation. To achieve this, chemically defined (elemental) diets consisting of small peptides and/or amino acids, with oligosaccharides and/or glucose, sometimes medium-chain triglycerides, and minerals and vitamins, have been used on the assumption that all these nutrients are absorbed proximally and do not reach the distal intestine. Alternatively, food has been excluded from the gut entirely by the use of parenteral nutrition.

So far, no controlled data have been obtained showing that these treatments do reduce inflammation. Unless justified for their nutritional benefit, their use should be reserved for special circumstances when other treatments are inappropriate or unsuccessful.

Exclusion diets

A few patients with colitis are helped by a milk-free diet, though at present it is not clear whether this benefit is due to exclusion of milk-protein or lactose. All patients with inflammatory bowel disease should be asked if milk apparently upsets them: if so, a trial of milk exclusion is indicated. A lactase tolerance test will indicate if lactase deficiency is present; besides measuring blood glucose levels, a note should also be made as to whether or not diarrhoea occurs during the test. In other patients a period of milk exclusion may be worth a trial if other treatments fail, but if there is no apparent benefit milk should again be allowed freely. There is no evidence at present that exclusion of other foods is helpful.

The addition of fibre and restriction of refined carbohydrate have been recommended as a treatment because epidemiological studies suggest that colitis and Crohn's disease may be associated with a highly refined diet. There are no controlled data so far to justify such dietary modification as a routine treatment.

Alteration of dietary composition

Failure to eat enough, diminished absorption from the small intestine, losses by exudation from inflamed mucosa and the systemic effects of chronic inflammation combine to produce nutritional deficiencies and metabolic abnormalities in many patients. Every patient's nutritional state should be assessed in terms of weight, height and specific haematological and biochemical deficits. The weight of adults should be expressed as a proportion of the usual (or optimal) value. During childhood and adolescence, weight and height should be plotted sequentially on a percentile chart so that both can be expressed in terms of the normal range for the same age and sex and so that growth rates can be determined.

Diet and supplements for replacement and growth

The daily intake of calories and protein can be expressed quantitatively by dietary assessment. This simple measure often shows that the patient is taking less than the 30–35 kcal/kg body weight needed to maintain weight, with no extra to regain weight or grow while allowing for the effects of inflammation. Further enquiry will reveal whether the reduced food intake is due to the poor appetite of systemic illness, the nausea and sense of fullness of chronic obstruction, or a wish to reduce bolus colic and/or diarrhoea. An appropriate increase in food intake may be achieved by suitable dietary supplements combined with drug or surgical treatment.

Calories and protein

Iron is commonly needed to replace blood loss, though sometimes the apparent iron deficiency is due to the failure of utilization which occurs in chronic disease. Vitamin B_{12} is needed by all patients in whom 100 cm or more of distal ileum have been resected. Folic acid may be needed by patients with

Specific deficits

small intestinal Crohn's disease. Blood transfusion, protein infusion, mineral and vitamin supplements may be needed in severe disease.

Diet for relief of symptoms

Diarrhoea. The use of a low residue diet as a treatment for diarrhoea is traditional but is not usually helpful. Patients may be encouraged to take a normal diet omitting any specific foods which appear to upset them. Certain patients with lactase deficiency are helped by milk exclusion (see above). Patients with severe malabsorption of fat due to small intestinal disease or resection benefit from a low fat diet.

Pain. Bolus colic due to the presence of strictures may be relieved by a simple low-residue diet, with small frequent meals, omitting such foods as nuts, mushrooms, fibrous fruit and vegetables, and meat containing lumps of gristle.

DRUG THERAPY

Drugs are used in inflammatory bowel disease for their anti-inflammatory effect, perhaps by an effect on chemical mediators of inflammation or on immune responses, for their antibacterial action and for their symptomatic effect on pain or diarrhoea.

Anti-inflammatory drugs

Corticosteroids

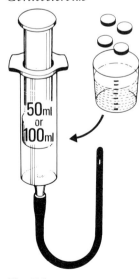

Corticosteroids have been shown by controlled trial to have a therapeutic effect in active ulcerative colitis and Crohn's disease. The most severely ill patients with acute colitis are treated with an intravenous infusion of prednisolone (60 mg daily) to ensure adequate tissue levels. Less severely ill patients with widespread inflammation of the intestine, or with systemic illness are given prednisolone by mouth, usually starting with a dose of 40–60 mg daily. Topical preparations may be used when inflammation is limited to the distal colon and rectum. The logic for use of topical treatment is that a high concentration of the drug comes into contact with the diseased mucosa but that systemic absorption is too small to cause side effects. Suitable vehicles are a suppository (for treatment of the rectum only), a retention enema of variable volume or a foam (for more proximal but limited disease). Retention enemas can be the commercially available disposable plastic-bag enemas (100 ml volume) or alternatively they may be made up by the patient using a dose of water-soluble corticosteroid tablets (prednisolone–21-phosphate, 10–40 mg or betamethasone phosphate,

Fig. 7.5

2–4 mg) and a volume of tap water (50–200 ml), both adjusted according to the extent and severity of the colitis and administered with bladder syringe and catheter (Fig. 7.5).

Sulphasalazine (Salazopyrin), a combination of sulphapyridine and 5-aminosalicylic acid, is poorly absorbed by the small intestine and split by bacteria to liberate the two constituents in the colon. Present evidence suggests that 5-aminosalicylic acid may be the active moiety, perhaps by depressing prostaglandin synthesis. Sulphasalazine has been shown to reduce inflammation in active ulcerative colitis and Crohn's disease affecting the distal small bowel and colon. Given over a prolonged period, it also reduces the relapse rate in ulcerative colitis. The drug can cause dyspepsia, nausea, malaise, skin rash and occasional haemolysis or a blood dyscrasia. For these reasons, a proportion of patients cannot take it or can take it only in a smaller dose than usual; nausea or dyspepsia may be avoided with the enteric-coated preparation.

Sulphasalazine

Azathioprine and 6-mercaptopurine are closely related chemically; they have an anti-inflammatory effect and also depress immune responses. Both drugs have been shown to reduce chronic inflammation, enable a maintenance corticosteroid dose to be reduced, and prolong remission in Crohn's disease. There is some evidence that azathioprine has similar effects in chronic ulcerative colitis. Both drugs can cause depression of the bone marrow, skin rash, febrile reactions and acute pancreatitis. The risks of treatment must, therefore, be weighed against the possible benefit. Regular blood counts are advisable to detect bone marrow depression, though this is unusual in the doses used for inflammatory bowel disease (2 mg/kg body weight).

Azathioprine and 6-mercaptopurine

Disodium cromoglycate has been reported to give benefit in some cases of ulcerative colitis but results are conflicting. Transfer factor, BCG, and levamisole have been tested without demonstrable benefit in Crohn's disease.

Other drugs affecting the immune response

There is no evidence at present that antibacterial drugs are useful for the treatment of ulcerative colitis. A wide range of antibacterial drugs seem to benefit some patients with Crohn's disease, perhaps by affecting secondary infection of the gut wall and surrounding tissues. Metronidazole is widely used for its particular effect on anaerobic bacteria.

Antibacterial drugs

217

Symptomatic treatments

Loperamide, codeine phosphate or diphenoxylate decrease stool frequency and water and electrolyte losses. The drugs are most useful in patients with an ileostomy or after ileorectal anastomosis. In colitis, these drugs rarely do good and can do harm; furthermore, it must be remembered that they only treat the symptom of diarrhoea and not the inflammation which causes it. If the proximal colon is normal, hard constipated stool may accumulate proximal to the diseased left colon and treatment with stool-softening or bulking agents may be necessary.

Cholestyramine may reduce diarrhoea after ileal resection when bile salts are not absorbed normally and so reach the colon.

Anticholinergic or other antispasmodic drugs are only useful in rare patients with co-existing irritable bowel syndrome; they may increase the likelihood of colonic dilatation in acute colitis.

SURGICAL TREATMENT

Indications

The indications for surgical treatment may be:

development of a dangerous acute complication, e.g. perforation, dilatation, severe haemorrhage

development of a chronic or sub-acute complication, especially in Crohn's disease, e.g. abscess, fistula, obstruction

failure of a severe acute attack of colitis to respond to drug therapy

chronic disability or ill-health, including growth retardation in young patients

rarely, the risk or development of a carcinoma, particularly in ulcerative colitis

Principles of surgical treatment

Definitive surgical treatment relies for its success on the removal of all or most of the inflamed intestine. Other procedures, such as drainage of an intra-abdominal abscess, are usually preliminary to a resection later. Anal lesions in Crohn's disease frequently require local surgical treatment.

The following types of abdominal operation may be undertaken:

Diversion procedures

Diversion procedures such as intestinal by-pass, with or without exclusion of the diseased segment, have been widely used, particularly in the treatment of Crohn's disease. However, inflammation tends to persist and even progress distal to the diversion. Even if inflammation subsides it tends to recur once continuity is restored unless the affected intestine is resected. Such procedures without resections are therefore usually reserved for occasional emergency use in a very ill patient when resection appears unsafe and time must be gained to improve the patient's general condition before definitive surgery.

Right hemicolectomy is the standard procedure for ileocaecal Crohn's disease; it is unsuccessful in right sided ulcerative colitis and inflammation generally recurs in the remaining distal colon. In Crohn's disease inflammation recurs, usually just proximal to the anastomosis, in about half the patients within ten years of operation.

Colectomy with ileorectal anastomosis when performed, for ulcerative colitis is essentially a compromise; since the rectum is usually inflamed, patients may still experience the symptoms of proctitis after operation, particularly urgency of defaecation and rectal bleeding, though their general health is restored by removal of the major part of the disease. The liquid or semisolid effluent from the ileum usually leads to the passage of 3–6 stools daily. The operation has much to commend it in young people when avoidance of a stoma is more important than complete relief from all symptoms.

There is a risk of carcinoma in the retained rectum and regular indefinite follow-up by sigmoidoscopy and mucosal biopsy is indicated. The operation should not be undertaken unless the patient realises the likely symptomatic limitations, the need for follow-up and the possible need for an ileostomy later.

This operation is undertaken in Crohn's disease when the distal colon and rectum are normal. It may also be performed, with the limitations described above, when the rectum is involved but the anus is normal or near-normal. Recurrence of inflammation either in the distal ileum and/or in the rectum occurs in about half the patients; even so, the symptoms may often be controlled by medical means and many patients with recurrent disease are still pleased with the results of the operation.

Proctocolectomy with ileostomy eliminates all inflamed intestine in ulcerative colitis and has proved to be a satisfactory treatment. Complications can arise from the ileostomy and some fastidious patients find the stoma difficult to accept. Considerable surgical ingenuity has been devoted to modifying the stoma so as to make it more acceptable. The ileal pouch with a continent nipple valve can be very successful but the high complication rate and the frequent need for more than one operation to achieve a satisfactory result limit its use. Recently an ileal pouch placed within the rectal stump denuded of

Resection with anastomosis

Excision of rectum with stoma

219

mucosa and opening at the anus has been devised but experience of this procedure is at present limited (Chapter 4).

Proctocolectomy and ileostomy is also used in Crohn's disease. Such patients may develop recurrent inflammation at the ileostomy or proximal to it. However, the results of the operation are usually very successful though delayed healing of the perineal wound is a problem in some patients. The risk of ileal recurrent disease is a contra-indication to the construction of an ileal pouch in Crohn's disease.

Excision of the rectum with colostomy can be very successful for anorectal Crohn's disease. The operation is sometimes performed for distal ulcerative colitis but the risk of inflammation in the proximal colon is so high that proctocolectomy with ileostomy is preferable.

Whenever the rectum is excised in inflammatory bowel disease the dissection should keep as close to the rectum and anal canal as possible. The fat behind the rectum is therefore preserved and the anal canal dissected in the intersphincteric space. The advantages of this are the small size of the pelvic wound and the lack of damage to the pelvic nerves responsible for bladder and sexual function.

INFLAMMATORY BOWEL DISEASE IN CHILDHOOD AND ADOLESCENCE

The major risk of inflammatory bowel disease in young people is retardation of growth and sexual development due to chronic inflammation, aggravated by decreased food intake and sometimes by corticosteroid therapy. Great emphasis should be placed on adequate nutritional treatment. Corticosteroid treatment should be used in such a way, for example by the use of single doses in the morning on alternate days, that side-effects are minimised. Retardation of development despite energetic medical treatment is an indication for surgical treatment after which there is often a period of rapid growth, though normal stature may never be achieved.

Children usually tolerate the illness and its treatment, including if necessary a stoma, very well. Their parents often become very anxious about the chronic nature of the disorder, the problems of drug treatment and the possibility of operation. Time and trouble are needed to gain their confidence.

INFLAMMATORY BOWEL DISEASE AND PREGNANCY

Fertility may be reduced in women who have undergone abdominal surgery or in whom Crohn's disease has led to inflammation in the region of the fallopian tubes. Reduced fertility among men taking sulphasalazine has been reported.

During pregnancy there does not appear to be an increased frequency of relapse of colitis, or worsening of active disease, but the danger of colitis to mother and fetus appears to be greater than the risks of treatment. Thus, although it is desirable to avoid drug treatment, particularly during the first trimester, no harm is usually seen from the use of sulphasalazine, topical corticosteroids and, if necessary, systemic corticosteroids.

Delivery is usually uneventful and women with an ileostomy often have a normal delivery unless previous perineal scarring makes Caesarian section advisable. There does appear to be an increased risk of a relapse of colitis during the puerperium.

THE CANCER RISK

Nearly all patients with colitis have heard of the cancer risk but keep the fear to themselves. It is encouraging for patients with distal colitis to hear that this is a needless worry, their risk of large bowel cancer is little, if at all, greater than a person without colitis. Positive reassurance can, therefore, be given to them and no special follow-up arrangements are needed unless the colitis becomes more extensive.

Patients who do have a greater risk than normal of developing cancer are the relatively small group with colitis involving most or all of the colon and a history of symptoms dating back ten or more years. The increased risk persists in the rectum if it is retained after surgical treatment.

Some clinicians advise all such patients to accept procto-colectomy to prevent cancer once the duration of symptoms exceeds ten years. Many patients are well and find this advice difficult to accept. Furthermore, the absolute number of cases of cancer arising in colitis is small.

Patients with extensive colitis or a retained rectum require meticulous follow-up.

Follow-up studies suggest that the individual risk is about 1 in 200 for each year between ten and twenty years, and thereafter 1 in 60 per year. These figures suggest that it is reasonable to keep patients under close observation, particularly as it is possible to detect dysplastic (precancerous) changes by mucosal biopsy.

Such dysplastic changes tend to be patchy and may be present in the colon but not the rectum. Regular colonoscopy, at perhaps two-yearly intervals, after the history exceeds ten years is, therefore, advisable so that multiple biopsies can be taken from different parts of the colon. Sigmoidoscopy and rectal biopsy is also worthwhile at 6–12 month intervals as almost half the cancers in colitis occur within reach of the sigmoidoscope.

Patients with precancerous changes (severe dysplasia) on repeated biopsies are advised to undergo colectomy; almost half of them will be found to have a small focus of carcinoma undectectable by colonoscopy or barium enema. With this follow-up policy surgical treatment is, therefore, restricted to those with a very high risk of carcinoma; any carcinoma present is usually small and the prognosis after colectomy is excellent. Precancer is an uncommon reason for colectomy, most operations for colitis are performed during an acute attack or because of chronic disability.

Statistically, there is an increased risk of carcinoma in Crohn's disease. Adenocarcinoma may occur in the terminal ileum after disease has been present for many years and occasionally in colonic Crohn's disease. In practice, the risk does not seem to be great enough to justify operation, though with increased length of medical follow-up the risk may in the future be found great enough to influence decisions about management.

CLINICAL MANAGEMENT OF ULCERATIVE COLITIS

The severity of ulcerative colitis varies greatly from patient to patient and from time-to-time in the same patient; the reason for the intermittent nature of the disease is not understood. Treatment varies according to the activity of the mucosal inflammation and its extent.

The *activity of the colitis* may be assessed clinically by the symptoms, physical signs, endoscopic appearance of the mucosa, by x-ray and by the evidence of laboratory investigations of acute inflammation and metabolic depletion. Symptoms of activity include anorectal bleeding, diarrhoea, abdominal pain (usually just preceding defaecation), malaise, anorexia and associated manifestations such as mouth ulcers, a red eye, erythema nodosum or acute arthritis. There may be weight loss, fever and abdominal tenderness. Endoscopically, active inflammation is shown by bleeding on lightly touching the mucosa (friability or contact bleeding) or spontaneous bleeding, and uncommonly by visible ulceration. On a plain abdominal x-ray the area of active disease is associated with an empty colon and perhaps an irregular outline between the luminal gas shadow and surrounding soft tissues. Barium enema may show a granular or ulcerated mucosa. A raised erythrocyte sedimentation rate, C-reactive protein or other acute phase reactants, with a low haemoglobin, total serum protein and albumin suggest active disease.

The *extent of the colitis* varies from involvement of the rectum only (proctitis) to involvement of any proportion of the colon proximal to, and in continuity with the rectum. The severity of an attack of colitis depends greatly on the extent of the disease. Patients with proctitis or proctosigmoiditis tend to pass solid stools, as well as liquid blood, mucus and pus, because the proximal colon absorbs water normally. Distal colitis is rarely associated with systemic disturbances and the patient does not feel ill.

Assessment of severity on clinical and radiological grounds is of paramount importance and will determine whether out-patient management is safe or admission indicated and also the most logical approach to treatment. Commonsense and repeated review of the patient's state is indicated; some cases need clinical reassessment every few hours with daily radiographs and blood tests, whereas others can be managed at home.

A patient with extensive colitis in the acute phase tends to pass only liquid stools and to show evidence of systemic disease. The extent can often be estimated with reasonable accuracy from the empty colon on a plain abdominal x-ray but if the patient is fit enough an unprepared barium enema (instant enema) gives more exact information.
The depth of ulceration determines the risk of colonic dilatation and perforation. Destruction of the mucosa with involvement of the underlying muscle correlates with dilatation of the colon and an irregular mucosal outline on plain abdominal x-ray.

Systemic features such as loss of appetite, weight loss, malaise, fever, rapid pulse rate, and/or severe abdominal tenderness, falling haemoglobin and low serum albumin are all evidence of a severe attack of colitis. The presence of one or more of these features should be taken seriously.

Acute colitis

The indications for immediate surgical treatment without preliminary drug therapy in very severe colitis are perforation or dilatation of the colon (the normal upper limit of the transverse colon is 5.5 cm) with an irregular mucosal outline (mucosal islands).

Very severe colitis requiring immediate colectomy

In such patients preliminary treatment is limited to fluid, electrolyte, blood and protein replacement. The operation performed is subtotal colectomy with ileostomy, the upper end of the rectum is brought out through the lower end of the wound as a mucous fistula (Fig. 4.15). Due to the destruction of muscle and possible adhesion of the surface to neighbouring structures as a result of full-thickness inflammation, there is an increased risk of rupture of the colon during operation. Spillage of liquid colonic contents may be averted, and the colon may become easier to handle, if an adequate incision has been made and liquid contents are emptied via a wide-bore tube introduced by an assistant through the anus and guided by the operator into the colon (the lithotomy–Trendelenburg position facilitates this manoeuvre). The risk of infection of the abdominal cavity or wound is high and the operation should be covered by anti-bacterial drugs active against aerobes (gentamicin) and anaerobes (metronidazole).

Severe colitis requiring potent drug therapy and collaboration between physician and surgeon

These patients with severe colitis have profuse fluid diarrhoea and usually evidence of systemic disturbance, but no dilatation of the colon on plain abdominal x-ray. Vigorous medical therapy includes replacement of losses (water, electrolyte, protein and blood) and a corticosteroid, such as prednisolone 60 mg daily, given by intravenous infusion. Sulphasalazine may be given if it does not cause or increase nausea. There is no evidence to support the use of antibiotics.

The indication for urgent surgical treatment is failure to respond to a regime of this type as judged by such features as:

persistent fever and/or tachycardia
persistent anorexia and malaise
severe abdominal tenderness
appearance of dilatation on repeated plain abdominal x-ray
falling body weight, haemoglobin or serum albumin

The timing of operation varies according to the clinical condition of the patient. If there is no improvement a decision is usually reached within a week of admission to hospital. If there is partial or transitory improvement decision may be delayed for 1–3 weeks. Since the postoperative mortality in elderly patients is particularly high, early, rather than late surgical treatment should be the rule for those over 60 years.

Moderately severe colitis usually responsive to drug therapy

Many patients are seen who have some systemic upset and troublesome diarrhoea, but who are not severely ill. Such patients usually respond to replacement therapy and a corticosteroid given by mouth, such as prednisolone 40 mg daily. Once general improvement has begun sulphasalazine should be introduced and corticosteroid retention enemas should be started when diarrhoea improves and the patient is able to retain them. The dose of oral corticosteroid should be progressively reduced and stopped over 1–3 months, treatment with corticosteroid retention enemas should then be continued until inflammation has settled. Sulphasalazine should be continued on a long-term basis (see below).

Mild distal colitis usually results in frequent soft stools rather than fluid diarrhoea but bleeding may be a feature; the patients feel well. They rarely need surgical treatment and most can be treated as outpatients without restriction of activities. The mainstays of treatment are sulphasalazine, often given for a prolonged period, and topical corticosteroid preparations given as necessary to control recurrent active inflammation. Commercially available 100 ml corticosteroid enemas are usually effective but the volume can be adjusted and steroid dosage increased if necessary by using a solution made up with water-soluble prednisolone tablets and administered using a 50 ml syringe and blunt-tipped tube (Fig. 7.5).

Mild distal colitis

Proctitis causes bleeding in the presence of formed or even constipated stool. Corticosteroid suppositories or aerosol foam are usually effective and sulphasalazine is not always required. A few unresponsive patients may benefit from arsenical suppositories (acetarsol BP 250 mg–Macarthys).

Proctitis

Chronic persistent colitis

A socially unacceptable illness is far more difficult to bear than one for which there is general sympathy; colitis induces a sense of isolation because the symptoms are socially taboo. One of the main disabilities is urgency of defaecation and a resulting fear of incontinence. The call to stool is often immediate, unexpected and insistent; incontinence cannot be avoided if a lavatory is inaccessible and is a source of great embarrassment. Patients, therefore, tend to find work at which there is ready access to a lavatory, they plan their journeys in relation to public toilets; they dread enclosed situations such as a car journey, bus ride or a supermarket. For this reason patients can become housebound, suitable work may be hard to find, social life may be sacrificed and activities for the whole family may be restricted. Add to this bowel frequency at night, a sense of constant tiredness, the embarrassment and fear of offensive stools containing blood, and it becomes evident why colitis can be such a social disability.

It is important to question patients with chronic symptoms about these aspects of the illness because they are reluctant to talk about details which they regard as shameful. A picture may emerge which shows that the current medical treatment is ineffective. Many of the symptoms are due to rectal inflammation. Prolonged topical corticosteroid therapy may greatly relieve the symptoms even though the colitis is extensive. Azathioprine appears to reduce chronic inflammation in some patients but must be used with care.

If medical treatment fails to enable the patients to lead a

reasonably normal life then surgical treatment should be considered even though the disease may be limited to the distal colon. When considering the advisability of colectomy with an ileorectal anastomosis it must be remembered that many of the symptoms arise from the diseased rectum and this operation may not relieve the disabling symptoms for which it is performed.

Colitis in remission

Consider the prognosis

A patient who has recovered from an acute attack of colitis is not cured, he is liable to further attacks. Severe acute colitis is a dangerous illness and the postoperative mortality after urgent colectomy undertaken because of failed medical treatment is rarely less than 10%. The mortality of elective colectomy, on the other hand, is low. It may therefore be advisable to recommend surgical treatment during a phase of remission for a few patients who have suffered recurrent severe attacks of colitis.

Reduce the risk of relapse

For most patients the aim is to reduce the relapse rate. Patients should be advised to avoid holidays in areas where bowel infections are specially common and to be particularly careful about the sources of food and water when travelling. Antibiotics by mouth should be avoided unless essential. In some patients relapses appear to be brought on by stressful situations and it is here that supportive pyschotherapy may help. In a few patients milk elimination may reduce the relapse rate.

The only drug known to reduce the relapse rate is sulphasalazine, usually given in a dose of 2 g daily. It seems wise to advise those patients who can tolerate the drug to continue it for about a year after the last attack, though a beneficial effect can be demonstrated over several years; prolonged treatment seems justified in patients with previously severe extensive or recurrent attacks.

Prepare for relapse

Patients need to know that a recurrence of symptoms is common and what to do if this happens. Having a reserve supply of drugs at home, for example a topical corticosteroid preparation and extra sulphasalazine, enables treatment to be started early and gives the patient confidence. The patient's doctor should be advised about appropriate treatment for a relapse. Special arrangements should be available for urgent outpatient appointments at hospital for patients with acute colitis.

The need for regular supervision of a small group of patients with extensive colitis has already been discussed.

The cancer risk

CLINICAL MANAGEMENT OF CROHN'S DISEASE

It is difficult to generalise about the treatment of Crohn's disease because of the variety of possible sites and structural complications of the disorder. In many patients active phases of disease appear to alternate with quiescent phases. Acute exacerbations may be due to activation of the primary disease, secondary infection of ulcerated areas with perhaps oedema, cellulitis or abscess formation, or a mechanical complication such as obstruction. Some of these situations are illustrated below (Fig. 7.6).

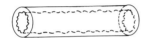

Mucosal inflammation and ulceration

(ANTI-INFLAMMATORY DRUGS ?SURGERY)

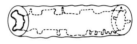

Full-thickness inflammation involving serosa and surrounding tissues

(ANTI-INFLAMMATORY, ANTI-BACTERIAL DRUGS ?SURGERY)

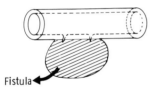

Fistula

Fissuring and ulceration leading to abscess or fistula formation

(SURGERY)

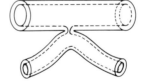

Fissuring and ulceration leading to internal fistula

(USUALLY SURGERY)

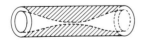

Fibrosis and thickening of intestinal wall leading to obstruction

(DRUGS — TEMPORARY RELIEF SURGERY)

Tags, ulceration, fistula and abscess

(ANTI-INFLAMMATORY AGENTS LOCALLY AND SYSTEMICALLY SURGERY)

Fig. 7.6 The problems of Crohn's disease (and their management).

Mucosal ulceration and inflammation may be helped by drug therapy, usually sulphasalazine and/or corticosteroids, with perhaps long-term azathioprine. Inflammation of the intestinal wall, perhaps involving the serosa and surrounding tissue, may respond to these drugs and also antibacterial drugs. A temporary obstructive episode may be relieved by drug therapy, presumably due to reduction in oedema and swelling of the gut wall, though surgical treatment is generally needed later. Abscesses usually need surgical drainage but since a chronic perforation is often the cause, an external enterocutaneous fistula commonly results. Such fistulae rarely close spontaneously or with bowel rest; resection of the underlying intestinal disease is required. Spontaneous internal fistulae between the diseased intestine and another viscus, usually another loop of intestine or the bladder, often need surgical treatment but occasionally close with medical treatment and sometimes cause so few symptoms that treatment is not needed.

Extensive small bowel disease

There may be extensive mucosal inflammation or multiple short segments of disease, often causing multiple strictures. Some patients remain well and symptom-free without drug treatment, despite severe radiological changes. Other patients with pain, malabsorption, or severe protein loss respond well to corticosteroids, perhaps with a low residue or low fat diet. Azathioprine may be needed to enable remission to be maintained and the corticosteroid dose to be reduced or stopped. Sulphasalazine is not usually effective; a short course of antibacterial drugs may apparently benefit acute exacerbations.

Surgical treatment is generally limited to resection, or bypass of short segments which cause obstruction. Occasionally extensive resection is needed with a jejunocolic anastomosis or jejunostomy. Fluid and electrolyte losses can then become a major problem, with losses of 2–3 litres of fluid daily containing about 100 mmol of sodium per litre. The intake of water and sodium can be increased by adding the maximum tolerable amount of salt to food and by drinking an electrolyte mixture containing glucose. Losses can be decreased by a strict low fat diet combined with codeine phosphate, loperamide and/or diphenoxylate in full doses and sometimes in combination.

Exceptionally, the remaining healthy intestine after a major resection is inadequate to maintain nutrition and fluid balance. In such patients parenteral nutrition, self administered as a long-term treatment at home, offers the only chance of health. Some of these patients find it better to take little or nothing by mouth, others use parenteral nutrition as a supplement to a reduced oral intake.

Terminal ileal and ileocolic disease

Patients with this, the commonest form of Crohn's disease, tend to develop obstructive symptoms or abscess formation. Drug treatment may defer, but does not usually avoid, the need for operation. Sulphasalazine and antibacterial drugs may be helpful. Corticosteroids should be limited to short courses.

Surgical treatment is usually needed and resection with anastomosis is possible in most cases. Postoperative bowel frequency is minimised if as much as possible of the right colon is conserved. Operation is often followed by long or apparently permanent relief of symptoms, particularly if the diseased segment is short. Unfortunately, no long-term drug treatment after resection has yet been found which reduces the recurrence rate.

Colonic disease

Acute attacks of this form of colitis behave and respond similarly to acute attacks of ulcerative colitis. In addition to the use of sulphasalazine and corticosteroids as already described for ulcerative colitis, antibacterial drugs and azathioprine may be useful. Some patients with Crohn's colitis appear to benefit from low-dose corticosteroids or from a very gradual dose reduction over several months, in contrast to the short courses usually advised in ulcerative colitis.

Surgical treatment, usually subtotal colectomy with ileostomy and mucous fistula, may be needed for acute disease with complications or acute attacks unresponsive to medical treatment. Protocolectomy or colectomy with ileorectal anastomosis may be needed for chronic disease.

Anorectal disease

Although severe lesions may cause gross structural changes, symptoms can be slight. Abscesses require surgical drainage and fistulae are best treated by a conservative surgical approach limited to the provision of free drainage and designed to conserve continence. Complex lesions may heal or become symptomless if the intestinal disease becomes quiescent. Antibacterial drugs, including metronidazole, can benefit acute infective episodes.

In some patients, the anal lesions are so severe that excision of the rectum is required. Provided that the inflammation is limited to the rectum and anus, the results from rectal excision with the formation of a left iliac colostomy are good.

Residual or recurrent disease after surgical treatment

Recurrent disease at an anastomosis or stoma may be treated medically with some success. Further surgical treatment may be needed for obstruction, pain or general ill-health. The risk of recurrent disease after a second or later resection appears to remain constant, so that about half the patients will develop further inflammation during the ten years after each successive operation.

Large unhealed anal or perineal wounds, sometimes associated with ulceration in the groins and natal cleft, may remain after anal operations or rectal excision. Usually these wounds heal slowly but not always completely, with meticulous nursing care. Topical steroid applications, such as betamethasone valerate cream, systemic corticosteroids and/or azathioprine sometimes seem to promote healing when no progress is made with frequent irrigations and surgical toilet.

REFERENCES AND FURTHER READING

Goligher JC. *Surgery of the anus, rectum and colon.* London: Ballierè Tindall, 1980.

Lennard-Jones JE and Powell-Tuck J. Drug treatment of inflammatory bowel disease. *Clinics in Gastroenterology* 1979; **8:** 187–217.

Lennard-Jones JE, Morson BC, Ritchie JK, Shove DC and Williams CB. Cancer in colitis: assessment of the individual risk by clinical and histological criteria. *Gastroenterology* 1977; **73:** 1280–9.

Ritchie JK. Results of surgery for inflammatory bowel disease: a further survey of one hospital region. *British Medical Journal* 1974; **1:** 264–8.

Watts JM and Hughes ESR. Ulcerative colitis and Crohn's disease: results after colectomy and ileorectal anastomosis. *British Journal of Surgery* 1977; **64:** 77–83.

8. Neoplasms

INTRODUCTION

Carcinoma of the large bowel is one of the commonest malignant tumours. In the United Kingdom, there are about 15 000 deaths a year from this disease and only carcinoma of the bronchus is more common. The incidence of colon cancer has risen steadily in the United States of America during the last 30 years where it is now the commonest solid tumour besides tumours of the skin. There is a slight preponderance of females affected by carcinoma of the colon; the reverse is true for carcinoma of the rectum.

The association between adenomas and carcinomas has been recognised for many years, and there is now much evidence indicating that many, if not most, carcinomas arise within a pre-existing adenoma. It is clear that genetic factors are important in the development of both these lesions but environmental influences also appear to play a major part. Epidemiological studies in the last 20 years have linked the incidence of large bowel cancer with cultural habits rather than with race or physical environment. There is some evidence both from epidemiology and experimental cancer models that high fat and low residue diets may predispose to the development of the disease. Other conditions of the large bowel, for example, inflammatory disorders of various types (ulcerative colitis, schistosomiasis) may also be predisposing factors. Little is known of the cellular events at the stage of transformation of normal colonic epithelial cells, but recent reports of altered mucin production by carcinomas and disturbances of the DNA regulation of colonic epithelium in familial adenomatous polyposis demonstrate that there are differences in cellular behaviour of large bowel neoplasms.

For many years the management of colon cancer has been by surgical resection. This is still the case today, but the results in terms of five year survival are no different now from what they were in the late 1940s. Many patients presenting for the first time have advanced disease and the average delay between onset of symptoms and diagnosis is of the order of one year. It is to be hoped that awareness among the public of suggestive symptoms will increase and that screening of the general population or selected subgroups may detect tumours at an earlier stage in the natural history; it will require large controlled trials to show whether this can be achieved or not. In the next few years the question may be answered as the incidence and types of cancer in screened compared to unscreened control populations become known.

AETIOLOGY

Interest in the causation of large bowel cancer has increased rapidly since the mid-1960s and there is considerable work in progress. The outline given here represents the consensus of opinion. Although there is very strong evidence for the adenoma-carcinoma sequence and it would be logical to study the aetiology of the precursor adenomatous lesion, this has proved difficult and most work has concentrated on the direct causation of carcinomas.

CARCINOMA

Epidemiology

Large bowel cancer is common in North-west Europe, North America and Australasia and is relatively rare in Africa, Asia and most of South America. Immigrants to the United States from low-risk areas such as Japan acquire, within a generation, the same risk as the host population. This indicates that environmental rather than genetic factors must be of overwhelming importance. The different racial populations of South Africa have grossly different incidences of the disease, as do the various religious sects in India and racial groups in Singapore. In these situations the groups compared all share the same physical environment (e.g. climate, air pollution) indicating that cultural factors are the key determinants.

Most epidemiologists have concluded that dietary agents are the major cause; there is, however, considerable disagreement on the component or components of the diet responsible. So far, meat, fish, animal protein, refined carbohydrate, dietary fibre deficiency, vitamins A and C, long chain polyunsaturated fatty acids and beer have all been suggested. Obviously fat and animal protein are highly correlated to each other; most epidemiological studies implicate either these foods or a low intake of fibre in the diet. Thus, although the incidence of large bowel cancer in South America is low, it is high in Argentina where meat consumption is high. Conversely, Seventh Day Adventists in the United States of America who adhere to a vegetarian diet have a low incidence. The epidemiological evidence for fibre deficiency is much less clear and by no means consistent.

Two mechanisms by which dietary factors could lead to large bowel cancer have been proposed. Both involve the gut bacterial flora, which is not surprising since the 1.5 kg of bacteria in the normal gut might be assumed to play some role.

The first mechanism requires the production by the gut bacteria of a carcinogen from some dietary component. The amount of carcinogen produced would depend on the amount of dietary component available, and the ability of the flora to produce the carcinogenic metabolite; as the colonic contents progressively dehydrate, the concentration of the carcinogen would increase. This would explain the higher frequency of carcinomas in the distal colon and rectum. The transit time is immaterial to this mechanism, since the concentration of the metabolite is the all-important factor.

There is some evidence to support this hypothesis. Studies in rats have shown that a high animal fat diet increases the numbers of experimentally-induced large bowel tumours compared to a low animal fat diet. There is also some indication that the faecal bile salt and cholesterol content is raised in patients with large bowel cancer. Hill, Drasar, Williams and their colleagues in 1975 have proposed that increased ingestion of cholesterol in the diet leads to increased bile acid output which by bacterial metabolism in the colon is turned into carcinogens or cocarcinogens.

With the second mechanism the production of carcinogens by the bacteria is again assumed, the risk of the disease depending on the rate of transit of the gut contents along the large bowel. The amount of carcinogen would be of secondary importance, the key factor being the opportunity for carcinogen and target to interact. Thus, with low dietary fibre content, transit time would be long and exposure to carcinogen greater. Tumour distribution along the large bowel would result from local stasis distally.

Both these mechanisms are tenable scientifically and are not mutually exclusive. At present the epidemiological data suggest the former to be the more important.

Genetic factors

There is an increased incidence of large bowel cancer in the close relatives of patients affected with the disease, cancer occuring in 15% of siblings and 10% of the children of index cases. These associations by no means exclude the environmental factors, however, and information on spouses is awaited.

Other predisposing factors

Inflammatory bowel disease

The incidence of large bowel cancer in ulcerative colitis is many times greater than normal. The underlying causative factors are unknown, but histopathological changes of severe dysplasia can be demonstrated in the mucosa of most patients with colitis who develop carcinoma. The risk increases with the duration of the disease, being insignificant up to ten years, 2 to 3% between 10 and 20 years and around 10% between 20 and 30 years. These rates apply to patients with extensive colonic involvement; in those with left colonic or distal colitis the risk is very low. Patients treated by colectomy with ileorectal anastomosis are also at risk of developing cancer in the rectal remnant; the incidence is 6% over a period of about 20 years.

In the last ten years it has become clear that Crohn's disease also predisposes to cancer (usually of the small intestine); although rare, the incidence is about 20 times the normal expectation. Chronic infection of the large bowel, for example amoebiasis and schistosomiasis, is also thought to be associated with large bowel cancer.

There is an increased incidence of cancer of the rectum in patients with radiation proctitis, over 50 cases having been reported, but large bowel cancer has not occurred more frequently then normal in people exposed to irradiation in atomic bomb explosions.

Immunological factors

Patients with advanced large bowel cancer often have poor cellular immunity and low lymphocyte counts in the peripheral blood. The presence of these deficiencies is associated with a poor prognosis compared to those who do not have them. There is also evidence that *in vitro* immunoreactivity (judged by lymphoblast–lymphocyte transformation and inhibition of leukocyte migration tests) is also depressed in these patients. Some have correlated these features with the stage of the disease. It may be, however, that these phenomena are the result of the malignant process and not involved with its cause. At the present time, the part played by immunology in the aetiology of large bowel cancer is unknown.

Large bowel cancer is associated with other malignant tumours. Thus, there is an increased incidence in patients with breast, ovarian and prostatic cancer. The reverse also applies; a patient presenting initially with a large bowel neoplasm is at greater risk of developing the others.

Tumours at other sites

Patients who have had a ureterosigmoidostomy may develop carcinoma at the site of the anastomosis. This is colonic in type and occurs after a period of about 20–30 years.

Ureterocolic anastomosis

ADENOMAS

The scanty evidence available suggests both a genetic and an environmental component in the aetiology of adenomas. It has been suggested that the genetic factor is a recessive gene (Veale, 1965) present in the same proportion of persons in low- and high-risk countries, the actual incidence of adenomas being determined by the environmental factor.

Putting the various theories together, the suggested aetiology of colorectal carcinoma involves a recessive genetic factor and an environmental factor to produce the precursor adenoma, with a further factor produced by gut bacteria to cause the development of malignancy in the adenoma. The actual incidence of adenomas and carcinomas is thought to be determined by the environmental factors, the genetic factor determining which persons within the population carry the tumours.

REFERENCES AND FURTHER READING

Hill MJ, Drasar BS, Williams REO, Meade TW, Cox AG, Simpson JEP and Morson BC. Faecal bile acids and clostridia in patients with cancer of the large bowel. *Lancet* 1975; **1**: 535–8.

Veale AMO. Intestinal polyposis. In: *Eugenics laboratory memoirs. Vol. 40*, London: Cambridge University Press, 1965.

Wynder EL, Reddy BS, McCoy GD, Weisburger JH and Williams GM. *Clinics in Gastroenterology* 1976; **5**: 463–82.

PATHOLOGY

Tumours of the large bowel are classified by their pathology. The majority are epithelial, those derived from connective or lymphoid tissue accounting for less than 1%. Tumours may

235

be benign or malignant, benign tumours being divided into neoplastic and non-neoplastic. Errors in diagnosis by the histopathologist may have serious consequences and it is important to have uniformity of nomenclature. The classification adopted here is that accepted by the World Health Organization (Morson, 1976).

BENIGN TUMOURS AND POLYPS OF THE COLON AND RECTUM

The classification of benign tumours and polyps is shown in Table 8a. Many of these lesions are polypoid, a polyp being the

Table 8a. *Classification of polyps of the large intestine*

Class	Varieties
Inflammatory	Inflammatory polyp
	Benign lymphoid polyp
Metaplastic (Hyperplastic)	
Heterotopic	Endometriosis
Hamartomatous	Peutz-Jeghers polyp
	Juvenile (mucus retention) polyp
Neoplastic	Adenoma – tubular
	– tubulovillous (papillary)
	– villous
	Adenocarcinoma
	Carcinoid tumour

clinical description of any elevated tumour. The term covers a variety of histologically different tumours and is not synonymous with a pedunculated adenoma. All types of polyps may occur as solitary lesions, synchronously in small numbers or as part of a polyposis syndrome. In established familial adenomatous polyposis more than 100 adenomas are present; adults with fewer than this number are not considered to have the condition (Bussey, 1975). Only the adenoma has any significant malignant potential and in the case of familial adenomatous polyposis cancer will inevitably develop; from a clinical point of view, therefore, the single most important distinction is between an adenoma and all other types of polyp.

Inflammatory polyps

Inflammatory polyps may occur after severe ulceration in any inflammatory process in the large bowel, typically in such conditions as long-standing ulcerative colitis, colonic Crohn's disease and schistosomiasis.

236

The polyps may arise as a result of undermining ulceration which partly elevates an area of mucosa, forming redundant tags of mucosa, often numerous, worm-like and up to several centimetres in length. The stroma contains much inflammatory granulation tissue and distorted tubules lined by the epithelium of normal colonic type. The surface of inflammatory polyps is commonly ulcerated and slough-covered, a feature shared with some juvenile polyps. Larger granulation tissue polyps may occur.

When carcinoma develops in long-standing ulcerative colitis it does not appear to derive from inflammatory polyps, the process usually occurring in non-polyploid mucosa. Inflammatory polyps, therefore, have no malignant potential.

Metaplastic (hyperplastic) polyps

These extremely common lesions are usually small (less than 10 mm diameter), pale, sessile nodules which are found only in the mucosa of the large bowel and particularly in the rectum (Fig. 8.1). Occasional examples may be larger than 1 cm and rarely a stalk is present. A reliable distinction from small adenomas is not always possible by naked eye inspection. Sometimes metaplastic polyps are sufficiently numerous to form metaplastic polyposis and there is a real danger of confusion with adenomatous polyposis unless biopsies are taken for histological examination. The histological appearances are characteristic with so-called 'saw-tooth' appearances of the elongated tubules which often show cystic dilatation but no epithelial dysplasia. Metaplastic polyps have no malignant potential.

Heterotopic polyps

The only relatively common example of a heterotopic polyp is endometriosis. This usually occurs within the bowel wall but rarely presents as a polypoid tumour of the large bowel and may lead to serious diagnostic difficulties for the pathologist and clinician unaware of its occurrence.

Hamartomatous polyps

Hamartomas are non-neoplastic localised tumour-like proliferations consisting of normal tissues arranged in an abnormal, disorganised fashion. Two types of polyp found in the large bowel come into this category; Peutz-Jeghers and juvenile polyps.

Peutz-Jeghers polyps occur more commonly in the small than in the large bowel and are also found in the stomach. They are usually multiple, but solitary examples are sometimes encountered in patients without any other features of the Peutz-Jeghers syndrome, which include circumoral and circumanal pig-

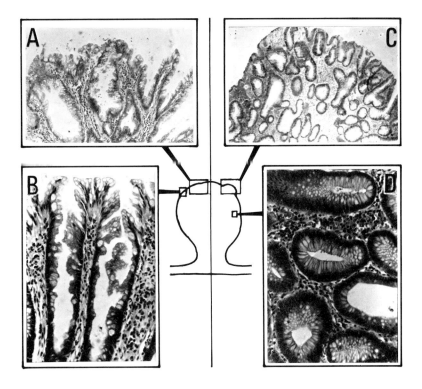

METAPLASTIC POLYP | **ADENOMATOUS POLYP**

Fig. 8.1 Structural difference between metaplastic and adenomatous polyps.

A Cystic tubules

B Saw-toothing of epithelium in elongated tubules

C Branching glands

D Hyperchromatic nuclei

mented freckles. Recently a rare form of ovarian tumour has been recognised as also being associated with the syndrome in some female patients.

The basic architectural arrangement of the Peutz–Jeghers polyp is of a tree-like fronded core of smooth muscle covered by normal epithelium (Fig. 8.2). Glandular structures may become misplaced to be intimately mixed with smooth muscle throughout the bowel wall and may be mistaken for infiltrating carcinoma; some reported cases of carcinoma supervening in Peutz–Jeghers polyps are probably examples of such an erroneous interpretation. For practical purposes Peutz–Jeghers

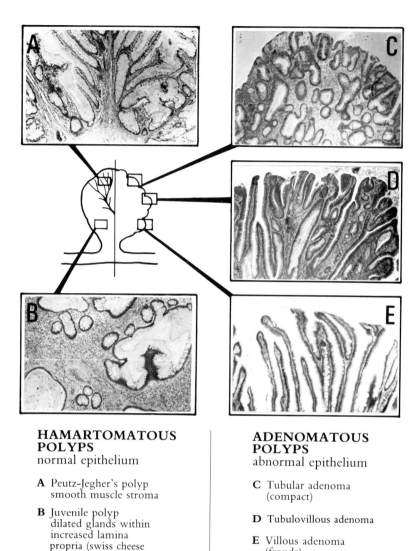

HAMARTOMATOUS POLYPS
normal epithelium

A Peutz-Jegher's polyp
smooth muscle stroma

B Juvenile polyp
dilated glands within
increased lamina
propria (swiss cheese
appearance)

ADENOMATOUS POLYPS
abnormal epithelium

C Tubular adenoma
(compact)

D Tubulovillous adenoma

E Villous adenoma
(fronds)

Fig. 8.2 Hamartomatous and adenomatous polyps.

polyps may be said to have very small malignant potential. Although there is a significant incidence of duodenal or small intestinal malignancy in these patients, it is not yet clear whether the malignancy has its origin within the hamartomatous polyps.

Juvenile (mucus retention) polyps are found predominantly in the large bowel, but may also occur in the small bowel or stomach. They may be solitary or multiple.

The head of a juvenile polyp is covered with normal mucosa and has a smooth, rounded contour, although in juvenile polyposis there may be a more convoluted surface. The pedicle may be long but is, nevertheless, very slender. It is composed of mucosa and some connective tissue, but lacks a component from the muscularis mucosae; torsion and 'auto-amputation' commonly follow as a result of this lack of support in the pedicle.

Juvenile polyps are composed of tubules lined by normal colonic epithelium set in an excessive amount of stroma formed from normal lamina propria (Fig. 8.2). Often the glands become cystically dilated by an accumulation of mucus and inflammatory exudate – hence, the alternative name of 'mucus retention polyp' and the 'Swiss cheese' appearance seen in sections of juvenile polyps. Juvenile polyps have no significant malignant potential.

Neoplastic polyps (adenomas)

Morphology

All forms of adenomas are part of a single neoplastic family and have in common a distinctive type of epithelium. In the World Health Organization classification they are divided into three categories, tubular, tubulovillous and villous, according to the architectural arrangement of the stroma and epithelium (Fig. 8.2). It should be appreciated that these patterns represent points on a spectrum of appearances ranging between the two extremes from the sessile villous adenoma to the typical pedunculated tubular adenoma; indeed these changes can all exist in a single adenoma. When an adenoma is pedunculated the stalk is covered by normal large bowel mucosa and includes an uninterrupted prolongation of the muscularis mucosae. Connective tissue, blood vessels and lymphatics in the submucosa of the head of the polyp are in direct continuity with the submucosa of the surrounding bowel, which is of great importance in considering the development of carcinoma in an adenoma. In all adenomas, the adenomatous epithelium is superficial to the muscularis mucosae and invasion of the muscularis mucosae is the criterion of malignancy.

Tubular adenomas have a pattern of branching tubules embedded in normal lamina propria. The tubular adenoma is usually divided into incomplete lobules which give the typical 'fissured' appearance on gross inspection.

Villous adenomas have a pattern of long, unbranched, finger-like processes which give a gross cauliflower-like appearance. There is no appreciable extension of muscularis mucosae into the villous processes (cf. Peutz-Jeghers polyps), which contain a sparse core of delicate connective tissue.

Tubulovillous (papillary) adenomas are usually intermediate in pattern between the above two types, with more branching villous processes having blunter tips; some are 'mixed' with tubular and villous portions.

The tubular adenoma is the most frequent form and although commonly pedunculated, may be sessile, especially when small. Conversely, although many are sessile, some villous adenomas are pedunculated. Villous tumours tend to be larger than those of tubular pattern (Table 8b) suggesting that as adenomas grow

Table 8b. *Size of adenomas of different histological types*

Histological type	Size		
	< 1 cm	1–2 cm	> 2 cm
Tubular	76%	20%	4%
Tubulovillous	16%	51%	33%
Villous	8%	29%	63%

they tend to adopt a more villous configuration (Muto, Bussey and Morson, 1975).

The beginnings of adenomas are observed most easily in familial adenomatous polyposis. The adenoma in this condition, and the adenocarcinomas which arise, resemble the much commoner solitary lesions in all detectable respects. However not only are there large numbers of adenomas at all stages of development, but also minute lesions invisible to the naked eye. If the large bowel mucosa from a case of familial adenomatous polyposis is sectioned horizontally in the plane of the mucosa, changes affecting tubules or even part of a tubule can be seen. Presumably, these single-tubule micro-adenomas bud and grow to form a small visible adenoma which later acquires a more tubular or villous configuration and may become stalked. The factors which determine both the pattern of an adenoma and the development of the stalk are unknown. So, too, are the factors which determine whether continued growth occurs or whether the adenoma remains static at a particular size.

Epithelial features

Regardless of the architecture the type of epithelium lining the tubules or covering the villous processes is the same. It is for this reason that all adenomas are considered to be one single type of neoplasm. Adenomatous epithelial cells are taller and more crowded than normal; their nuclei occupy relatively more of the cell volume and are hyperchromatic with increased mitotic activity.

The degree of resemblance to normal epithelium varies. Loss of this resemblance is referred to as dysplasia. As dysplasia increases there is greater variation in nuclear size, shape and depth of staining and a decrease in the mucin content (Fig. 8.3). Mitotic figures increase in frequency and may be abnormal.

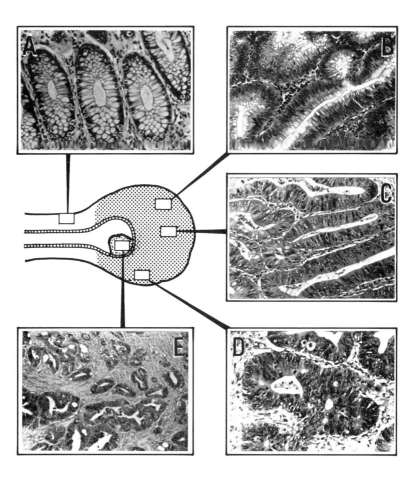

Fig. 8.3 Morphology of adenoma – adenocarcinoma sequence.

A Normal epithelium

E Invasive carcinoma

B Mild dysplasia
C Moderate dysplasia
D Severe dysplasia

There is progressive 'loss of polarity' of the cells, the nuclei losing their normal uniform position at the base of the cells, and the glands become irregular and poorly formed, with intraglandular bridging.

The appearance of severely dysplastic adenomatous epithelium may closely resemble areas of some infiltrating adenocarcinomas. As long as these changes remain localised above the level of the muscularis mucosae, however, it is incorrect to make a diagnosis of malignancy. Some authorities refer to such severe dysplasia as 'carcinoma-in-situ' or 'focal carcinoma'.

Used in pathological reports, these terms may be confusing and lead to incorrect assumptions on the part of the clinician. The diagnosis of carcinoma arising in an adenoma can only be made when dysplastic epithelium is seen to be invading across the muscularis mucosa into the submucosal plane (Fig. 8.3), where it has access to submucosal lymphatics with the potential for metastases to regional lymph nodes. The mucosa and lamina propria of the large bowel, both normal and adenomatous, contain no lymphatic channels. The type of intramucosal carcinoma characterised by invasion of the lamina propria by malignant mucinous (signet-ring) cells seen so commonly in the stomach is a rarity in the large bowel and is encountered mainly in the context of ulcerative colitis, when it is associated with premalignant dysplasia.

The principles governing the diagnosis of carcinoma are the same for sessile as for pedunculated tumours. The presence or absence of a pedicle in the adenoma determines only the ease with which complete local excision may be accomplished by the clinician.

Pseudocarcinomatous invasion or *'misplaced adenoma'* is the histological description of an entirely benign phenomenon in which adenomatous tissue may be seen within the submucosal structures beneath the head of the adenoma. The appearance is thought to be a result of torsion and consequent partial infarction of the tip of an adenoma allowing its epithelium to be misplaced to the submucosa. The situation is comparable to the formation of submucosal inclusion cysts in chronic ulcerative colitis (colitis cystica profunda). Histologically the displaced glands are immediately surrounded by normal lamina propria and not the desmoplastic (fibrous) reaction of infiltrating carcinoma. They also lack the severe degree of epithelial atypia usually associated with carcinoma. Surrounding haemosiderin desposition, which is generally marked, indicates previous haemorrhagic infarction. Differentiation between this appearance and carcinoma is important not only for the individual patient but for the compilation of accurate data on adenomas and malignant change.

The risk of malignancy is influenced by the histological type, size and degree of differentiation of the adenoma. The incidence of malignant change within the different histological types of adenoma is shown in Table 8c. This shows an almost ten-fold increase of the presence of malignancy in villous compared to tubular adenomas.

Although there is a risk of malignancy developing in any adenoma (about 10% overall), this increases with increasing size of tumour. It rises steeply for tumours larger than 2 cm in

The risk of malignant change

243

Table 8c. *Frequency of malignant invasion in adenomas*

Histological type	Surgical series percentage with carcinoma				Colonoscopic series percentage with carcinoma			
	<1 cm	1–2 cm	>2 cm	Total	<1 cm	1–2 cm	>2 cm	Total
Tubular	1%	10%	35%	5%	1%	3%	10%	2%
Tubulovillous	4%	7%	46%	23%	0%	4%	11%	6%
Villous	10%	10%	53%	41%	0%	5%	38%	18%

diameter but, even in those less than 1 cm across, there is a small but definite risk.

The histological type and size are not independent of each other and the relative risk of malignancy when these factors are considered together is also shown in Table 8c. Both are also related to the degree of dysplasia, the third factor influencing malignant change (see Table 8d). These figures derive from a

Table 8d. *Relationship of dysplasia in adenomas to the frequency of malignant change*

Grade of dysplasia	Percentage with carcinoma
Mild	6%
Moderate	18%
Severe	35%

large surgical series (Muto, Morson and Bussey 1975). Comparable data from a colonoscopic polypectomy series (Gillespie, Chambers, Chan et al., 1979) shows similar trends but about half the malignancy rate (5% overall).

Carcinoma found within a surrounding adenoma is usually moderately or well differentiated. In these circumstances, there is less than 1% risk of metastasis to the regional lymph nodes having already occurred. Major surgical treatment following local excision is, therefore, probably unjustified since the five year survival for these selected lesions is over 90% (Morson, Bussey and Samoorian, 1977). In the very uncommon instance of poorly differentiated carcinoma occurring in a clearly recognisable adenoma, the risk of nodal metastases rises to about 10% and major surgery is justified.

The adenoma–adenocarcinoma sequence

There is a great deal of evidence to indicate that adenomas have a potential to undergo malignant change. The common finding of cancer within adenomas has already been discussed. Severe dysplasia confined to an adenoma is cytologically indistinguishable from well-differentiated carcinoma. Adenomas and carcinomas share similar histochemical and chromosomal aberrations. Many early carcinomas contain areas of benign adenomatous tissue, but the frequency of this association is lower in more advanced carcinomas; this suggests that the original adenoma becomes destroyed as the carcinoma grows and there is strong evidence in support of the thesis that adenomas are the main predisposing lesion in carcinoma of the large bowel.

Apart from the comparatively rare situation of malignant change in chronic ulcerative colitis, no early carcinomas (of a few mm diameter) have been seen except within adenomas. Despite great opportunity for its detection, carcinoma *de novo* has not been observed histologically.

Patients with multiple adenomas have a higher risk of developing carcinoma either synchronously or metachronously, the risk reaching 100% in patients with familial adenomatous polyposis. In about 20% of patients presenting with large bowel cancer, synchronous adenomas are present. The distribution of carcinomas within the large bowel is similar to that of adenomas, the majority of both lesions being found in the distal colon and rectum.

The geographical distribution of adenomas and carcinomas is also similar; both are rare in African negroes and in Japanese in their own countries, while both are common in Western Caucasians and are more common in Japanese living in the West or eating 'Westernised diets'.

The peak age incidence of detection of carcinomas occurs about five years later than that of adenomas, both in the general population and those afflicted with familial adenomatous polyposis, suggesting a temporal progression.

There is also evidence to suggest that removal of adenomas reduces the incidence of carcinoma. In the rectal stump of patients with familial adenomatous polyposis after ileorectal anastomosis, fulguration of remaining adenomas results in a marked lowering of the expected rate of cancer of the rectal stump. In a group of over 18 000 normal subjects a programme for detection and removal of rectal adenomas resulted in a rectal cancer rate of seven times lower than would have been expected in the non–screened population (Gilbertsen, 1974); although this study lacked a defined control group, the results strongly suggest that adenomas can progress to carcinomas.

The pathology of adenomas determines their management. *Practical* Both the clinician and pathologist must therefore observe some *considerations* simple rules:

> Small fragments of large pedunculated polyps obtained by biopsy forceps are of little help because malignant change may be missed in the sampling. The relationship of one fragment to the

245

remainder of the polyp is unknown and completeness of excision cannot be determined.

Pedunculated polyps should, therefore, be treated by complete excision with an attempt to preserve the lesion, if not intact, than at least in a few large pieces.

The entire lesion, including the stalk (if any) should be examined by the pathologist.

The specimen should be orientated so that sections may be cut in the correct plane for proper assessment. Several sections at different levels through the specimen should be examined histologically. This is especially important when initial examination reveals severe dysplasia, since there is a high chance that subsequent sections will reveal invasive cancer in another part of the polyp.

A pathological report on an adenoma should contain the following information: Histological type; size; degree of dysplasia; presence or absence of a stalk; presence or absence of malignancy; involvement or not by carcinoma if present, of the line of resection; histological grade of carcinoma when present.

MALIGNANT TUMOURS OF THE COLON AND RECTUM

Adenocarcinoma

The great majority of large bowel malignant tumours are adenocarcinomas. There are several uncommon histological variants, some of which will be discussed. Definite conclusions about their behaviour and prognosis are difficult to draw because the sparsity of such cases precludes the collection of sizeable series within a particular centre.

In the preceding section the probable development of adenocarcinoma within adenomas was discussed and much of the pathology of adenocarcinoma described. Emphasis has been put on this aspect of the large bowel cancer, first because of its fundamental importance and, secondly, because the concept of the adenoma-adenocarcinoma sequence deserves wide recognition.

Over 60% of adenocarcinomas occur in the sigmoid colon or rectum and about 20% in the right side of the colon. They may be polypoid or sessile, ulcerated or non-ulcerated. Frequently the whole circumference of the bowel is involved, resulting in a malignant stenosis which may cause obstruction; this occurs more often in left-sided lesions. The typical carcinoma of the large bowel is a raised lesion with central ulceration and everted edges.

The tumour spreads by local invasion and by distant dissemination into blood vessels or lymphatics or into the peritoneal cavity. Penetration of the muscularis mucosae is followed by invasion across the submucosa into the muscularis propria. Invasion continues to the outer surface of the bowel to penetrate the overlying serosa or, where this is absent, the fascia propria. Extramural spread then takes place into surrounding fat and connective tissue and may involve other organs. During this progression, lymphatics and veins in the submucosa and outside the bowel wall may become invaded. Involvement of lymph nodes by the tumour progresses in a gradual manner from nodes closest to the growth, along the course of the lymphatic vessels to those placed centrally.

Preparation and examination of operative specimens

The basic purpose of the histopathological examination of operation specimens, particularly those removed for malignant disease, is not merely to make a diagnosis, but to obtain as much information as possible for assessing prognosis and the need for further therapeutic measures. The collection of this information is facilitated by suitable preparation of the specimen prior to fixation.

The specimen should be sent immediately after removal to the pathology department where it is washed through with water to remove faecal content. Relatively straight segments of intestine are opened along the antimesenteric border. Slight deviation to avoid cutting into the tumour does not matter. The specimen is then pinned out on a cork board, stretching the specimen just sufficiently to remove most of the mucosal folds. Immersion in 10% formaldehyde solution usually completes fixation in 24–48 hours. If the specimen is curved as at one of the flexures, or is involved by adhesion or fistula with other loops of intestine, it is often useful to distend it with fixative to enable the gross anatomy to be more easily defined.

The first part of the examination consists of careful inspection of the specimen and recording of the shape, size and position of all abnormalities present, including in addition to the main primary lesion, any polyps, mucosal nodules, ulcers or diverticula etc. which are also present. The prefixation preparation of the specimen makes these lesions easier to see. The initial inspection together with palpation helps considerably in deciding what areas should be taken for microscopical examination. The three main methods of spread, by direct continuity, lymphatics and veins, are investigated. The extent of spread into and through the bowel wall can be observed by incising the tumour at the level of deepest invasion which is usually the point of deepest ulceration. Ideally, all lymph nodes found either by anatomical dissection or by slicing of the mesentery should be examined microscopically. Any submucosal thickening, especially if cord-like, at the margin of the growth or distended veins within the mesentery or arising from the direct continuity spread should be sectioned to confirm venous invasion by carcinomatous tissue.

It is useful to prepare a diagram on which the results of the examination can be marked. Such a diagram is easily made by the use of carbon paper covered by a sheet of plastic material on which the specimen is placed. An accurate outline of the specimen and its anatomical features can be traced on to a sheet of paper with a blunt probe and the histopathology findings added subsequently (Fig. 8.4).

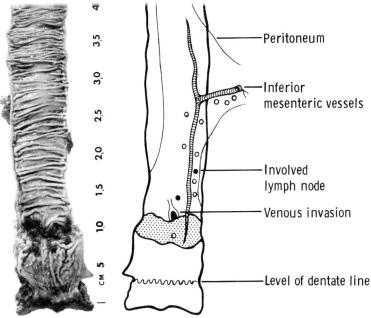

Fig. 8.4 Carcinoma of the rectum – an operative specimen (luminal aspect) and diagram (external aspect).

While agreeing with the desirability of so detailed an examination, some pathologists would argue that this is not practical in a busy department. However, much can be done by inspection of the specimen and microscopical examination limited according to the available facilities; it is not essential to section a lymph node which is obviously invaded by carcinoma but a record of its existence and position helps in assessing the prognosis.

Pathological stage   In 1932 Dukes published a system of pathological staging for operable carcinoma of the rectum which is recognised as a valuable prognostic indicator of survival and its principles are universally understood. It was soon applied to colonic as well as rectal growths. Other systems of pathological staging have since been proposed but Dukes' classification remains as practical and useful as any.

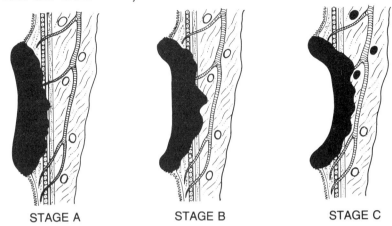

STAGE A   STAGE B   STAGE C

Fig. 8.5
Dukes' classification.

The stages of the Dukes' classification are (Fig. 8.5):

A. Spread by direct continuity into submucosa or muscle, but not beyond, and without lymph node involvement.
B. Spread beyond the muscle coat into pericolic or perirectal tissues, but without lymph node involvement.
C. As stage A or B but with metastasis to regional lymph nodes. Stage C is subdivided into:
    C1 where involved nodes do not extend up to the point of surgical ligature of the vascular pedicle;
    C2 where the node at or immediately below the ligature is involved (Fig. 8.6).

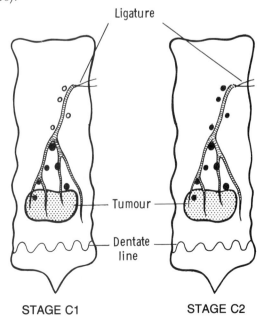

STAGE C1   STAGE C2

Fig. 8.6
Dukes' classification.

There is no *stage D* in Dukes' classification. This is occasionally and incorrectly added by others to denote cases with distant metastasis. The relative frequency of tumours of different Dukes' stages is shown in Table 8e.

Table 8e. *Dukes' classification*

Stage	Proportion of cases
A	15%
B	40%
C	45%

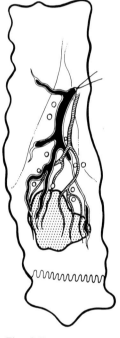

It is now clear that invasion of veins in and around the tumour is also an important pathological determinant of prognosis. Not only is survival poorer when venous invasion is present, but it is worse when veins outside the bowel wall are involved than when intramural veins only are invaded (Table 8f, Fig. 8.7). There is also an association between the presence of venous invasion and the pathological stage of the tumour (Tablot, Ritchie, Leighton *et al.*, 1980).

Table 8f. *The comparison of survival with intramural and extramural venous invasion*

Venous invasion	Five year survival (%)
Intramural	64%
Extramural – thin walled vein	40%
– thick walled vein	19%

Fig. 8.7

The Dukes' staging system can obviously only be applied to a carcinoma following surgical removal and pathological examination. It is, therefore, unusable as a guide to operability or to the type of operation possible. With the increasing numbers of conservative operations and local excisions for rectal cancer there is a need for a clinical staging system prior to operation.

Histological grade

Another important indicator of prognosis in colorectal cancer is the histological grade of tumour, originally classified by Broders (1925). It is determined (somewhat subjectively) by such features as degree of tubule formation; variability in size, shape and staining of nuclei; orderliness of arrangement of cells and their nuclei within tubules; number of mitotic figures. The grading is generally accepted as a reproducible and accurate guide to prognosis, which complements the staging; the relative frequency of the different grades is given in Table 8g.

Table 8g. *Histological grade*

Stage	Proportion of cases
Well differentiated	20%
Moderately differentiated	60%
Poorly differentiated	20%

Distant metastases

Metastases are common in large bowel cancer and are the most important cause of death. The liver is involved in over 60% of patients with disseminated disease, the lungs being the second most common site. The distribution of metastases at autopsy in a series of patients dying with large bowel carcinoma is shown in Table 8h. In Malmö where these data were

Table 8h. *Frequency of metastases at different sites from Berge, Ekelund, Mellner et al, (1973)*

Site of metastases	Colon	Rectum
Brain	6%	8%
Lung	48%	64%
Liver	76%	62%
Peritoneum	49%	25%
Skeleton	12%	19%
Ovary	17%	4%
Number of patients	239	134

obtained, over 80% of people dying had a postmortem examination and the figures are, therefore, as accurate as any available (Berge, Ekelund, Mellner *et al.*, 1973).

Ulcerative colitis and carcinoma of the large bowel

The only observed exception to the adenoma-adenocarcinoma sequence as the mechanism of development of large bowel cancer is the precancer – cancer sequence of chronic ulcerative colitis. Carcinoma is a well-recognised complication of long-standing extensive ulcerative colitis and the cumulative risk with a history in excess of 20 years is approximately 5–10%. Nevertheless, it accounts for only a very small proportion (less than 1%) of all cases of large bowel carcinoma. The importance of cancer in colitis lies in the morphologically recognisable precancerous phase. Control of cancer by prevention must therefore be the aim in ulcerative colitis, as it is in adenomatous polyposis where the possession of multiple adenomas defines the precancerous phase.

Precancerous changes in the large bowel mucosa of ulcerative colitis were described by Morson and Pang (1967), who detected them in 9% of specimens from colectomies performed in patients with ulcerative colitis for various reasons and in all of those containing a carcinoma. Just as a spectrum of dysplasia may be found in a population of adenomas, culminating in severe dysplasia before invasive malignancy occurs, so a similar spectrum of epithelial dysplasia is seen in chronic ulcerative colitis. Changes range from mild to severe dysplasia; the latter is called *precancer* and is equivalent to *carcinoma-in-situ* (Fig. 8.8).

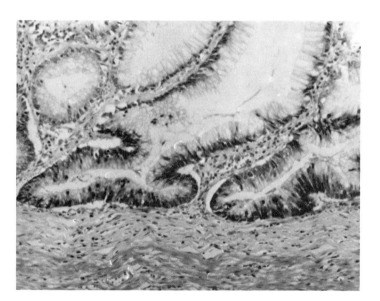

Fig. 8.8 Severe dysplasia in chronic ulcerative colitis.

This name should not be taken to indicate that such changes *necessarily* will progress to invasive carcinoma any more than severe dysplasia in an adenoma will. Severe dysplasia is, however, consistently and significantly associated with carcinoma whether it has developed contiguously or at a distance. Precancer in ulcerative colitis may occur in flat or only slightly irregular mucosa and in patchy ill-defined areas as well as more obvious polypoid areas. It should be appreciated, therefore, that precancerous mucosa often cannot be identified by the naked eye or by radiography (in contrast to adenomas); biopsies are mandatory for its reliable detection or exclusion.

Carcinomas developing in ulcerative colitis tend to be a atypical in their gross and histological appearances. Often the lesion is a flat or slightly elevated non-ulcerated plaque. Occasionally, an established infiltrating carcinoma is invisible to the naked eye, being not only non-ulcerated but also non-elevated within the surrounding mucosa. The distribution of carcinomas in ulcerative colitis differs slightly from that of more conventional carcinoma. In colitis the carcinomas tend to be proximally situated more often and only 55% are in the rectosigmoid region, as compared with 75% for the usual carcinomas.

Other types of malignant tumour

Mucinous (colloid) and signet-ring cell carcinoma

Although all adenocarcinomas of the bowel show some degree of mucin secretion, occasional tumours produce such a vast excess that large pools of mucus are seen lying free in the tissues. Small clumps and individual carcinoma cells float in these mucus 'lakes'. Sometimes the carcinoma cells have a signet-ring appearance and no clear distinction is possible between mucinous (colloid) and pure signet-ring cell carcinoma. Both types are rare in the large bowel except as tumours complicating ulcerative colitis. The derivation of carcinomas from adenomas in this condition is not established. Mucinous carcinoma is often the type of carcinoma which arises in perirectal fistulae.

Squamous metaplasia in adenocarcinoma

Small foci of squamous metaplasia are sometimes seen within the glands, both of adenomas and adenocarcinomas. When these are a prominent feature of the latter, the tumour may be called an adeno-acanthoma. It does not seem justifiable however to regard this as any different from pure adenocarcinoma, since it behaves in an identical manner.

Adenosquamous carcinoma

Adenosquamous carcinoma is quite different pathologically and in its behaviour. In such tumours there are areas both of adenocarcinomatous appearance and of infiltrating squamous carcinoma, which has all the features of invasive squamous carcinoma at other sites in the body. The prognosis seems to be poor. The rare example of an apparently pure squamous carcinoma of the colon or rectum may, in fact, be adenosquamous carcinoma which has been inadequately sampled.

253

Both adeno-acanthoma and adenosquamous carcinoma in the rectum must be distinguished from the muco-epidermoid carcinoma which occurs in the anal canal (see below).

Undifferentiated (small cell) carcinoma

Despite its name, this type of carcinoma does not appear to behave in an aggressive fashion and relatively large tumours may be removed before local nodal or distant metastasis has occurred. They are only undifferentiated in the sense that mucin secretion and well-formed tubules are not in evidence. There is a certain uniformity of the cells and their particular arrangement in small groups suggests an affinity with carcinoid tumours. Special stains for carcinoid tumours are generally negative, however, and the carcinoid syndrome does not occur.

Carcinoid tumours

The tumours of the large bowel which come into this category do not generally resemble the typical mid-gut carcinoid tumour as found in terminal ileum or appendix. The term carcinoid tumour might seem inappropriate but it is sanctioned by long and widespread usage, and the alternative 'endocrine cell neoplasm' is somewhat clumsy.

Although all carcinoid tumours are potentially malignant there is a distinct and recognisable variety, often found in the rectum, which is of small size and behaves in a benign fashion. Such tumours are essentially submucosal in location, with only a very small mucosal component. The overlying mucosa is intact and the tumour forms a smooth sessile nodule, usually less than 2 cm in diameter, projecting into the lumen of the bowel. Many are asymptomatic, incidental findings on rectal examination. Microscopically, they are composed of uniform cells arranged in anastomosing cords giving a festooned appearance (Fig. 8.9). They are not known to contain or secrete

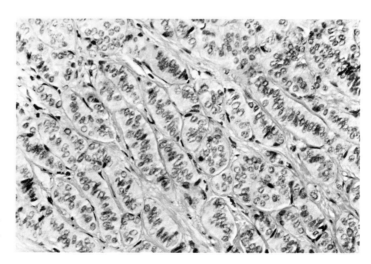

Fig. 8.9 Carcinoid tumour showing festooned appearance.

5-hydroxytryptamine (5-HT) and are not associated with the carcinoid syndrome.

In the rectum, these small carcinoid tumours are easily excised in the submucosal plane and if removal is judged to be complete on microscopic examination, no further operative treatment is required.

Large exophytic or ulcerated tumours of carcinoid type are obviously not in the above category and clinically appear malignant *ab initio*. They often behave in an aggressive fashion with local invasion and distant metastasis. Microscopically there is a range of possible appearances from a ribboned arrangement of cells similar to the benign variety, to a highly cellular malignant tumour with an appearance closely akin to oat-cell carcinoma of the bronchus. This is not surprising, since the oat-cell bronchial carcinoma is a malignant endocrine cell neoplasm of fore-gut origin.

TUMOURS OF THE ANAL CANAL AND ANAL MARGIN

Tumours in the anal region account for 3–4% of all malignant tumours of the large intestine. The mean age of patients affected is about 60 years. The anal canal is lined mainly by a 'transitional-type' epithelium (Chapter 11), which gives way to non-keratinising squamous epithelium at the anal verge. Neither region has any of the specialised appendages (e.g. hair or sweat follicles) of the external skin surface. Melanocytes, however, are present in the epithelium of the anal margin and to a lesser extent of the anal canal.

The tumours which arise in this region derive mostly from either this 'transitional-type' or squamous epithelium. Malignant melanoma also occurs. Tumours of accessory structures, such as anal glands, are very rare.

Benign tumours

Squamous papillomata

Squamous papillomata (condylomata acuminata) are exophytic excrescences found both at the anal margin and in the anal canal. Most are probably viral and have, in addition to their papillary structure, the other microscopic features which suggest a viral origin, i.e. vacuolated cells and inclusion bodies. When situated in the anal canal, viral warts often appear as rather flat, pale plaques and may not be recognised clinically for what they are. There are extremely rare examples of squamous carcinoma developing in viral warts, but the evidence for squamous papilloma being precancerous is tenuous.

Giant condyloma

Giant condyloma is a different and rare lesion which extensively involves the anal canal and verge. Histologically it is similar to the viral wart but behaves as a low grade malignant tumour despite this bland appearance. Even the local recurrences after excision retain the very well differentiated appearance of the squamous epithelium.

Malignant tumours

Malignant tumours in about 70% of cases involve the anal canal while 30% occur at the anal margin. There appears to be a sex difference in these two sites; tumours of the anal margin are more common in males while more females develop carcinoma of the anal canal. Anal margin carcinoma is considered to be similar to epithelioma of the skin occurring at other sites.

These tumours invade the submucosa or subcutaneous tissue and continue through the anal sphincter into the fat of the ischio-rectal fossa and the muscles of the pelvic floor. Lymphatic spread occurs both to the postrectal and to the inguinal nodes.

There are several histological types, including squamous cell, basaloid, muco-epidermoid, adenocarcinoma, malignant melanoma and basal cell carcinoma.

Squamous cell carcinoma

Squamous cell carcinoma (epidermoid carcinoma) may develop in squamous papillomata around the anal verge. It can rarely occur within such precancerous skin conditions as Bowen's disease. Squamous carcinoma may be graded histologically according to Broders' system. The prognosis is related to the grade of tumour and the grade also influences the likelihood of lymphatic metastasis to regional lymph nodes.

Basaloid carcinoma (cloacogenic carcinoma)

Basaloid carcinoma arises from the epithelium lining the anal canal and may conveniently be regarded as a variety of squamous carcinoma peculiar to this location. The term basaloid carcinoma is derived from the appearances of the tumour cells which resemble the cells of the basal layer of the epidermis. Unlike basal cell carcinoma, basaloid carcinoma of the anal canal may metastasise to lymph nodes. It is graded as well-, moderately- or poorly-differentiated and the grade of tumour determines prognosis.

Muco-epidermoid carcinoma

Muco-epidermoid carcinoma resembles squamous carcinoma, but is generally not well keratinised. This tumour tends to occur close to the squamocolumnar junction of the upper anal canal and lower rectum. It must be distinguished histologically from an adenoacanthoma or an adenosquamous carcinoma in the lower rectum.

The prognosis is similar to that of moderately-differentiated squamous carcinoma of this region.

Adenocarcinoma may be of rectal type, arise from the anal glands or complicate a long standing fistula-in-ano.

Adenocarcinoma

Malignant melanoma of the anus is a highly aggressive neoplasm which is often polypoid in this region, rather than ulcerated. It usually arises high in the anal canal and may encroach upon the lower rectum and be mistaken for a rectal adenocarcinoma. The difficulty in diagnosis is compounded by lack of melanin pigmentation in many examples; typical melanosomes are seen on electron microscopy. If fresh tissue is available the enzyme activity of DOPA-oxidase should be demonstrable. The prognosis is very poor, dissemination is rapid and widespread and the tumour often proves fatal within a few months.

Malignant melanoma

Benign pigmented lesions, i.e.. intradermal naevi, are also occasionally seen in the anal canal.

Basal cell carcinoma of the anal margin resembles basal cell carcinoma found elsewhere on the external skin surface in all respects, being only locally invasive and radiosensitive. It must be distinguished histologically from a basaloid carcinoma which arises in the anal canal.

Basal cell carcinoma

REFERENCES AND FURTHER READING

Berge T, Ekelund G, Mellner C and Wenckert A. Carcinoma of the colon and rectum in a defined population. *Acta Chirurgica Scandinavica* 1973; supplement 438.

Broders AC. The grading of carcinoma. *Minnesota Medicine* 1925; **8:** 726–30.

Bussey HJR. *Familial polyposis coli.* Baltimore and London: The Johns Hopkins University Press, 1975.

Dukes CE. The classification of cancer of the rectum. *Journal of Pathology and Bacteriology* 1932; **35:** 323–32.

Gillespie PE, Chambers TJ, Chan KW, Doronzo F, Morson BC and Williams CB. Colonic adenoma – a colonoscopic survey. *Gut* 1979; **20:** 240–5.

Gilbertsen VA. Proctosigmoidoscopy and polypectomy in reducing the incidence of rectal cancer. *Cancer* 1974; **34:** 936–9.

Morson BC. *Histological typing of intestinal tumours.* Geneva: World Health Organization, 1976.

Morson BC and Pang LSC. Rectal biopsy as an aid to cancer control in ulcerative colitis. *Gut* 1967; **8:** 423–34.

Morson BC, Bussey HJR and Samoorian S. Policy of local excision for early cancer of the colorectum. *Gut* 1977; **18:** 1045–50.

Muto T, Bussey HJR and Morson BC. The evolution of cancer of the colon and rectum. *Cancer* 1975; **36:** 2251–70.

Talbot IC, Ritchie S, Leighton MH, Hughes AO, Bussey HJR and Morson BC. The clinical significance of invasion of veins by rectal cancer. *British Journal of Surgery* 1980; **67:** 439–42.

MANAGEMENT OF BENIGN TUMOURS AND POLYPS

Polyps of the large bowel are very common and may be found in about 10% of patients attending a rectal clinic. Before the advent of the double contrast barium enema many of these lesions would have been missed, but with the increasing use of this technique more are being found. The introduction of colonoscopy has also increased the diagnostic yield but its greatest impact has been in the treatment of polyps. In former days, polyps beyond the reach of the rigid sigmoidoscope were removed surgically either with a resection or through a colotomy. This operation has become a rarity since most colonic polyps can be safely removed at colonoscopy.

GENERAL PRINCIPLES

The management of large bowel polyps can be divided into four parts: diagnosis, removal, follow-up, family genotyping. These are considered with particular reference to adenomas.

Diagnosis

Diagnosis comprises four stages: identification of the polyp; determination of numbers present; assessment of size and morphology; determination of histological type.

Identification

A polyp may be seen either at sigmoidoscopy or, if more proximal, on the barium enema examination. The symptoms caused by an adenoma are indistinguishable from those of a carcinoma. Almost 50% of cases occur within 25 cm of the anal verge, 5% in the caecum and ascending colon, and the rest are distributed between these sites. The rigid sigmoidoscope

258

should, therefore, in theory reach the majority but in practice the rectosigmoid region can only be passed in 60% of patients, hence the growing interest in fibre-sigmoidoscopy. Polyps lying immediately above a valve of Houston can easily be missed and especial care should be taken in examining these parts of the rectum. Blood in the lumen is a most important warning sign and if the sigmoidoscopy (or preferably fibre-sigmoidoscopy) is normal this observation must be followed by a double contrast barium enema and, if this is negative, by diagnostic colonoscopy.

The double contrast barium enema is much more able to identify polyps than the conventional single contrast barium examination. Over 90% of polyps greater than 5 mm in diameter are shown and the examination is particularly accurate in visualising lesions in the right colon. The one area of weakness is the sigmoid loop, where up to 30% of polyps under 10 mm may not be shown. The diagnostic accuracy in all parts of the colon of the single contrast barium enema for polyps of this size is only of the order of 50–60%.

Colonoscopy as a diagnostic procedure will identify those polyps not seen on the barium enema, and is particularly accurate in the distal colon. The two techniques together should provide 100% accuracy in diagnosis, and the combination of fibre-sigmoidoscopy and double contrast barium enema is probably the 'best buy' for polyp diagnosis.

Determination of numbers present

Large bowel polyps are frequently multiple. There is, furthermore, a greater chance of a large bowel carcinoma being present in a patient with one or more adenomas. An incidental adenoma is present in about 20% of patients with a carcinoma. It is important to determine the number and site of polyps, not only to identify them for removal, but also to consider the possibility of multiple polyposis, particularly familial adenomatous polyposis. Patients with this disorder have in excess of a hundred adenomas in the large bowel (often several thousand are present), whereas patients without this dominant hereditary predisposition rarely have more than 20.

For these reasons, full radiological examination of the colon using the double contrast technique must be undertaken in a patient found to have a polyp, and if the x-rays previously taken are substandard, diagnostic total colonoscopy is indicated.

Assessment of size and morphology

The relationship between size and the likelihood of malignant change within an adenoma has already been discussed. Morphology is also important in this respect, sessile adenomas being more likely than pedunculated to contain foci of carcinoma.

These considerations influence the method of removal, although in most cases endoscopic assessment is indicated to make a definite decision since the radiological appearance can be misleading. Thus, pedunculated polyps in any part of the large bowel can be removed endoscopically, snaring the stalk with a wire loop to coagulate and divide it with diathermy. On the other hand, a sessile lesion over 2–3 cm diameter is often unsuitable technically for diathermy snare excision and because of its high chance of malignant change should be considered for surgical removal unless the patient is a very poor operative risk. Whether the operation should be a local excision or involve removal of a length of bowel depends on the site and size of the lesion, and on clinical factors. Adenomas within 10–12 cm of the anal verge can be assessed by digital examination of the rectum. Often they are difficult to feel owing to their soft consistency but when malignant change has occurred, the finger is well able to detect areas of hardness indicative of invasion. A careful digital examination is therefore essential. The radiological features of malignant polyps have already been discussed (Chapter 1).

Determination of histological type

The histology of the polyp is crucially important in management, since adenomas are premalignant but polyps of other histological types do not have this potential. A partial biopsy of a polyp is a mistake for two main reasons. First, if it proves to be adenomatous the histopathologist is not able to tell whether malignant invasion of the muscularis mucosae has occurred since he does not have enough material and, secondly, after a partial removal it may on subsequent examination be more difficult to find the lesion in order completely to remove it. Histological examination should therefore follow complete removal. There are exceptions to this principle: when a non-pedunculated lesion is strongly suspected to be a carcinoma and in the diagnosis of familial adenomatous polyposis; in both cases, the treatment to be adopted depends on histological confirmation of the lesion. At colonoscopy an obvious lipoma may require neither biopsy nor removal. Proof of probable non-neoplastic inflammatory polyps in a patient with colitis can be established with a few representative biopsies.

Removal of colonic polyps

Before the development of colonoscopic removal, patients were submitted to a laparotomy and removal of the polyp through a colotomy. The operation carried a low but significant mortality and a faecal fistula through a leaking colotomy wound developed in about 5% of cases. It was sometimes difficult to find the polyp despite good x-ray pictures and multiple polyps required multiple colotomies.

Now over 95% of colonic polyps can be removed endoscopically at colonoscopy, usually on an outpatient basis. The incidence of bleeding and perforation of the colon is around 2% and 0.2%, respectively. Up to 10% of polyps over 2 cm diameter may bleed: patients with such large polyps should be admitted with blood for transfusion available. Surgery is rarely necessary when bleeding occurs, severe bleeding being controllable by angiographically administered pitressin. Almost all pedunculated polyps can then be removed with the diathermy snare; even most sessile lesions up to about 25 mm diameter can also be excised using this technique by applying gentle traction to raise a false pedicle or by piecemeal removal. Removal of multiple polyps can be undertaken at one sitting, small polyps under 5 mm can be destroyed using diathermy-biopsy forceps by which the base is coagulated and a biopsy retrieved in the forceps; this technique is referred to as 'hot biopsy'. A large polyp in the distal bowel can often be snared and brought down to the level of the lower rectum by intussusception through traction on the snare. Surgical excision under direct vision is then possible.

Removal of rectal polyps

Pedunculated polyps, as in the colon, can all be removed using the diathermy snare. This can be performed at colonoscopy after the removal of more proximal lesions, or through the rigid sigmoidoscope, if the barium enema has shown the lesion to be solitary.

The accessibility of the rectum to clinical examination and to peranal or transanal surgical techniques affords more opportunity for conservative surgery than is possible in the colon. Thus, it is possible with some accuracy to know beforehand whether malignant change has occurred in a rectal lesion, and if a local excision is decided upon this can be carried out through the anus taking a surrounding margin of normal tissue. The peranal approach allows large sessile adenomas to be removed by the technique of submucosal excision. The entire lesion is thereby delivered to the histopathologist with little disturbance to the patient. Sessile lesions of the upper rectum, rectosigmoid and even the sigmoid colon can often be brought down to the level of the lower rectum or anal canal usually under general anaesthesia and by applying traction with long forceps or a snare wire, to cause intussusception of the more proximal bowel. They can be excised under direct vision.

Almost all adenomas of the rectum from the small to the extensive can be removed without a major abdominal operation.

Follow-up

Patients who have had an adenoma are at greater risk of developing metachronous adenomas and adenocarcinomas of the large bowel. A 30–40% incidence of adenomas and a 3% incidence of carcinomas has been found at eight years follow-up. There is, furthermore, a risk of local recurrence after excision of sessile rectal adenomas, amounting to about 20–30% over a five year period (Thomson, 1977). A regular system of follow-up is therefore desirable for these patients but in view of the large numbers of adenomas treated this policy must be carefully thought out if it is not to be too great a burden on medical services.

A double contrast barium enema performed every three years, preferably combined with fibre-sigmoidoscopy, will be adequate protection for patients with very few previous adenomas. 'High-risk' patients with numerous adenomas or previous malignancy may require more frequent checks. All patients should be instructed to report change in bowel habit or blood loss at any time.

Family genotyping

For many years registers of patients affected with familial adenomatous polyposis have been in existence. Genealogies (family trees) of the families of these patients have been compiled, from which the dominant mode of inheritance of the disease has been shown (Fig. 8.10). This policy has also enabled

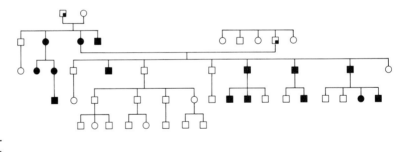

Fig. 8.10 Familial adeno-matous polyposis – a family tree. The dominant mode of inheritance.

□ Male   ○ Female   ▣ Died of bowel cancer   ● Familial adenomatous polyposis coli

members of succeeding generations to be screened. It is one of the few examples of effective cancer prevention, since affected individuals can be identified and treated before large bowel cancer occurs.

An increased familial incidence of large bowel cancer *not* associated with familial adenomatous polyposis has been recognised for many years. In some of these families, the risk appears to be very high, the distribution of affected cases indicating a recessive mode of inheritance. A careful family history is part of the management of any patient with a large bowel adenoma; a high familial incidence of adenoma or carcinoma should prompt the screening of other members of the family.

NON-ADENOMATOUS POLYPS

Inflammatory polyps usually require no specific treatment, any management being directed at the causative colitis. Most are small or worm-like, often capped with characteristic white slough. Occasionally larger polyps, composed of granulation tissue, are best removed by snare polypectomy to avoid anxiety.

Metaplastic (hyperplastic) polyps are found on routine proctosigmoidoscopy in at least 10% of patients. They are rarely greater than 5 mm across and usually appear as shiny hemispherical lesions. Occasionally they are pedunculated. Metaplastic polyps are of no pathological significance and probably do not cause symptoms. It is, however, impossible on appearance to distinguish a metaplastic polyp from an adenoma and they should be removed entirely for histological examination. When the histology is confirmed and provided no other type of pathological lesion has been found, no further follow-up is needed.

Often they are multiple and sometimes examination of the colon reveals them in great numbers. The possibility of metaplastic polyposis should be recognised, since it may cause confusion with adenomatous polyposis but does not require surgery.

Juvenile polyps may be solitary or multiple and usually present in childhood or adolescence; juvenile polyposis occasionally occurs. The question of cancer risk is uncertain but, if it exists, the risk must be very low. A juvenile polyp may only declare itself with a brisk bleed from the remaining stalk after having undergone spontaneous 'auto-amputation'.

A double contrast barium enema is indicated to define the number of polyps present and snare-polypectomy is usually easy because of the narrow stalk. Multiple polypectomies are rapidly· possible at colonoscopy because it is unnecessary to retrieve more than a few samples for histology. Surgery is never indicated.

Peutz-Jeghers polyps occur as part of a Mendelian-dominant inherited disorder. Large bowel polyps are only part of the problem presented since symptoms are frequently due to the small bowel lesions, presenting with abdominal pain due to intussusception. Less commonly the lesions may bleed or cause anaemia. The finding of pigmented lesions around the mouth and anus and within the buccal cavity makes the diagnosis.

Radiological investigation of the whole intestine should be carried out, including barium small bowel follow-through and enema examinations.

Intestinal obstruction or intermittent intussusception require surgery to avoid infarction of small intestine. This is likely to involve removal of polyps at different sites along the small bowel through multiple enterotomies. Several operations may be required at intervals of a few years if further large polyps develop in the small intestine. Those in the stomach, duodenum and colon are easily removed by endoscopic polypectomies, mainly to avoid anaemia. Carcinomas have been reported in the duodenum but surveillance is probably unnecessary.

TECHNIQUES OF POLYPECTOMY

Colonoscopic polypectomy

A prerequisite for efficient and safe rectal or colonic polypectomy by any means is successful bowel preparation. This is necessary in order to see the lesion properly, and to avoid both electrical current leakage and the additional possibility of an explosion hazard. Colonic bacteria ferment amino-acids and carbohydrates to methane and hydrogen respectively and unless the whole bowel has been completely cleansed carbon dioxide should be insufflated (extreme care being taken to aspirate and re-insufflate several times) before electrocoagulation (Cotton and Williams, 1980).

Polypectomy is usually quick and easy, since 90% of polyps are under 2 cm diameter and have relatively thin stalks. What is less easy is to ensure that the snare loop is accurately placed a short way down the stalk (so that the pathologist gets a proper assessment of the base of the polyp) and then to ensure that full electrocoagulation has occurred before cutting through with the polypectomy snare wire. The electrosurgical unit is used on low power (25–75 watt range) and on a coagulation or blended current setting. Any fibre-optic scope is suitable for polypectomy, usually using one of the convenient commercially-available snare loops; with the low power setting used the procedure is extremely safe and controlled. Only very thick (over 1 cm) stalks or broad-based (over 2 cm) polyps present significant risk of haemorrhage or perforation respectively, and these should be left to an experienced endoscopist. Above the rectum the majority of small (2–7 mm) polyps prove to be adenomatous and are quickly biopsied and destroyed using the 'hot-biopsy' technique with purpose-made insulated biopsy forceps transmitting electrosurgical current through the pulled-up polyp base (Fig. 1.43).

Piecemeal removal of many large polyps is possible by repeated snare polypectomies if surgery is clinically contra-indicated. Partial removal of a large lesion, especially if malignancy is suspected, will give the pathologist a 'snare-loop biopsy' without any risk to the patient. The tissue-damaging effect of electrocoagulation will sometimes destroy the base of an apparently unremoved lesion, so that a check examination may be wise before subsequent operation.

Multiple polyps may necessitate repeated passage of the instrument in order to retrieve the specimens accurately for the pathologist, although if more than five to ten polyps are seen it is important to look for (and biopsy) other smaller polyps in case partial colectomy is the more logical long-term management. The smaller polyps may only be made visible using a dilute dye (washable blue ink) to show up surface detail – the 'dye-spray technique'.

Peranal techniques

Submucosal excision

After preparation of the bowel with two phosphate enemas the patient is anaesthetised, placed in the lithotomy position and an anal self-retaining retractor passed. If the polyp is easily accessible, no form of traction is necessary. If not, the tumour may be brought to a lower position in the rectum by means of stay sutures placed around it or by traction on tissue forceps applied to the mucosa in its vicinity. Owing to the mobility of the rectal wall, tumours as high as 15 cm from the anal verge can often be brought down to the level of the anorectal ring. Using this method, it may even be possible to deliver sigmoid adenomas by intussusception to a position sufficiently accessible to carry out submucosal excision.

An adrenaline-saline solution (1:300 000) is injected from a syringe into the submucosa underlying the tumour (Fig. 8.11). This raises the mucosa and tumour from the rectal wall muscle. An incision into the mucosa about 5 mm from the lower edge of the tumour is made with sharp scissors and this is continued on each side around its perimeter. The mucosa bearing the tumour is then separated from the rectal wall by further scissor dissection during which fibres of the circular muscle will be seen (Fig. 8.12). The excised specimen should be removed in one piece if possible. It is desirable to pin it out on a cork slab before fixation (Fig. 8.13) since this orientation is most helpful to the pathologist in his assessment as to whether invasion of the muscularis mucosae has occurred. The rectal mucosal defect is usually left to heal by secondary intention but can be closed with sutures (Fig. 8.14). Bleeding points are coagulated with the diathermy. This technique can be used to remove sessile tumours of the rectal mucosa involving the entire circumference extending to its upper reaches but it may be necessary to reline

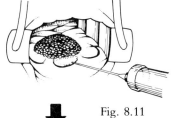

Fig. 8.11

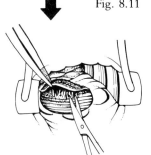

Fig. 8.12

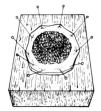

Fig. 8.13

265

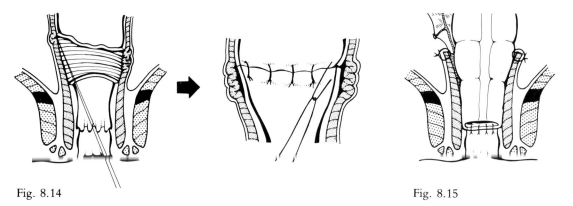

Fig. 8.14   Fig. 8.15

the rectal muscle tube with colon to avoid stricturing (Fig. 8.15) (Parks, 1966).

Full thickness
excision

There may be some doubt from the pre-operative assessment that a sessile tumour is entirely benign and in these circumstances it is safer to carry out a full thickness excision in preference to submucosal removal. This technique differs only in taking the circumferential incision through all layers of the rectum, removing thereby the tumour on a plaque of rectal wall. The defect is sutured after taking care to stop bleeding from the exposed perirectal fat. This technique is only suitable in those parts of the rectum not covered by peritoneum.

Diathermy snare

The principle is similar to colonoscopic snare excision. In the rectum this may be carried out through a rigid sigmoidoscope. A wire snare mounted on a rigid insulated shaft is placed around the pedicle. The snare is closed by means of a slide on the handle of the shaft and current is then applied. The polyp must be retrieved and the site of its removal inspected for bleeding.

Diathermy
fulguration

With the techniques of removal available, there should be little need for this method of treatment. It is used to control symptoms of extensive lesions in patients considered too infirm to tolerate any other form of local therapy, to destroy small areas of residual or recurrent adenoma after local excision or adenomas developing in the rectal stump of patients with adenomatous polyposis after colectomy with ileorectal anastomosis. There is no place for diathermy destruction as a first line of treatment in the fit patient since the lesion cannot be examined by the pathologist.

266

FAMILIAL ADENOMATOUS POLYPOSIS

Familial adenomatous polyposis is a general neoplastic disorder of the intestine and although the large bowel is predominantly affected, lesions occur in the stomach, duodenum and small intestine in a significant proportion of cases. The main risk is large bowel carcinoma but duodenal and ampullary carcinomas have been reported. It is inherited as a Mendelian-dominant, males and females being equally affected, and there is no racial predisposition. Familial adenomatous polyposis can also occur sporadically, without family history, presumably by mutation; there is, however, usually a family history of large bowel cancer occurring in young adulthood or middle age suggesting pre-existing adenomatosis (Bussey, 1975).

Multiple intestinal adenomas may be associated with benign mesodermal tumours, such as desmoid tumours and osteomas; epidermoid cysts also occur (Gardner's syndrome). Intra-abdominal desmoid tumours can cause serious problems because, although non-metastasising, they invade locally to involve the intestinal mesentery and are then unresectable.

Natural history

It is rare for affected individuals to develop adenomatous polyps before adolescence but polyps are usually visible on sigmoidoscopy by 15 years and will almost always be visible before the age of 30. Carcinoma of the large bowel occurs in all patients if followed for long enough; one or more cancers will already be present in two-thirds of those presenting with symptoms.

The average age of clinical presentation is 36 years with a reported range from four to over 70 years. Patients may be symptomatic or asymptomatic.

Symptomatic patients are either new propositi or those belonging to affected families who have not attended a screening clinic; they are likely already to have a cancer. Their symptoms are the same as those that occur in non-familial large bowel neoplasia. Polyps are seen on sigmoidoscopy, the diagnosis of adenomas is made histologically on biopsies and the number and distribution of polyps (or cancers) shown on air contrast barium enema. If in doubt colonoscopy is performed with further biopsies to establish the number and histological type of polyps; with at least 100 adenomas the diagnosis can be made with confidence and it is essential not to misdiagnose one of the non-neoplastic forms of polyposis.

Asymptomatic patients are usually members of affected families attending a screening clinic and found to have one or more polyps on sigmoidoscopy. There is no means of knowing whether an individual is affected unless adenomas develop and, although this is unlikely if there are no adenomas by the thirtieth year, screening should be continued for life. If the diagnosis is made during adolescence, operation is normally deferred until socially convenient, usually at 17–18 years, since there is no significant risk of carcinoma before this age.

Treatment

Treatment is the same for all affected patients. It consists of three parts:

Total colectomy with ileorectal anastomosis.
Regular follow-up.
Screening of the family.

Colectomy with ileorectal anastomosis is the usual operation since this avoids an ileostomy in a young patient. The rectum is subsequently cleared of polyps by electrosurgical snaring or fulguration and the patient is examined by sigmoidoscopy at three-monthly intervals thereafter. It is helpful to know the distance of the anastomosis from the anal verge; this distance should be recorded at the original operation and should not be greater than 15 cm.

Recurrent rectal adenomas are removed or fulgurated *per anum*. Areas suggesting malignant change should be biopsied.

Despite this policy a proportion of patients develop carcinoma in the rectal stump. The risk of carcinoma in the St. Mark's series of 140 cases was 10% over a period of 30 years (Bussey, 1979) and this experience suggests that with regular surveillance of the rectum the policy of colectomy with ileorectal anastomosis is reasonable at the present time. However, an incidence of carcinoma in over 50% of patients followed for over 20 years after ileorectal or ileosigmoid anastomosis has been reported from the Mayo Clinic (Moertel, Hill and Adson, 1970) where proctocolectomy with ileostomy has become the primary procedure in the last ten years. To remove the risk of cancer without stoma formation the ideal procedure may prove to be some form of sphincter-saving proctocolectomy such as the ileal pouch with an anal anastomosis (Chapter 4).

Examination of blood relatives, including cousins, nephews and nieces is essential. Family trees should be constructed (Fig. 8.10) and a register of affected families maintained. Children at risk should be seen for sigmoidoscopy or fibresigmoidoscopy every two years from the thirteenth year and followed indefinitely, although with less frequent visits, after thirty years. Barium enema or total colonoscopy are only needed if adenomas are found distally.

REFERENCES AND FURTHER READING

Bussey HJR. *Familial polyposis coli*. Baltimore and London: The Johns Hopkins University Press, 1975.

Bussey HJR. Familial polyposis coli. *Pathology Annual* 1979; **14:** 61–81.

Cotton PB and Williams CB. *Practical gastrointestinal endoscopy*. London: Blackwell, 1980.

Moertel CG, Hill JR and Adson MA. Surgical management of multiple polypsis. The problem of cancer in the retained bowel segment. *Archives of Surgery* 1970; **100:** 521–6.

Parks AG. Benign tumours of the rectum In: Rob C, Smith R and Morgan CN, eds. *Clinical surgery: abdomen, rectum and anus* London: Butterworths, 1966; 541–8.

Thomson JPS. Treatment of sessile villous and tubulovillous adenomas of the rectum. *Diseases of the Colon and Rectum* 1977; **20:** 467–72.

Todd IP, ed. *Colon, rectum and anus. (3rd ed. Operative surgery)*, London and Boston; Butterworths, 1977.

MANAGEMENT OF MALIGNANT TUMOURS – SURGERY

At the present time the best chance of cure for a patient with cancer of the large bowel is obtained by a radical surgical operation, that is, one which aims to remove the growth and an adequate margin of normal tissue and the related lymphatic field. Occasionally removal of the tumour without removal of any circumferential part of the bowel wall suffices for a very early malignant tumour, such as a pedunculated polyp with malignant change. Radiotherapy alone will occasionally result in cure, but the results of radical surgery have proved to be so good that few would recommend radiotherapy as an alternative to surgery in an operable case.

PRE-OPERATIVE ASSESSMENT

The treatment of large bowel cancer requires major abdominal surgery and the age and general condition of the patient must be taken into account before deciding whether that patient is fit to undergo such procedures. Usually this is best done in conjunction with an anaesthetist, but sometimes the opinion of a general physician will be required when there are cardiac, respiratory or metabolic problems. Sometimes the operation can be deferred for a week or two in order to correct cardiac failure or stabilise a diabetic state.

Apart from the general condition of the patient, the surgeon must try before deciding about operation to assess the spread of the tumour and, in particular, to determine if there is such widespread dissemination that laparotomy may not be justified; for instance, if there is evidence of gross ascites, lymph node involvement in the neck, gross hepatic enlargement or complete fixity of the tumour. Pre-operative investigations should also include a chest x-ray looking for evidence of pulmonary metastases, and in some cases a liver scan may be advisable. In cases where large or fixed tumours are present at the pelvic brim or within the pelvis, a pre-operative intravenous urogram is advisable to see if there is any displacement of the ureters or pressure on them leading to hydronephrosis. Occasionally a pre-operative cystoscopy may be valuable.

In every case of large bowel cancer both a pre-operative sigmoidoscopy and a double contrast barium enema are necessary in order that second tumours in the bowel may be firmly excluded. In over 20% of patients with large bowel cancer an adenoma is present somewhere else within the large bowel and in approximately 3% of cases a second primary cancer is also present.

It is important to prepare the bowel before surgery. This consists first of mechanical clearance and, secondly, the use of antibacterial agents aimed to reduce the bacterial population in the lumen (Chapter 4).

COLONIC CARCINOMA

Growths of the right colon are best approached through a long right paramedian and those in the left half through a long left paramedian incision. A careful laparotomy is performed to exclude co-existing disease. The liver is examined for metastases and, if possible, a direct view obtained of any nodules within it, since small cysts may be mistaken for secondary deposits in the liver. Examination of the whole colon is made for multiple primary growths, though the pre-operative barium enema should have determined this point. Para-aortic and regional lymph nodes are examined and finally an assessment of the mobility of the primary tumour is made. The decision can now be made whether to go ahead with removal of the tumour

270

or whether some lesser palliative procedure is all that is possible.

If it is decided to go ahead with resection, both the growth and sufficient colon on each side are mobilised. Turnbull, Kyle, Watson *et al*., (1967) have advocated that all the vessels leading from the tumour should be ligated and divided before any mobilisation of the tumour is undertaken, in order to prevent dissemination of malignant cells. It is by no means clear that this 'isolation technique' leads to better survival rates (Hawley, 1974) and sometimes it makes the operation more difficult and more hazardous. It has not been adopted generally. After adequate mobilisation the vessels of the mesocolon are then divided so as to remove a wide area of vascular and lymphatic field. It is less important to remove a wide area of bowel around the primary tumour and probably a margin of 5–8 cm on each side of the tumour is sufficient.

Resection for carcinoma of the caecum and ascending colon is the standard right hemicolectomy, removing the last few centimetres of terminal ileum, caecum, ascending colon, hepatic flexure and a little of the right transverse colon, with ligation of the ileocolic and right colic arteries at their origins from the superior mesenteric. Hepatic flexure growths require resection of that area of bowel, ligating the right and middle colic arteries and relying on the ascending left colic to supply the distal colon. Transverse colon growths require ligation of the middle colic artery at its origin, which may involve removal of much of the transverse colon but ensuring good supply to both ends remaining. Growths of the splenic flexure and left colon need ligation of the left branch of the middle colic and of the ascending left colic arteries at their origins, while growths of the sigmoid colon require ligation of sigmoid arteries at their origin from the inferior mesenteric.

A more radical removal for growths of the left and sigmoid colon involves ligation of the inferior mesenteric artery at its origin from the aorta. Here, mobilisation of the splenic flexure is necessary in order to carry out an anastomosis with a good blood supply between the left part of the transverse colon and the upper part of the rectum, which is supplied by the inferior and middle haemorrhoidal arteries. After adequate mobilisation and removal of the specimen, the two ends of bowel are brought together without tension after ensuring that both ends to be anastomosed have a good blood supply. If these conditions are not fulfilled, further mobilisation is necessary; an anastomosis under tension or with impaired blood supply to either end of bowel is likely to leak.

There is some risk that exfoliated carcinoma cells in the lumen of the colon, adjacent to the tumour, may become implanted on the suture-line in the bowel. Suture-line recurrence occurs in up to 5% of patients in various reported series. Some of these cases appear to result from growth into the lumen from local recurrence outside the bowel wall. Nevertheless, it is worth attempting to reduce the risk of implantation at the time of surgery by irrigating the two ends of bowel with distilled water or a cancericidial solution, such as 1% cetrimide or perchloride of mercury (1:1000). It would seem that these preparations can do little harm and may prevent some suture-line recurrences.

End-to-end anastomosis is most conveniently carried out by the open method. Some surgeons prefer a single layer technique using interrupted non-absorbable material placed as mattress sutures to invert the bowel. Others prefer to use a two layer inverting anastomosis, most usually with an outer layer of interrupted seromuscular silk sutures and an inner layer of continuous catgut taking the full thickness of bowel. Differences in size between the two ends of bowel to be joined can usually be overcome, but sometimes one end may need to be trimmed or enlarged before the anastomosis can be started. On completion of the anastomosis the defect in the mesentery is closed by continuous catgut or interrupted silk sutures. The abdomen can then be closed. The use of drains is a matter of individual preference. Many surgeons do not drain intra-peritoneal anastomoses, but some prefer to do so, bringing the drain out through a stab incision for a few days (Chapter 4).

RECTAL CARCINOMA

Choice of operation

The early operations for rectal cancer by limited perineal amputation or sleeve resections done through the postrectal space were inadequate cancer operations which led to a high local recurrence and a low cure rate. Over 70 years ago, Miles published his researches into the spread of rectal cancer and emphasised the importance of extensive removal of the lymphatic field (Miles, 1908). He advocated a combined abdominal and perineal operation, removing the entire rectum and anal region with ligation of the vessels and lymphatic field at the level of the aorta. Miles believed that there was extensive spread of tumour cells in the lymphatics distal to the tumour, as well as proximal to it and, therefore, advocated a combined excision in every case. However, the work of Dukes and others during the 1930s showed that lymphatic and intramural spread beyond 2 cm below the tumour were extremely rare, occurring in only about 2% of cases. Even in these it rarely extended to more than 2.5 cm and then only in cases with advanced spread or with high grade tumours. It was, therefore, realised that for growths in the upper rectum an adequate cancer operation could be

272

undertaken with preservation of the lower rectum, thus preserving the anal sphincter. The most widely used restorative operation is the anterior resection. Other forms of sphincter-saving operations are technically more difficult, have a high complication rate and do not give quite such good functional results. Nevertheless, they have a place in surgical practice in certain cases.

Careful pre-operative examination should assess the size of the rectal tumour, the distance of its lower edge from the anal verge and its degree of clinical fixity. A biopsy will give the surgeon some guide as to whether the tumour is well or poorly differentiated. An anterior resection is usually possible for tumours above 10 cm, depending to some degree on the obesity and sex of the patient. Growths in the lower third of the rectum certainly require an excision, whereas growths between 7 and 10 cm may sometimes be treated by restorative procedures, and others by excision of the rectum. If a tumour is reported to be of a high grade malignancy, restorative procedures may be unwise unless local conditions are found to be very favourable at operation, owing to the high chance of local recurrence. Over the last 15 years, there has been a trend towards using the restorative resection increasingly for growths involving the mid-rectum, which does not appear to have vitiated the five year survival rate.

Restorative resection

It is usually possible to carry out an anterior resection, with a sutured anastomosis from the abdomen, with tumours above 10 cm in women and perhaps a little higher than that in men, but the technical difficulties depend largely on the build of the patient. For growths at about that level no definite decision about what will be done should be made until the abdomen has been opened and the growth assessed directly. It may be found, for instance, that the tumour is larger than expected or appears to be disseminating locally. Under such conditions it may be unwise to do an anterior resection and preferable to do an excision of the rectum. On the other hand, a growth initially thought to be amenable to only total excision of the rectum may, after mobilisation, be found suitable for a restorative operation.

For growths between 7 and 10 cm from the anal verge an anterior resection is often still possible using a hand-sutured anastomosis. A low abdominal anastomosis may, however, be made easier by the use of a circular stapling device (Fig. 4.10) although it does not, *per se,* enable an anastomosis to be performed any lower than was possible using previous established techniques. Thus, it is also possible to excise the entire

rectum and restore intestinal continuity by a peranal anastomosis, or by sacro-abdominal or abdomino-anal pull-through
techniques. The essential question to consider with these low
anastomoses is the radicality of the operation. A 5 cm length of
rectum below the tumour was recommended as a safe margin of
excision in the early days of anterior resection (Goligher, Dukes
and Bussey, 1951). In recent years, on occasions, this has
become reduced. Whether local recurrence rates will increase as
a consequence remains to be seen.

Anterior resection

There is a distinction between high anterior resection with
the anastomosis lying above the peritoneal reflexion and low
anterior resection in which it is performed below the reflexion.
The incidence of some degree of anastomotic dehiscence is
about five times greater with the latter. The growth should be
mobile without evidence of local spread and the pre-operative
biopsy should have shown the tumour to be of average or low
grade of malignancy.

The patient is placed on the operating table in the lithotomy-
Trendelenburg position (Fig. 4.5). The abdomen is opened, the
vascular pedicle ligated and the rectum mobilised below the
tumour. In order to ensure an adequate length of proximal
colon to bring down to the distal rectum without tension it is
usually necessary to mobilise the splenic flexure. Limitation of
length tends to be due to blood vessels, particularly the inferior
mesenteric artery and its lower left colic branch. These may
require division, leaving the colon supplied by the marginal
artery. The marginal artery is, therefore, vital and great care
must be taken not to damage it. An adequate blood flow can be
inferred if it is seen to be pulsating. The point of proximal
division is selected to allow a sufficient length of bowel to reach
the rectum. This is usually in the region of the mid to upper
sigmoid colon. Clamps are applied and the bowel is divided. A
right-angled clamp is then placed across the rectum 5 cm below
the lower margin of the tumour and the rectum washed out
through the anus by an assistant so that all faecal matter and any
malignant cells that may have exfoliated from the surface of the
growth are removed. Solutions such as distilled water or
perchloride of mercury (1:1000) may be used. The rectum is
divided below the clamp and the specimen removed.

Resection with
peranal anastomosis

Most of the abdominal operation is done as for the low
anterior resection. It is almost always necessary to mobilise the
splenic flexure. After removal of the specimen, the proximal
colon is passed through the anal canal to a second surgeon. An
anastomosis of interrupted sutures is carried out by the perineal

operator through the dilated anal canal between colon and anal canal (Fig. 4.14). This anastomosis is often technically rather difficult.

Following this operation there is a greater risk of some degree of anastomotic breakdown and of pelvic haematoma and sepsis, and it is, therefore, usually wise to carry out a transverse colostomy. If all goes well the colostomy can be closed within a few weeks.

The actual technique that a surgeon uses to accomplish excision of the rectum will depend largely on his own training and experience and on the facilities and help available to him. The following two techniques are those most usually practised today.

Excision of the rectum

For a synchronous combined excision of the rectum the patient is positioned on the operating table in the lithotomy – Trendelenburg position so that both an abdominal operator and a perineal operator can work at the same time. The abdominal operator explores the abdomen, ties the vascular pedicle and mobilises the rectum from above, whilst the perineal operator dissects the anal canal and rectum from below. After removal of the rectum the abdominal operator closes the pelvic peritoneum, establishes the colostomy in the left iliac fossa and closes the abdomen. The perineal operator, meanwhile, either closes the perineum loosely round a drain in the sacral hollow or carries out primary suture of the perineal wound with suction drainage to the presacral space.

Synchronous combined excision

This technique is to be preferred, for all aspects of the operation can be carefully controlled throughout, especially with regard to blood loss. It is particularly suitable where there are large adherent growths, as the two surgeons are often able to help each other in their safe removal. The procedure does, however, require the special table fittings for correct positioning of the patient and the simultaneous presence of two operating teams.

Abdominoperineal excision of the rectum (Miles operation) is probably more widely practised throughout the world than any other. The operation is done mainly from the abdomen, with early ligation of the vascular pedicle and full mobilisation of the rectum down to the pelvic floor. The bowel is divided in the sigmoid colon and the proximal end brought out as a

Abdominoperineal excision

terminal colostomy. The distal sigmoid and mobilised rectum are pushed into the pelvis and the pelvic peritoneum closed before closing the abdomen. The patient is then turned on his side and the operation completed through a perineal approach removing the anal canal and lower rectum, closing the perineal wound loosely with a large drain in the pelvic cavity.

This operation has stood the test of time and is usually easily accomplished, but it may sometimes be difficult in a fat patient to push the specimen below the pelvic peritoneum and close the latter satisfactorily.

Special problems

Liver metastases

The presence of metastatic deposits in the liver is not normally a contraindication to removal of the primary tumour, and this is usually still advisable for palliative reasons. Many such patients have lived in reasonably good health for as long as 18 months or two years. The occasional patient may survive three or four years.

Extended operations

Primary tumours of the colon may be adherent to surrounding structures, such as stomach, small gut, omentum, pelvic viscera or the abdominal wall, and it may sometimes be necessary to excise all or part of the related viscus. Not infrequently, the adhesions are inflammatory and not due to malignant infiltration, so that the prognosis after such radical excision is often much better than might have been expected at the time of operation.

Other viscera may also need to be removed *en bloc* with the rectum when the primary tumour is locally adherent. In the female the posterior vaginal wall, the uterus, tubes and ovaries can be removed without greatly increasing the hazards of the operation. In the male, part of the bladder base and the vesicles can sometimes be excised with the primary tumour. It is where such extended operations are necessary that the synchronous combined operation will be found particularly valuable.

An extension of the operation which appears logical and desirable may be achieved by ligating the inferior mesenteric artery at its origin from the aorta, rather than at the level of the aortic bifurcation as originally described by Miles. The 'high ligation' removes an extra 2–4 cm of vascular and lymphatic pedicle, increasing the amount of lymphatic and vascular clearance. Many surgeons only practise high ligation when there are definite indications; i.e. when a pre-operative biopsy has shown an anaplastic tumour, or when palpable lymph nodes extend up to the origin of the artery. Others use it routinely when performing a radical resection. There is little information on the benefit or otherwise of this manoeuvre in terms of five year survival.

A further extension of the operation advocated by some surgeons is that of pelvic lymphadenectomy; i.e. removal of the lymph nodes along the common and internal iliac arteries. However, this step increases the hazards of the operation and considerably increases the postoperative morbidity particularly with regard to urinary function. Again, it is doubtful whether long-term survival is increased. Though this procedure is justified in the occasional case, it should not become part of the routine operation for excision of the rectum.

Loaded bowel

Ideally, patients coming to elective operation for bowel carcinoma should have a virtually empty colon after suitable mechanical preparation with laxatives or washouts. This is not always achieved, however, and many patients, particularly those with constricting tumours, are found at laparotomy to have a moderately loaded bowel proximal to the lesion. If faecal loading is gross it may be better to abandon the operation, establish a proximal colostomy and return in two or three weeks' time to remove the tumour under better operation conditions. Alternatively, the bowel may be washed out on the operating table by using a suitable apparatus so that it may be done aseptically, or the surgeon may feel justified in proceeding to resection with anastomosis, taking particular care to avoid contamination at the time and establishing a proximal colostomy at the end of the operation.

If contamination from the lumen of the bowel does occur during the anastomosis it is advisable to wash the affected area of peritoneum with chlorhexidine (1:5000) so that all particulate matter is removed from the peritoneal cavity. Antibacterial agents should be given if this has not already been done. The area of anastomosis and probably the subcutaneous tissues of the wound should also be drained.

Temporary defunctioning loop colostomy

A temporary colostomy should be considered in operations where either the chance of anastomotic dehiscence is high or where the consequence of dehiscence would be particularly serious. The following circumstances are examples of the need for such a colostomy: low colorectal or colo-anal anastomosis, where the anastomosis has been particularly difficult, where there is a degree of obstruction, in cases with gross faecal loading and in extended pelvic resection including bladder and uterus.

The colostomy is closed usually after a period of several weeks, provided the anastomosis has healed and any pelvic sepsis has resolved. If the delay is too long, there is a possibility that the anastomosis will become narrow, lacking the dilating effect of passing faeces.

Local excision

A purely local excision of the lesion may be justified for small protuberant carcinomas in the lower rectum, particularly in patients who are very elderly or in some other way at increased risk from major surgery. The policy of local excision as a curative procedure relies on the fact that there is a low incidence of lymph node metastases of between 5 and 10% with these smaller carcinomas. A suitable growth has the following features. It should not measure more than 3 cm across, it must be mobile and there should be no palpable extrarectal spread or enlarged postrectal lymph nodes. High-grade tumours and those occupying the circumference of the bowel are excluded.

A local excision involves the removal of the growth with a surrounding margin of normal full thickness rectal wall. It can usually be carried out by operating through the dilated anus by aid of special retractors, but sometimes a trans-sphincteric approach from behind, as described by York Mason (1977) may be preferable. The defect in the rectal wall is closed by primary suture. The excised specimen must be submitted to the most careful examination by the pathologist. If it is reported that the tumour is of high-grade of malignancy or has not been completely excised, then a radical operation should be considered.

ANAL CANAL AND ANAL MARGIN CARCINOMA

Choice of operation

Before deciding about the treatment, the tumour must be carefully assessed, if necessary by examination under anaesthesia. The surgeon not only needs to know the histological nature of the tumour but the extent of its local spread, whether there are palpable lymph nodes behind the rectum which would indicate involvement of the superior haemorrhoidal nodes and whether there are nodes palpable in the inguinal region.

Treatment depends on the pathological nature of the tumour as shown by biopsy. Anal canal carcinoma should be treated by synchronous combined excision of the rectum. The perineal skin should be excised widely, the fatty contents of the ischiorectal fossa must be removed and the levator ani muscles divided close to the pelvic wall.

Unless very extensive, squamous cell carcinoma of the anal margin is a relatively more benign disease and is best treated by wide local excision. The lower half of the internal sphincter, together with a part of the adjacent external sphincter and the surrounding ischiorectal fat, should be excised with the tumour. It is, of course, necessary to preserve the upper half of both sphincter groups in order to maintain anal continence. The large wound so produced may be easily covered by a skin graft or may be left open to heal by secondary intention. If extensive, the growth should be removed by radical excision of the rectum.

Involved inguinal nodes should be treated by bilateral block dissection of the groins, the five-year survival being less than 20% in these patients. It should not be used as a prophylactic measure in patients with clinically uninvolved nodes since survival is not improved and the operation itself has a morbidity. These latter patients should be followed at monthly intervals after the primary operation and block dissection carried out if metastatic nodes subsequently develop. Their appearance is most likely within the first six months of primary treatment. With this policy, five year survival rates of over 40% can be obtained.

Inguinal lymph nodes

Radiotherapy has an important place in the management of squamous carcinoma of the anal canal (see following section).

Radiotherapy

RESULTS

The operative mortality after radical surgery is around 5% with little difference between restorative procedures and total excision of the rectum in most reported series; it rises to above 10% when these operations are used as palliative treatment. Despite operability rates of over 90% in specialist centres, 20% of patients have incurable disease when first seen; this rises to above 30% in district general hospitals. These patients rarely live for more than a year although survival for three years or more with disseminated disease occasionally occurs. The survival after radical excision of large bowel cancer depends on the pathological stage and histological grade of the tumour. It is worse in patients who present with intestinal obstruction or perforation and also in young adults and negroes. Corrected five-year survival for the Dukes' stages and histological grades are shown in Table 8j and 8k (Lockhart-Mummery, Ritchie and Hawley, 1976). Treatment failures are due to the development of disseminated disease or local recurrence or to both. Reported rates of local recurrence range from around 10 to over 20% and are higher after removal of high grade tumours. There appears to be no difference either in five-year survival, or local recurrence after restorative operations or total rectal excision when used to treat tumours of similar pathological types.

Colon and rectum

279

Table 8j. *Survival after radical surgery for carcinoma of the large bowel*

Stage	Corrected five-year survival
A	95–100%
B	65– 75%
C1	30– 40%
C2	10– 20%

Table 8k *Survival after radical surgery for carcinoma of the large bowel*

Grade	Corrected five-year survival
Well differentiated	80– 90%
Moderately differentiated	60– 70%
Poorly differentiated	25– 30%

The five-year survival of tumours treated by local excision is over 90% where excision is complete, but it must be remembered that these comprise a small group of selected carcinomas.

*Anal canal
and anal margin*

The crude five-year survival for well-differentiated squamous carcinoma is about 80%, for moderately differentiated 50% and for poorly differentiated tumours less than 30%. With involvement of local nodes, survival falls from 60 to 20–30%. The prognosis is slightly better for tumours of the anal verge compared with those in the anal canal; thus overall five year survival for anal canal cancer is about 40% compared to over 50% for cancer of the anal margin.

REFERENCES AND FURTHER READING

Dukes CE. The spread of cancer of the rectum. Introduction to the treatment of carcinoma of the rectum by radium. *British Journal of Surgery* 1930; **17**: 643–69.

Goligher JC, Dukes CE and Bussey HJR. Local recurrences after sphincter-saving excisions for carcinoma of the rectum and recto-sigmoid. *British Journal of Surgery* 1951; **39**: 3–15.

Hawley PR. Carcinoma of the colon. *British Journal of Hospital Medicine* 1974; **11**: 211–16.

Lockhart-Mummery HE, Ritchie JK and Hawley PR. The results of surgical treatment of carcinoma of the rectum at St. Mark's Hospital from 1948–1972. *British Journal of Surgery* 1976; **63**: 673–7.

Mason AY. Trans-sphincteric resection: In: Todd IP, ed. *Colon, rectum and anus*. (3rd ed. operative surgery) London and Boston: Butterworths, 1977: 178–90.

Miles WE. A method of performing abdominoperineal excision for carcinoma of the rectum and of the terminal portion of the pelvic colon. *Lancet* 1908; **2**: 1812–13.

Turnbull RB, Kyle K, Watson FR and Spratt J. Cancer of the colon. Influence of the no-touch technic on survival rates. *Annals of Surgery* 1967; **166:** 420–7.

MANAGEMENT OF MALIGNANT TUMOURS – RADIOTHERAPY

The role of radiotherapy in the management of colorectal cancer has been evaluated with increasing interest since the introduction of megavoltage x-ray machines. Equipment of this type (Linear Accelerators, Betatrons and Telecobalt machines) provide high energy, deeply penetrating beams of radiation that may readily be concentrated around deep-seated tumours within the abdomen or pelvis while sparing overlying skin and other normal tissues.

The belief that gastro-intestinal adenocarcinomas are radio-resistant is quite erroneous. In the past, radiotherapy has tended to be used only for the treatment of large and inoperable cancers. With such advanced tumour the probability of obtaining a complete response with acceptable doses of radiation was negligible. It is now known that there is no consistent difference in the radiosensitivity of normal and tumour cells. The apparent differences in responsiveness are principally a reflection of the range of proliferation rates of cells within tissues since mammalian cells normally die after radiation damage only when required to divide. Intestinal epithelium, with its high cell turnover, will quickly demonstrate radiation damage, while adenocarcinoma (with a slower rate of cell division) will respond more slowly. It has been shown that rectal adenocarcinoma takes an average of six months to regress completely following x-ray therapy compared to three months for squamous cancers of comparable size arising elsewhere (Rider, 1975). This slow regression is often mistaken for radio-resistance.

While surgery remains the treatment of choice for cancers of the large bowel, radiotherapy can be of value in the primary management of inoperable tumours or in patients unfit for surgery. It may also have an adjuvant role in the management of operable cancers and may be used to good effect in the palliation of patients with locally advanced cancers.

Primary treatment

High dose radiotherapy is required for good local tumour control, and this can be done with a low morbidity. Williams and Horwitz (1956) reported a series of 220 patients with inoperable rectal cancer treated by high dose megavoltage radiation alone; 5% survived five years, suggesting that radiotherapy can be curative. Rider (1975) obtained a 29% five-year survival (almost twice as good as in historical controls) in 38 patients with inoperable rectal cancer.

Primary radiotherapy has also been given to well differentiated superficial cancers of the rectum by intracavitary low voltage irradiation. Papillon (1975), who first described this technique, has reported a five-year survival of 78%. Similar results using this technique have been obtained by others but, of course, surgical methods such as local excision or electrocoagulation may be equally effective in this selected type of cancer. It certainly demonstrates, however, that adenocarcinoma does respond to radiation with negligible morbidity. In order further to improve the results of radiotherapy in rectosigmoid cancer it has been suggested that added 5-fluorouracil might increase local tumour control; there is no good evidence for this without an increase in normal tissue morbidity and its use is no longer advised.

Adjuvant treatment (radiotherapy and operation)

The theoretical aim of pre-operative radiotherapy is to reduce the number of viable cells in the tumour with the hope of diminishing the chance of dissemination at operation and reducing the incidence of local recurrence and metastases. A trial at Memorial Hospital, New York, showed no difference in five-year survival in patients treated by low-dose pre-operative radiotherapy (2000–2500 rads in 10 daily fractions) compared to those treated by surgery alone (Stearns, Deddish, Quan et al., 1974) but this study did not consist entirely of randomly allocated patients. Shortly after, the Veterans' Administration conducted a randomised controlled trial with a similar protocol (Roswit, Higgins and Keehn, 1975). In 414 patients subjected to abdominoperineal excision the irradiated group had a significantly higher five year survival rate of 41% compared to 28% in the control group; there was no benefit to the patients who had other forms of resection. The proportion with lymph node metastases was lower in the irradiated group (24% compared to 38%) although it is not certain whether this was due to the irradiation. An improved survival after high dose pre-operative radiotherapy (4500 rads in 25 daily fractions) has been reported by Kligerman (1975) but the number of patients in this study was small. Further evaluation of pre-operative adjuvant radiotherapy is required.

Immediate postoperative high dose radiotherapy for residual cancer has not been popular because of the high morbidity, especially radiation enteropathy. Its role has not been well defined and it is not recommended as a routine form of primary management.

Palliative treatment

Radiotherapy can provide worthwhile symptomatic palliation of patients with recurrent or inoperable rectal and rectosigmoid cancers (Arnott, 1975). Pain from local pelvic infiltration is completely relieved in about 60% of patients. Rectal discharge and bleeding can be alleviated in about 30% of patients with advanced rectal cancer for a time following palliative radiotherapy. It is less easy to achieve resolution of perineal recurrence, but doses of 4000 rads in 20 fractions in four weeks should produce a marked reduction of tumour volume in about 50% of patients.

Carcinoma of the anal canal and anal margin

Squamous cell carcinoma of the anus can be successfully treated by interstitial radiotherapy, external beam irradiation or a combination of both methods. Curative radiotherapy should normally be restricted to relatively small cancers suitable for radio-nuclide implantation. Techniques involve the use of radium or caesium needles, iridium-192 and tantalum-182 wire or gold-198 grains. External beam therapy may also offer very good control of secondary lymph nodes in the groins.

REFERENCES AND FURTHER READING

Arnott SJ. The value of combined 5-fluorouracil and x-ray therapy in the palliation of locally recurrent and inoperable rectal carcinoma. *Clinical Radiology* **26:** 177–82.

Kligerman MM. Pre-operative radiation therapy in rectal cancer. *Cancer* 1975, **36:** 691–5.

Papillon J. Intracavitary irradiation of early rectal cancer for cure. A series of 186 cases. *Cancer* 1975; **36:** 696–701.

Rider WD. Is the Miles operation really necessary for the treatment of rectal cancer? *Journal of Canadian Association of Radiologists* 1975, **26:** 167–75.

Roswit B, Higgins GA and Keehn R. Pre-operative irradiation for carcinoma of the rectum and rectosigmoid colon: Report of a National Veterans Administration Randomised Study. *Cancer* 1975; **35:** 1597–602.

Stearns MWJ, Deddish MR, Quan SHQ and Leaming RH. Pre-operative roentgen therapy for cancer of the rectum and rectosigmoid. *Surgery, Gynecology and Obstetrics* 1974; **138:** 584–6.

Williams IG and Horwitz H. Primary treatment of adenocarcinoma of the rectum by high voltage roentgen rays (1000 kV). *American Journal of Roentgenology, Radium Therapy and Nuclear Medicine* 1956; **76:** 919–28.

MANAGEMENT OF MALIGNANT TUMOURS – CHEMOTHERAPY

Cytotoxic drugs have been used either to treat advanced surgically incurable disease or as an adjuvant to curative surgery with hope of producing a response and improving survival. In large bowel cancer a response is judged to have occurred if the size of measurable tumour mass is reduced by more than 50%. The response rate of a given drug (expressed as a percentage) is the proportion of patients who will have a response. Evaluation of a response can only be made where tumour size can be measured and this may explain some of the differing rates of response reported for many of the agents tested.

Survival can be expressed either by the proportion of patients surviving a certain period of time (for example one or five year survival) or by the time taken for 50% of patients to die (median survival). The effect of a drug on survival can only adequately be assessed when compared to a control group of untreated patients. Many studies have been uncontrolled or have used statistics from historical controls, i.e. from past experience, and there are objections to this form of comparison as time differences and problems of selection are introduced.

At the present time, response rates are generally below 25% and there is no evidence that survival is improved. For these reasons the use of these drugs should be confined to scientific investigation and patients should be treated only as part of a clinical trial.

Single agent chemotherapy

5-fluorouracil is the most active single agent with a response rate of about 20%. Several other drugs have activity in colon cancer (e.g. nitrosureas and mitomycin C), but none superior to 5-fluorouracil (Moertel, 1975).

Different routes of administration of 5-fluorouracil have been studied. There appears to be little difference between a weekly injection of 5-fluorouracil and a five day course given monthly. Though infusions of 5-fluorouracil give less toxicity and less bone marrow depression no therapeutic advantage is seen when compared to bolus injections of 5-fluorouracil. For convenience of patients bolus injection offers considerable advantage and is the method of choice. Oral 5-fluorouracil was tried in the hope that this method of administration would be an advantage in patients with hepatic metastasis. However oral absorption is unreliable and this route gives inferior results and should be abandoned.

Hepatic artery infusion of 5-fluorouracil is associated with an increased morbidity and time spent in hospital and has not been shown to be more effective (Grage, Vassilopoulos, Shingleton *et al.*, 1979).

Patients who have an objective response to 5-fluorouracil have a longer survival than non-responders, but there is no difference in the proportion of patients surviving 30 months.

Combination chemotherapy

In some studies combination chemotherapy has resulted in an increased response rate compared to 5-fluorouracil used as a single agent (Moertel, 1975; Baker, Talley and Vaitkevicius, 1976). In a randomised study (Moertel, 1975) patients receiving a combination of 5-fluorouracil, methyl CCNU and vincristine had a response rate of 43.5% compared to 19.5% for 5-fluorouracil alone.

Other investigators however have failed to demonstrate this increase in response rate (Lokich, Skarin, Mayer *et al.*, 1977) with combination chemotherapy. Those studies which demonstrated an increased response rate to combination chemotherapy were not associated with an increase in survival over 5-fluorouracil alone, but were associated with an increase in toxicity.

It appears that new agents will have to be found before significant improvement in chemotherapy of advanced disease takes place.

Immunotherapy alone or in combination with chemotherapy has not yet been demonstrated to have any advantage over chemotherapy alone.

Adjuvant therapy

Controlled studies have now been published in which 5-fluorouracil was compared to placebo in patients who had had curative surgery or were left with minimal residual disease.

In two studies reported by the Veterans Administration Group (Higgins, Humphrey, Juler *et al.*, 1976) patients were randomised to surgery alone or surgery plus 5-fluorouracil. There was a slightly better survival in patients receiving 5-fluorouracil but this was not statistically significant.

A randomised study by Lawrence, Terz, Horsley *et al.* (1978) showed no benefit from adjuvant 5-fluorouracil at five years follow up for patients undergoing curative surgery for colonic cancer.

Studies of combination chemotherapy with and without immunotherapy as an adjunct to surgery, are at present under way in several centres and the results of these studies are awaited.

REFERENCES AND FURTHER READING

Baker LH, Talley RW and Vaitkevicius VK. Phase III comparison of the treatment of advanced gastrointestinal cancer with bolus weekly 5-FU vs. methyl CCNU plus 5-FU. *Cancer* 1976; **38**: 1–7.

Grage TB, Vassilopoulos PP, Shingleton WW, Jubert AV, Elias EG, Aust JB and Moss SE. Results of a prospective randomised study of hepatic artery infusion with 5-fluorouracil versus intravenous 5-fluorouracil in patients with hepatic metastases from colorectal cancer. A central oncology group study. *Surgery* 1979; **86**: 550–5.

Higgins GA, Humphrey E, Juler GL, Le Veen HH, McCaughan J and Keehn RJ. Adjuvant chemotherapy in the surgical treatment of large bowel cancer. *Cancer* 1976; **38**: 1461–7.

Lawrence W, Terz JJ, Horsley JS, Brown PW and Romero C. Chemotherapy as an adjuvant to surgery for colorectal cancer. *Archives of Surgery* 1978; **113**: 164–8.

Lokich JJ, Skarin AT, Mayer RJ and Frei E. Lack of effectiveness of combined 5-fluorouracil and methyl CCNU therapy in advanced colorectal cancer. *Cancer* 1977; **40**: 2792–6.

Moertel CG. Clinical management of advanced gastrointestinal cancer. *Cancer* 1975; **36**: 675–82.

9. *Vascular Disorders*

VASCULAR MALFORMATIONS

Vascular malformations are a rare cause of intestinal blood loss which may be overlooked at proctosigmoidoscopy or be invisible during routine investigations.

Pathology

The terms haemangioma, arterio-venous malformation, naevus and telangiectasis have been used by different authors to describe the lesions. Solitary or multiple telangiectases, usually in the right colon, have been called angiodysplasia. The descriptive term vascular malformation used here implies no particular aetiology.

Histologically it is not always possible to conclude whether the lesions are neoplastic, hamartomatous or degenerative. Interpretation is sometimes made more difficult by secondary pathological changes due to thrombosis and local extravasation.

For practical purposes vascular malformations can be small or large.

Small vascular malformations (telangiectases, angiodysplasia) are mucosal lesions, up to 1 cm diameter, single or multiple. They may occur anywhere in the intestine but in the colon they are usually on the right side, more frequently in the elderly. They may also exist in company with oral and cutaneous lesions (hereditary telangiectasia, Osler-Rendu disease) or very rarely with similar lesions in the limbs (Weber-Klippel disease).

Large vascular malformations (cavernous or giant haemangioma) involve the whole thickness of the intestinal wall and sometimes adjacent structures, usually starting in the rectum and extending for a variable distance proximally.

Diagnosis

Bleeding is the commonest presenting symptom. Sometimes it can be torrential, but more often there is a long history of small repeated haemorrhages. Frequently there is a history of bleeding in childhood, a most useful feature in diagnosis, although presentation may not occur until the third decade of life. Often the patient has had previous operations for bleeding lesions such as duodenal ulcer or haemorrhoids or a mistaken diagnosis of ulcerative colitis may have been made.

The lesion is often seen on proctosigmoidoscopy or colonoscopy as a red patch or an area of dilated, tortuous submucosal vessels with a bluish tinge (prominent but straight veins are a normal finding of no significance). The smallest vascular malformations may be invisible or missed behind haustral folds. A plain abdominal radiograph may show the presence of calcified phleboliths in large venous malformations. Barium studies are unhelpful and even contra-indicated because of the masking effect of residual barium on subsequent angiography. Selective arteriography will often identify and assess the extent of the lesion; delayed films or venography may be necessary to demonstrate a venous abnormality. Arteriography is particularly useful during active or massive bleeding when endoscopy may be difficult; isotope scanning with the gamma camera is non-invasive and has also been used for localisation of the bleeding site.

Management

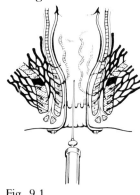

Fig. 9.1

Hereditary telangiectases are too widely distributed for excision to be of value, but those that are accessible to fibre-endoscopy can sometimes be successfully electrocoagulated using insulated forceps through the endoscope; the patient is then managed conservatively with oral iron and occasional blood transfusion. Endoscopic electrocoagulation is also successful for many small solitary malformations; active bleeding has been arrested by the technique of arteriographic embolisation. If these techniques and conservative management prove inadequate, as in patients with multiple vascular malformations of the right colon, resection may be necessary.

The more diffuse rectal haemangioma is successfully treated surgically, using one of the pull-through operations, avoiding total rectal excision and covering the abnormality of the lower rectum with a layer of normal colon. The mucosa of the rectum is excised after infiltrating the submucosa with an adrenaline/saline solution (1 : 300 000) (Fig. 9.1). The rectum is subsequently relined with normal colon by performing a peranal colo-anal sleeve anastomosis (Jeffery, Hawley and Parks, 1976) (Fig. 9.2).

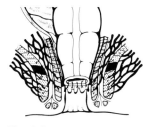

Fig. 9.2

REFERENCES AND FURTHER READING

Jeffery PJ, Hawley PR and Parks AG. Colo-anal sleeve anastomosis in the treatment of diffuse cavernous haemangioma involving the rectum. *British Journal of Surgery* 1976; **63:** 678–82.

ISCHAEMIC DISEASE

The gastro-intestinal tract is supplied by the three visceral branches of the aorta: the coeliac axis and the superior and inferior mesenteric arteries. Roughly speaking, the proximal half of the large bowel is supplied by the superior mesenteric artery and the distal half by the inferior mesenteric and internal iliac arteries (Fig. 9.3), but studies have shown that this ana-

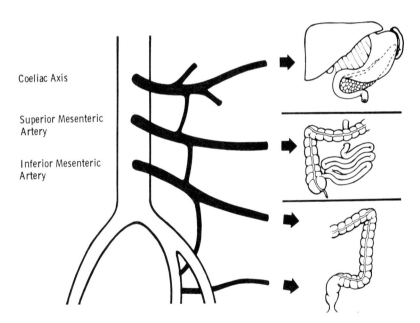

Coeliac Axis

Superior Mesenteric Artery

Inferior Mesenteric Artery

Fig. 9.3 The distribution of the three main aortic branches.

tomy is very variable because of the different ways in which the three main routes of supply may connect. There are no complicated vascular arcades as are found in the small bowel mesentery: their place is taken by the marginal artery, and the viability of a segment of colon following occlusion of a major vessel depends to a great extent on the configuration of this artery. It is frequently absent or poorly developed at the splenic flexure, where the superior and inferior mesenteric territories join, so that it is here that ischaemic damage is most often seen.

From the marginal artery arise two sets of vessels, the *vasa recta* and *vasa brevia*, which penetrate alternate aspects of the bowel wall and communicate in a rich submucosal plexus, from which penetrating branches run up between the crypts to supply the mucosa. Arteriovenous anastomoses exist in this part of the bowel, though their functional significance is not clearly understood.

There are few quantitative studies of colonic bloodflow in man, and most statements about its quantity and distribution are by analogy from experimental animals. The relationship of blood pressure to bloodflow in the intestine is not linear; in other words within the physiological range the flow does not vary much with alterations of pressure at the origin of the main vessel, but at extremely low pressures there is rapid fall-off in flow, perhaps due to the input pressure becoming less than the critical closing pressure of the intestinal arteriole. A kinked or distended loop has a diminished blood supply, which may explain why after major vascular occlusion the intestinal changes are often patchy, the extent of necrosis varying from one segment to another. Furthermore, obstructing lesions of the colon tend to induce ischaemia in the proximal distended bowel, and these changes may on occasion present clinically or be seen histologically.

CAUSES

Surgical interruption of the blood supply

Ligation of the inferior mesenteric artery at its origin from the aorta is frequently practised by surgeons performing radical operations for large bowel carcinoma and also in the resection of aortic aneurysms. This manoeuvre may result in ischaemia to the left side of the colon in a small proportion of patients; an incidence of 1–2% has been reported by Johnson and Nabseth (1974) following aortic reconstruction.

Angiographic injury

The colon can be damaged following free or selective abdominal angiography, but it is uncertain whether the contrast medium or the trauma of cannulation is to blame, or indeed whether the inferior mesenteric artery is blocked at all as a result of the angiography. Experimental work suggests that the gut is very tolerant of concentrated angiographic media, and the more recently introduced of these agents are probably much less toxic than those in use at the time of the original studies.

Spontaneous thrombosis of the colonic vessels

The inferior mesenteric artery is frequently narrowed or blocked at its origin by an atheromatous plaque and this is usually well-compensated by the development of collateral pathways. If the compensatory mechanisms fail, the colon is damaged and there are many recorded examples of this occurring as a result of acute occlusion of the artery. The changes described vary from gangrene to the more familiar changes of 'thumb printing', mucosal ulceration and stricture formation (see below). These features have all been produced in the laboratory.

Small vessel disease

Often, the causative lesion is at a subradiological level, in the intramural vessels. As in the small bowel, any condition which produces inflammation of minor arteries may result in mucosal damage. These include primary vascular disorders such as polyarteritis and Buerger's disease, systemic lupus erythematosus, rheumatoid arthritis, dermatomyositis, Wegener's granuloma, anaphylactoid purpura and Dagos' disease. Necrosis of the colon occasionally complicates renal transplanation and radiotherapy, particularly in the treatment of uterine carcinoma.

Atheromatous emboli from the aorta, and intimal thickening occurring in diabetes mellitus, have also been incriminated. It seems entirely logical that such conditions could lead to colonic ischaemia, but direct evidence for this is lacking.

Low flow states

When its blood supply fails the resulting inflammatory damage in the colon will be more rapid and more metabolically harmful than a similar process in the small gut, due to the presence of pathogenic bacteria. Clostridia, which can be found in the colon in one third of normal people, are of particular importance. Under certain circumstances particularly virulent strains of Clostridia can induce necrosis in a colon with a normal blood supply. As in the small bowel, predisposing factors include cardiac failure (particularly in association with digitalis intoxication), hypertension, diabetes mellitus, and any condition which leads to disseminated intravascular coagulation.

Intestinal obstruction

Blood flow in the wall of the intestine is affected by intraluminal pressure, radial muscle tension and diameter, quite apart from vascular influences (Fig. 9.4). The characteristic radiological and pathological changes of ischaemic colitis occur frequently in the segment of bowel immediately proximal to an obstructing carcinoma (so-called 'stercoral' ulceration). Sometimes the clinical effects of the ischaemic lesion may be sufficiently severe to mask the presence of the tumour. Other factors

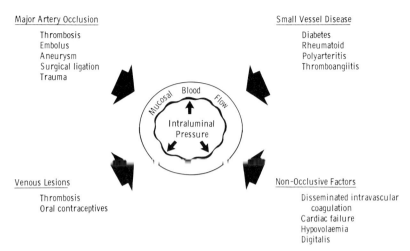

Major Artery Occlusion

    Thrombosis
    Embolus
    Aneurysm
    Surgical ligation
    Trauma

Small Vessel Disease

    Diabetes
    Rheumatoid
    Polyarteritis
    Thromboangiitis

Mucosal Blood Flow

Intraluminal Pressure

Venous Lesions

    Thrombosis
    Oral contraceptives

Non-Occlusive Factors

    Disseminated intravascular
      coagulation
    Cardiac failure
    Hypovolaemia
    Digitalis

Fig. 9.4 Factors leading to ischaemia of the colon.

leading to obstruction of the lumen of the large bowel, such as prolapse, volvulus, adhesions, or narrowing of the site of a colostomy may in the same way give rise to local ischaemic change.

Venous occlusion

Experimental studies demonstrate that, although interruption of the inferior mesenteric vein or one of its major tributaries produces very little effect, extensive venous thrombosis, such as results from injections of thrombin into colonic veins, leads to a haemorrhagic type of infarction, with gross oedema (Marcuson, Stewart and Marston, 1972). As this lesion matures, it comes to resemble the late results of arterial occlusion.

By the time x-rays can be taken and histological material is available, it may be impossible to decide whether the original causation of the infarct was on the arterial or the venous side. Circumstantial evidence to incriminate oral contraceptives (known to have a selective influence on venous thrombosis elsewhere in the body) is not hard to come by, though no colon has ever been proven to have been damaged as a direct result of such medication. The earlier reported series (Marston, Pheils, Thomas and Morson, 1966) of patients with ischaemic colitis included no premenopausal females, whereas those reported since the introduction of oral contraceptives have included a limited number of young women. This evidence cannot be taken to be more than suggestive and indeed the incidence of the condition in young men appears to be on the increase.

Infarction of unknown origin

It is important to realise that some cases of colonic infarction have no associated vascular block. This parallels what occurs in the small bowel, where it is well-recognised that in about one third of cases of fatal mesenteric infarction, the vessels appear normal at autopsy.

EFFECTS OF ACUTE COLONIC ISCHAEMIA

When, through one of the mechanisms described above, the blood supply to a loop of colon is suddenly interrupted, necrosis begins at the innermost layer of the mucosa and spreads outwards. The delicate capillary plexus is weakened and leaks plasma and blood into the interstitium, while bacterial invasion of the intestinal wall occurs and results in a profuse poly-morpho-nuclear exudate. The outcome of the ischaemic damage depends on both general and local circumstances. The haemoglobin level and the presence or absence of heart disease with its associated peripheral vasoconstriction, are important factors in influencing the fate of the colon. Additionally, the size of the blocked vessel and the duration of the occlusion, the pattern of collaterals present in the individual patient and the bacterial population of the gut may be critical.

In severe prolonged ischaemia progressive destruction of the colon occurs ending in full thickness necrosis, sloughing and rupture. At the other end of the scale a transient episode of ischaemia will result in superficial congestion and inflammation which may resolve completely and be followed by no histo-logical abnormality, as the collateral supply dilates. An inter-mediate state exists in which the remaining blood supply to the bowel is insufficient for the needs of the more specialised tissues, the mucosa and muscle, but at the same time enough remains to preserve overall viability. In these cases there is a brisk inflammatory response to start with, which is followed by ulceration of the mucosa and gradual replacement of the muscle layers with fibrous tissue. This may result in a stricture of the bowel, which may be annular and thus easily confused with a neoplasm. If a large vessel is affected the resulting stricture may occupy most of the length of the large bowel, and then will produce difficulty in the differential diagnosis from ulcerative colitis and Crohn's disease.

In practice, two quite separate clinical situations are encountered; namely gangrene of the colon, and ischaemic (non-gangrenous) colitis.

Gangrene of the colon

Clinical features

The patient is characteristically middle-aged or elderly and often has a background of degenerative cardiovascular disease

293

such as hypertension, episodes of left ventricular failure and myocardial infarction. He is characteristically under treatment with digitalis, diuretics and potassium supplements. There is no pre-existing history of bowel disturbance and the onset of the present illness is sudden and dramatic, with severe generalised abdominal pain, colicky at first but rapidly becoming diffuse and constant. Almost all patients vomit early in the course of the illness, and diarrhoea is a very frequent feature, although bleeding is unusual.

Over the course of the next few hours this clinical picture gives way to one of progressive abdominal distension, accompanied by thirst, restlessness, air-hunger, and all the symptoms of peripheral circulatory collapse.

Due to the obvious severity of the illness, early medical attention is sought. It is obvious from the most superficial examination that the patient is gravely ill. He is typically pale, sweaty and dyspnoeic, with tachycardia and arterial hypotension. The central venous pressure is low.

On examination of the abdomen there are the signs of a widespread peritonitis with diffuse tenderness, rigidity and absent bowel sounds. Rectal examination may reveal dark blood.

The underlying condition is virtually impossible to diagnose on the clinical picture alone. The usual impression is of a mesenteric embolus, peritonitis secondary to rupture of a hollow viscus, acute strangulation obstruction, or fulminating pancreatitis.

Radiological appearances

In the very early stages of the illness, the plain film of the abdomen will be normal. After a few hours, the prominent feature is progressive dilatation of the large and, later, the small bowel, suggesting toxic megacolon or volvulus. A barium enema is clearly inappropriate because of the severity of the illness. The place of emergency aortography is debatable; the only positive advantage to be gained is to exclude the possibility of a mesenteric embolus. The abdominal signs are such, however, that no surgeon would be dissuaded from immediate exploration, even by the demonstration of a normal aortogram.

Laboratory findings

As in all other forms of acute intestinal ischaemia, early leucocytosis is the rule. There is progressive haemoconcentration with a rise in packed cell volume, accompanied by metabolic acidosis with elevated blood urea and potassium. The serum enzymes follow no very consistent pattern, but changes in transaminases, amylase and lactic dehydrogenase levels may occur, as in other forms of acute abdominal disease. In particular, the intestinal iso-enzyme of alkaline phosphatase, which on theoretical grounds might be expected to show a considerable rise, is usually normal.

The first phase of treatment follows the standard lines for any patient suffering from a severe intra-abdominal catastrophe. The treatment is not specific for colonic gangrene, since the diagnosis has not yet been made. The clinician is presented with a collapsed, dehydrated, elderly patient, with poor myocardial reserve and signs of peritonitis. The first essential is to replenish the circulating volume by local administration of crystalloid solution (Ringer lactate or Hartmann's) and colloid (plasma or dextran), so as to bring down the packed cell volume and raise the central venous pressure. Oxygen is given by mask, a nasogastric tube passed and the stomach evacuated, an analgesic premedication given and preparation is made for immediate emergency exploration of the abdomen (Fig. 9.5). It is most

Management

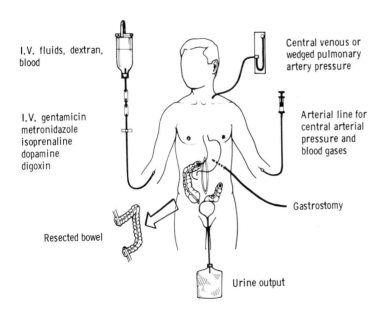

I.V. fluids, dextran, blood

I.V. gentamicin
metronidazole
isoprenaline
dopamine
digoxin

Resected bowel

Central venous or wedged pulmonary artery pressure

Arterial line for central arterial pressure and blood gases

Gastrostomy

Urine output

Fig. 9.5 The management of gangrene of the colon.

important to measure the urinary output and a urinary catheter should be inserted in all patients.

In a case of unexplained peritonitis, most surgeons will have opened the abdomen with a small right paramedian incision, which can be extended upwards and downwards according to

Operative technique

295

what is found. In this instance, it will be immediately obvious on opening the peritoneum that a length of colon (and indeed sometimes of small bowel) has undergone ischaemic necrosis. The appearance of the bowel varies from livid red through purple to black or even dark green, and the length involved may extend for any distance between the rectosigmoid and the caecum. It is, however, unusual to find involvement below the distal sigmoid colon. The incision is enlarged and a check made of the peritoneal contents, to exclude any other abnormality. The mesenteric vessels are then inspected and palpated, and are usually found to be pulsatile up to the margin of the colon.

The affected bowel is mobilised in the usual way, but must be handled with great gentleness to avoid tearing its fragile wall, and producing massive peritoneal contamination. The vessels at the base of the mesentery are ligated and a length of colon resected between non-crushing clamps, well wide of the abnormal area. The mucosa is then inspected carefully, and the clamps released, in order to confirm that there is arterial bleeding from the cut ends. Usually, the mucosal damage is considerably more extensive than would be suspected from outside, and it may be necessary to cut the bowel back still further, in order to be certain of having removed all ischaemic tissue.

No attempt is made to achieve a primary anastomosis. The proximal end of the bowel is exteriorised in any convenient position on the abdominal wall, and the distal end either brought out in the same way, or closed and dropped back, according to the length and position of the bowel affected. The peritoneal cavity is then washed out with saline, and the wound closed with appropriate drainage. A gastrostomy tube may be inserted for postoperative gastrointestinal decompression, thus avoiding a nasogastric tube.

Results

It is generally agreed that colonic gangrene carries a mortality of 80–90%, which is scarcely surprising in that this dangerous condition usually occurs in people who are already suffering from degenerative cardiovascular disease. Nonetheless, the figures are biased by the fact that the diagnosis is usually made only at a late stage in the operation, or at autopsy. Given modern methods of pre-operative resuscitation, followed by application of well-tried surgical principles, there is every reason to suppose that this very high death rate can be reduced. Metabolic disturbances are common to all acute abdominal conditions, and the surgery of the acute abdomen, aided by efficient muscular relaxation, supplementary oxygen, fluid replacement and antibiotic therapy, has now lost much of its danger.

Ischaemic colitis is the non-gangrenous form of the disease, which varies from a transient episode of inflammation to a massive fibrous stricture of the bowel causing complete obstruction.

For detailed accounts of the pathology, the reader is referred to the writings of Morson (1972).

The clinical features depend on the stage of the disease at which the patient presents. Typically the patient is a middle-aged or elderly male with evidence of arterial disease elsewhere in the body but without preceding gut symptoms. The onset is acute and the first symptom is generally a sharp pain in the left iliac fossa spreading across the abdomen and up into the epigastrium. This is followed by the passage of a small motion mixed with dark blood. The bleeding is quite characteristic: it differs from the massive bright exsanguination which occasionally complicates diverticular disease, and from haemorrhoidal bleeding, which is smaller in amount, bright red and unmixed with the stool. In ischaemic colitis the bleeding is moderate in amount, dark, mixed with stool and may contain clots.

If examined at this stage of the disease the patient is generally not grossly ill or shocked though the temperature and pulse are raised. The constant abdominal finding is of extreme tenderness in the left iliac fossa and in the pelvis, with dark blood on the fingerstall following rectal examination.

Examination with the rigid sigmoidoscope does not usually bring the lesion into view as the area affected lies above the reach of the instrument. However, the diagnosis is sometimes made by this means. The appearances described are of irregular heaped-up bluish-purple mucosa, with oedema and contact bleeding. Colonoscopy is likely to be extremely useful in the early diagnosis of the disease, especially as the histopathological examination of biopsies may be diagnostic. As yet, insufficient experience has accumulated, but at the same time no complications or disasters have been reported.

A plain x-ray will on occasion delineate an area of large bowel where the intraluminal gas shadow demonstrates 'thumb printing' (Fig. 9.6). At a later stage in the disease, there may be signs of small bowel obstruction, with dilatation of the ileum and fluid levels.

The place of angiography remains controversial. While there are many reports in the literature of radiologically demonstrated

Ischaemic colitis

Clinical features

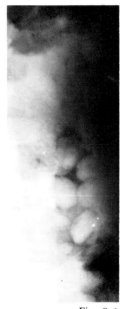

Fig. 9.6

Endoscopy

Radiological appearances

arterial blocks, non-occlusive disease appears to be more frequent, so that a negative angiogram does not exclude the diagnosis. It is certainly not required as a routine examination in every case.

The barium enema, however, is most useful. The changes are characteristic (Fig. 9.7); an abnormal segment of colon is seen,

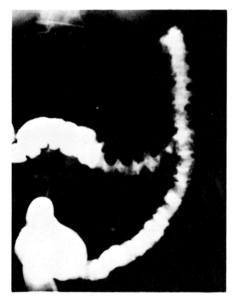

Fig. 9.7 Characteristic site and radiological appearances of ischaemic colitis.

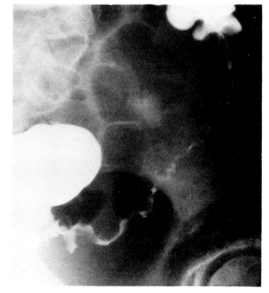

Fig. 9.8 Complete narrowing in ischaemic colitis.

which is, as a rule, clearly demarcated from the adjoining bowel and usually situated around the splenic flexure. This segment is always narrowed, and the narrowing varies from slight to complete obstruction (Fig. 9.8). Its length may be from a few centimetres to involvement of the whole of the tranverse and descending colon. The normal haustral pattern is lost and rigidity of the segment may be demonstrated by screening or serial films. In detail the following features are seen: polypoid change, mucosal irregularity, tubular narrowing and sacculation. Polypoid change – called 'thumb printing' by Boley, Schwartz, Lash and Sternhill (1963) – consists of rounded filling defects in the barium filled colon (Fig. 9.9). Mucosal irregularity presents either as smooth ridges projecting into the lumen, or else as craters of varying size, extending into the wall. Sacculation consists of smooth outpouching of the colonic wall. Generally speaking, polypoid change and mucosal irregularity are seen earlier in the course of the disease.

If a short stricture has developed it may be very difficult to distinguish this from an annular neoplasm. The main distinguishing points are the absence of 'shouldering' and 'half-shadowing', which are so characteristic of carcinoma. Ischaemic proctitis can occur and cause confusion with other causes of rectal inflammation.

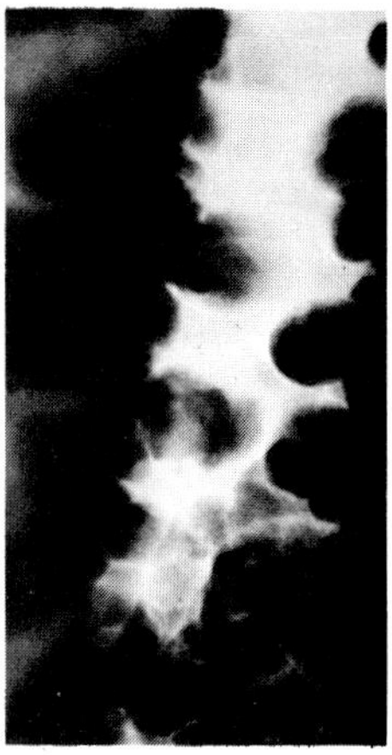

Fig. 9.9

Laboratory findings

Laboratory studies give rather nonspecific results. There is almost invariably a polymorph leucocytosis (15 000 per mm^3, or more), and the serum enzymes may be raised in a rather inconsistent fashion, as in colonic gangrene.

Differential diagnosis of ischaemic colitis

In a typical case presenting as an emergency, the diagnosis should be straightforward, particularly if there is associated rectal bleeding. The main conditions with which it can be confused are:

Infective gastro-enteritis
Acute large bowel Crohn's disease and ulcerative colitis
Complicated diverticular disease
Carcinoma of the large bowel
Perforation of a hollow viscus
Acute pancreatitis
Left sided renal colic
Leaking abdominal aortic aneurysm

It is quite likely (but unproveable) that many episodes of abdominal pain and diarrhoea, particularly in the older age groups, diagnosed as gastro-enteritis or diverticular disease, in fact represent transient episodes of ischaemia. A helpful feature which may distinguish ischaemia from these conditions is the presence of the characteristic dark rectal bleeding, though this occurs only in some two thirds of cases. Often, the diagnosis is not made immediately, but comes to light only with the barium enema examination.

When seen later in the course of the illness, the condition may closely resemble Crohn's disease or ulcerative colitis. The most important distinguishing features are the characteristic age group of the patients, the association with degenerative cardio-vascular disease, and the distinctive radiological appearances and their distribution.

Management

From the practical point of view, it may be said that when the patient has been assessed it becomes possible to draw a fairly accurate distinction between what is *probably* ischaemic colitis, where continued observation and further assessment is justified, and what is probably some form of purulent peritonitis or haemorrhagic condition, where immediate exploration of the abdomen is mandatory. The crucial diagnostic step is to obtain a barium enema at the earliest possible opportunity, because the appearances are so characteristic.

Once the diagnosis has been established, treatment should in almost every case be expectant. The patient is rested in bed, given intravenous fluids, according to the degree of peritoneal irritation, and monitored by daily leucocyte counts and packed cell volume readings. It may be wise to give antibiotics, as it has been established that such therapy mitigates the effect of colonic ischaemia in the experimental laboratory, but no controlled clinical trials have been performed.

On this expectant regime, there are three possible sequelae. These are:

Progression to gangrene
Resolution (formerly described as 'transient ischaemia')
Stricture formation

For a patient with acute nongangrenous ischaemic colitis to develop gangrene of the colon is, fortunately, extremely rare. In a personal series it occurred only twice in 122 cases. The usual course of events is for the pain, bleeding and diarrhoea to settle rapidly over the course of a few days, or perhaps a week or two, and for a subsequent barium enema to show a normal colon, or one with minimal involvement (Marcuson, 1972). In about a third of all cases, a fibrous stricture develops but this is frequently quite asymptomatic, and does not require treatment.

Indications for operation

The indications for operation are:

Gangrene
Persistent bleeding due to deep ulceration
Obstruction
Uncertain diagnosis, e.g. malignancy

The only strictures which require operation are those which cause distress by persistent bleeding, cramps, diarrhoea or other obstructive symptoms, or which could be neoplastic.

Surgical resection of an ischaemic stricture of the colon does not differ in any important respect from operations carried out for cancer or diverticular disease. Special care should be taken over the vascularity of the resected ends, but provided that the mucosa is pink and healthy with pulsatile vessels up to its margins, no particular difficulty is encountered, and the incidence of anastomotic breakdown is not high.

In summary, ischaemic disease of the colon is now a well-recognised and established clinical condition, which may occur spontaneously or follow interference with the vasculature. Two quite distinct forms of the illness occur, and it is rare, though not unknown, for one to progress to the other. In the first place there is full-thickness necrosis of the colonic wall, which presents as an abdominal catastrophe, requires urgent excisional surgery, and carries a high mortality. The milder form of the illness presents as an acute left-sided peritonitis, usually associated with diarrhoea and rectal bleeding, and can safely be treated expectantly. About half the patients managed in this way will develop a fibrous stricture in the colon, but only a minority of these give rise to symptoms which are bad enough to warrant operation.

REFERENCES AND FURTHER READING

Boley SJ, Schwartz S, Lash J and Sternhill V. Reversible vascular occlusion of the colon. *Surgery, Gynecology and Obstetrics* 1963; **116:** 53–60.

Johnson WC and Nabseth DC. Visceral infarction following aortic surgery. *Annals of Surgery* 1974; **180:** 312–18.

Marcuson RW, Stewart JO and Marston A. Experimental venous lesions of the colon. *Gut* 1972; **13:** 1–7.

Marcuson RW. Ischaemic colitis. *Clinics in Gastroenterology* 1972; **1:** 745–63.

Marston A, Pheils MT, Thomas ML and Morson BC. Ischaemic colitis *Gut* 1966; **7:** 1–10.

Marston A. *Intestinal ischaemia.* London: Edward Arnold, 1977.

Morson BC. The pathology of ischaemic colitis. *Clinics in Gastroenterology* 1972; **1:** 765–6.

10. *Paediatric Problems*

CLINICAL ASSESSMENT

In the assessment of children with anorectal problems it is important to remember that aetiological factors may antedate birth. Furthermore, congenital abnormalities are often multiple; oesophageal atresia, congenital heart disease, urinary tract anomalies and low spinal abnormalities, for example, occurring in association with anorectal anomalies.

HISTORY

In the neonatal period distension, vomiting and the passage of explosive stools may suggest Hirschsprung's disease, constipation supervening at a later stage. Similar symptoms, persisting 24–48 hours, may accompany temporary myenteric dysfunction, particularly in a premature child. Excessive straining indicates anal stenosis, in which ribbon-like stools may be passed. Complete obstruction at birth occurs in the severe forms of anorectal anomaly.

In childhood, abdominal pain occurs in faecal loading, functional bowel disorders and organic disorders such as Crohn's disease. Peri-anal pain occurs with fissure, peri-anal abscess, diarrhoea and soiling.

As in adult life, bleeding from the distal and proximal bowel can be distinguished by its nature. Fissures and large bowel polyps are common causes whereas ulcerative colitis, vascular malformations and the solitary ulcer syndrome are less frequently encountered. Intussusception can produce the characteristic redcurrant jelly stool, although its absence does not exclude the condition. The passage of mucus not associated with bleeding is unusual but may be a presenting feature of fissure, prolapse and polyps.

Pruritus ani, if predominantly nocturnal, suggests the presence of threadworms (*Enterobius vermicularis*) but itching may occur with other anal disorders and bowel dysfunction.

The frequency, consistency and size of stool may help to diagnose malabsorption or the various types of constipation. In patients with soiling a normal stool passed in an abnormal situation is unlikely to have an organic cause, whereas the child who soils spontaneously requires investigation to exclude an organic cause.

EXAMINATION

The more obstructive anorectal anomalies and severe types of Hirschsprung's disease lead to a rapidly developing, tense, abdominal distension in the neonatal period. Anal stenosis, low anomalies with fistulous openings and the less obstructive types of Hirschsprung's disease result in the more gradual development of distension. Long-standing distension may produce splaying of the costal margin. Lesions of the lower rectum and anal canal causing incomplete obstruction may result in enlargement of the rectum, even to the costal margin, with little dilatation of the colon.

Abdominal Examination

Examination of the child's back is important since pits, hairy patches or lipomata may indicate underlying spinal dysraphism. The presence of a normal sacrum should be confirmed as sacral agenesis may be associated with neurogenic disorders.

Examination of the back

The clinician must be aware of a potentially painful lesion before digital examination, if the child's co-operation is to be retained. Anal skin tags indicating fissure, warts, abscess and fistula and peri-anal excoriation should therefore be looked for before passing a finger. Examination under anaesthetic may be necessary. Haemorrhoids are extremely rare in childhood and should not be confused with haemangioma. Anal manifestations of Crohn's disease should be borne in mind.

Anorectal Examination

The diagnosis of most anal anomalies is usually obvious in the new-born but may be delayed. An ectopic anus lies anteriorly and may be stenosed.

The normal anal canal of a full-term child usually admits the little finger. In Hirschsprung's disease and congenital constipation anal tone is usually normal. The anal canal may apparently feel longer than normal in children with' short segment Hirschsprung's disease where the finger passes into the tense, distended rectum above it. Polyps in the lower rectum may be palpable. The examining finger should also exclude sacral agenesis and the rare anterior meningocoele. Proctoscopy and sigmoidoscopy in children is probably best done under anaesthesia.

INVESTIGATIONS

Stool examination

Stools are examined for parasites, bacteria and viruses. Infestations with protozoa and helminths are common. Diarrhoea may be due to infections with Salmonella, Shigella and coliform bacteria as well as viruses such as *hepatitis virus A*.

Stool containing reducing sugars with a persistent pH of 5 suggests a mono- or di-saccharide intolerance. Temporary lactase or sucrose isomaltase deficiency is not uncommon after the relief of intestinal obstruction.

For the identification of threadworm infection a strip of adhesive tape is applied to the peri-anal skin and then pressed on a glass slide; ova may be seen under the microscope.

Fibrocystic disease should be suspected where a child passes large pale frothy stools. A high stool content of protein suggests the diagnosis which is confirmed by reduced trypsin activity in the stool and a high sodium concentration of sweat (60 mmol/l).

Radiology

Plain films of the abdomen are important in the diagnosis of neonatal intestinal obstruction and megacolon in later childhood. Supine and erect or lateral decubitus views should be taken.

A barium enema examination may be indicated in patients with low bowel obstruction, rectal bleeding, some anorectal anomalies and malrotation.

It is dangerous to introduce hypotonic solutions into the enlarged colon owing to the possibility of water intoxication. This can be reduced by suspending the barium in normal saline and introducing it in small quantities into unprepared bowel. In Hirschsprung's disease this method shows the 'cone', that is the transition from the distal segment into the dilated proximal segment (Fig. 10.1). A lateral view of the rectum to show short or ultra-short segment disease is also important.

In neonatal intestinal obstruction the diagnosis of Hirschsprung's disease will be the primary consideration, but other forms of large bowel obstruction must be excluded. Premature children, or children who have been subject to anoxic episodes in the perinatal period, may present with temporary, functional, large bowel obstruction. This group may include 'mucus plug', 'meconium plug' and the small left colon syndrome. The appearances on the barium films of these other disorders may be difficult to differentiate from Hirschsprung's disease, particu-

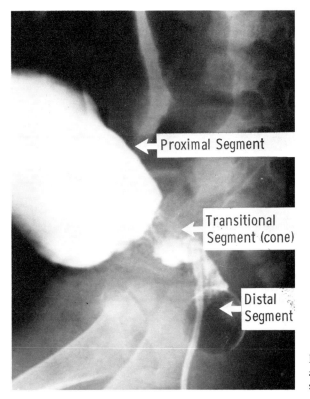

Fig. 10.1 Radiological appearances of Hirschsprung's disease.

larly where an apparent cone may lie at the splenic flexure. In the older child, the indication for a barium enema examination is usually to distinguish Hirschsprung's disease from other causes of megacolon or in the diagnosis of anorectal bleeding. Large bowel polyps occur predominantly in the rectum but may be situated more proximally (Fig. 10.2). Small angiomatous malformations are difficult to demonstrate, unless projecting into the lumen. Lymphoid hyperplasia, which may be associated with rectal bleeding in childhood, may also be shown on barium enema. In inflammatory bowel disorders a barium enema is needed to define the extent of the disease, as in the adult.

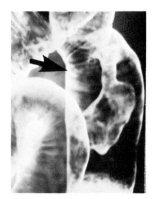

Fig. 10.2

The indications for endoscopic examination are the same as in the adult. Owing to the difficulty in obtaining the child's co-operation, this often requires a general anaesthetic and can usually be undertaken on a day-case basis.

Proctoscopy, sigmoidoscopy and colonoscopy

305

Biopsy

Biopsies may be readily taken during the various endoscopic procedures. In suspected Hirschsprung's disease, precision in the selection of the site of the biopsy is necessary owing to the possibility of short and ultrashort segment disease. Though mucosal biopsies are acceptable to laboratories used to dealing with Hirschsprung's disease, most still require a full thickness specimen (Todd, 1977). Acetylcholinesterase and non-specific esterase stains greatly facilitate the diagnosis.

Anorectal physiology

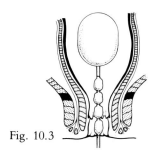

Fig. 10.3

Tests to record the pressure profile of the anal canal and lower rectum may confirm the diagnosis of Hirschsprung's disease. A probe which may be used for this purpose has been described by Lawson and Nixon (1967) and is illustrated in Fig. 10.3. The recordings of anal pressure include a resting trace, the response to rectal distension, the response to stimulation of the peri-anal skin and to movement of the probe in the anal canal.

REFERENCES AND FURTHER READING

Lawson JON and Nixon HH. Anal canal pressures in the diagnosis of Hisrchsprung's disease. *Journal of Paediatric Surgery* 1967; **2:** 544–52.

Todd IP. Intractable constipation and adult megercolon. In: Todd IP. ed. *Colon, rectum and anus* (3rd ed. Operative surgery). London and Boston: Butterworths, 1977: 268–70.

CONGENITAL ANOMALIES

NORMAL DEVELOPMENT

Information on the development of the anorectum and urinary tract, which are intimately related, is available from two sources, the study of normal embryos and known anomalies.

In the four millimetre (4 week) embryo the hindgut connects with the allantois and develops a proximal dilatation. With the entry of the mesonephric ducts the dilatation becomes a cloaca. At five weeks the postallantoic hindgut diverticulum appears in the dorsal portion of the cloaca. The caudal, convex surface of the dilatation comes into proximity with the ectoderm behind the body stalk to form the cloacal membrane. Two folds grow in to form the urogenital septum which separates the cloaca into two parts. At seven weeks the cloacal membrane is divided into a ventral urogenital membrane and a dorsal anal membrane to form the 'primary perineum'. A proctodeal pit develops in this dorsal portion of the membrane and deepens to meet the downwards extension of the primitive rectum. At the same time the sinovaginal bulb forms, destined to become the lower part of the vagina and its opening migrates caudally to open on to the vulva. The ureters are formed from outgrowths of the mesonephric ducts which migrate cranially to meet the metanephros.

At the same time, the external genitalia develop from genital folds on each side of the cloacal membrane appearing in the seventh week. The perineal body forms at about the same time from a condensation of mesenchyme in the urorectal septum. The nerve supply (S.2, 3, 4) of the external anal sphincter muscle suggests a different segmental origin from that of the pelvic floor (S.3, 4, 5). It is suggested that the mesenchyme migrates from dorsal rather than ventral myotomes. The medial portions of the levator ani are considered to be homologous with the 'rectus column' from which the rectus abdominis muscles are derived.

There appear to be two portions to the internal sphincter, upper and lower. The lower derives from a 'cloacal sphincter' which develops into the lower internal anal and urethral sphincters. The upper portion appears to originate from the smooth muscle of the primitive rectum.

These determinant steps are complete by the tenth week of intra-uterine life. Failure or arrest of development in these early stages result in the various congenital anomalies.

ANOMALIES

Classification

In 1971, an international classification of anorectal anomalies based on the relationship of the hindgut to the pelvic floor was proposed (Stephens and Smith, 1971). The abnormalities were broadly sub-divided into three groups;

Low, where the bowel passes through the levator ani (translevator)
Intermediate, where the bowel enters the levator ani but is arrested at this point, and
High, where the bowel is held up above the levator ani (supralevator).

To this was added a miscellaneous group including a number of uncommon variants which do not fall readily into the basic classification (Table 10a; Fig. 10.4).

In the intermediate and high groups there may be an associated fistula between the gut tube and the vaginal vestibule, and very rarely the urinary system in females, and between the gut tube and the urinary system in males. In some anorectal

Table 10a. *Classification of anorectal anomalies*

Low (translevator)

Normal anal site	covered anus – complete anal stenosis
Perineal site	covered anus – incomplete (anocutaneous fistula)
	anterior perineal anus
Vulval site	vulvar anus
	anovulvar fistula
	anovestibular fistula

Intermediate

Anal agenesis without fistula		
with fistula	*male*	rectobulbar
	female	rectovestibular
		rectovaginal (low)
Anorectal stenosis		

High (supralevator)

Anorectal agenesis without fistula		
with fistula	*male*	recto-urethral
		rectovesical
	female	rectovaginal (high)
		rectovesical
		rectocloacal
Rectal atresia		

Miscellaneous

Imperforate anal membrane
Covered anal stenosis
Anal membrane stenosis
Vesico-intestinal fissure
Duplications of anus, rectum and genito-urinary tract
Combination of deformities from the basic types
Perineal groove
Perineal canal

anomalies there may be a degree of narrowing of the anus or anorectum which in the extreme case can be completely obliterated (atresia). Other deformities, for example reduplication, fall outside this classification.

Clinical features

The presentation depends on the type of disorder and the severity of the occlusion of the gut tube. Atresia and agenesis present with neonatal obstruction, whereas anal stenosis may not be apparent for some months; it may present as soiling and constipation in the infant or older child (see following section).

Low (translevator)

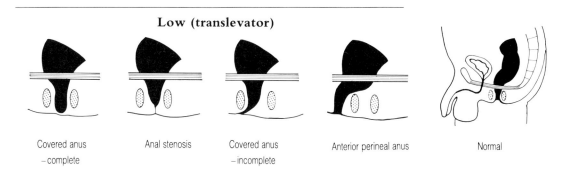

Covered anus
– complete

Anal stenosis

Covered anus
– incomplete

Anterior perineal anus

Normal

Intermediate

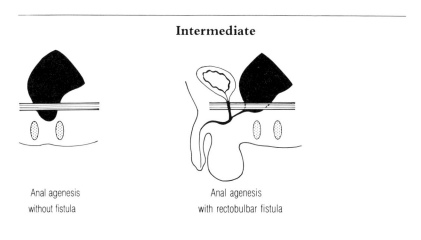

Anal agenesis
without fistula

Anal agenesis
with rectobulbar fistula

High (supralevator)

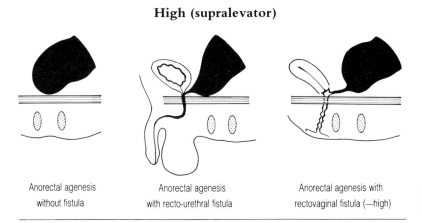

Anorectal agenesis
without fistula

Anorectal agenesis
with recto-urethral fistula

Anorectal agenesis with
rectovaginal fistula (—high)

Fig. 10.4
Anorectal anomalies.

Fistulae into the urinary tract may lead to the passage of meconium or flatus *per urethram* or cause vaginal soiling when they enter the vagina.

The anus may be stenosed, ectopic or both. In cases of agenesis a midline skin dimple in the perineum may be seen, and indicate the site of anal sphincter musculature.

309

Radiological assessment

A plain x-ray of the abdomen will show the degree of distention and determine whether gas has reached the distal bowel. A film with the child inverted with marking of the anal skin dimple may distinguish between a high and a low anomaly. Gas held up above the ossified ischium or above a line between the pubis and the last ossified segment of the spine indicates a high anomaly but meconium retained in the rectal stump or air escaping through a large fistula may make the interpretation of this x-ray difficult. Contrast radiographs of fistula tracks may be very helpful.

Operative treatment

The aims of treatment are to provide relief of intestinal obstruction, an adequate anal opening at, approximately, the normal site, a mechanism that will enable the child to close this opening by providing an adequate surrounding musculature, adequate anal and rectal sensation and an adequate reservoir for retention of the stool.

A defunctioning loop colostomy should be made if the obstruction cannot be relieved by dilatation of the stenosis or where extensive surgery for high and intermediate anomalies is proposed.

In patients with low anomalies gentle anal dilatation continued over a few months is often all that is required, although a cut-back operation to treat covered anus is sometimes necessary. Delay in diagnosis may lead to megarectum which may then require prolonged treatment.

In patients with intermediate and high anomalies a compromise has to be made between the need for adequate mobilisation of the bowel on the one hand and the preservation of the voluntary muscle and sensory nerves on the other.

Most surgeons make a perineal, or perineal and sacral approach, combined with an abdominal dissection. Many intermediate anomalies, particularly those without fistulae, may be corrected via sacral and perineal approaches without an abdominal dissection.

Sacral approach

An incision is made over the lower sacrum and coccyx dividing the superficial sphincter, disarticulating the sacrococcygeal joint and dividing the anococcygeal raphe. This brings the operator into the retrorectal space. The dissection is carried forward over the upper surface of the anococcygeal raphe, in front of the V of the puborectalis and down to the upper surface of the skin dimple.

Perineal approach

A cruciate incision, centred on the anal dimple, allows mobilisation of four skin flaps, after the detachment of the fibres of the levator ani muscle. A sling of Penrose tubing can be passed from the sacral to the perineal wound and acts as a guide for the subsequent dilatation and pull-through.

The aims of this part of the operation are to mobilise sufficient bowel to bring it down to the perineum and to divide a rectourethral or rectovaginal fistula. The distal bowel can be mobilised by close dissection around the rectal stump and the fistula divided. This type of dissection, most suited to the high anomalies, is considered inadvisable by some surgeons who feel it puts the pelvic nerve plexuses at risk. The alternative is to divide the bowel muscle above the peritoneal reflection, coring out the mucosa from the distal stump and ligating the fistula from within. An opening is then made in the muscle stump and the mobilised bowel is brought down through the resulting muscle tube. The muscle layers of the pulled-through rectum can then be sutured to the peri-anal subcutaneous structures, the rectal mucosa being opposed to the skin flaps.

Abdominal approach

Postoperatively, the new anus will require gentle dilatation, continued for about three months. It should be of adequate size before the colostomy is closed. Close observation over many years is necessary to ensure that there is no obstruction at the site of anastomosis to cause rectal dilatation and further loss of sensation. This may require further anal dilatation or anoplasty.

REFERENCES AND FURTHER READING

Hamilton WJ, Boyd JD and Mossman HW. *Human embryology.* Cambridge: Heffer, 1972.

Smith ED. The identification and management of anorectal anomalies. The factors ensuring continence. *Progress in paediatric surgery* 1976; **9:** 7–40.

Stephens FD and Smith ED. *Anorectal malformations in children.* Chicago: Year Book Medical, 1971.

CHRONIC CONSTIPATION AND SOILING

The vast majority of children who present with soiling have marked faecal retention. The rectum distends and there may be impairment of rectal sensation as a result. The child may have

Pathogenesis

a reduced or even absent desire to defaecate which, by leading to further rectal loading, sets up a vicious circle. There may be an obvious obstructive cause for the retention, for example Hirschsprung's disease, congenital anal stenosis, neurogenic lesions and fissure. In other cases, however, no physical lesion can be found. Sometimes there is a past reason for rectal distension which persists after the cause has disappeared. Examples of this include transitory functional obstruction in the newborn, resolving fissures and mild degrees of anal stenosis. In a few cases, soiling may occur without faecal retention. This may be due to impaired sensation of the anal canal. It is then often associated with disturbances of micturition.

Psychological disturbances are often present in children with constipation and soiling. These are usually secondary to the bowel abnormality. The soiling child may have a profound effect on the family. Psychological symptoms improve dramatically when the constipation and soiling is treated. In 25% of patients there is a family history of similar trouble amongst close relatives. Cretinism, Chagas' disease and side effects of drugs, such as vincristine in children being treated for neuroblastoma, are general causes of constipation. There is an association between mental deficiency, constipation and soiling; anoxia may have damaged both the myenteric plexus and cortical nerve cells in the brain.

Clinical assessment

Symptoms from a congenital obstructive lesion may be long delayed. Anal stenosis is rarely noted before the third month. Symptoms in short-segment Hirschsprung's disease, 'congenital constipation' or anal achalasia may not start until six months or a year and appear to follow changes in diet or activity, altering the consistency of the stool. Pain on defaecation and passage of bright red blood suggests the diagnosis of an anal fissure. The fissure may be primary, however it may be an event in a long-standing history of constipation due to other causes.

It is open to question that a child with a normal anorectum can 'hold back' sufficiently to cause chronic constipation, as a normal child has considerable difficulty in holding a volume of greater than 150 ml.

As some drugs cause constipation, a careful drug history should be taken. The child may already have been treated for constipation by medicines including laxatives, suppositories and enemas. There may have been previous manual evacuations. Occasionally the child has had previous surgical treatment for an anorectal anomaly.

Most children with chronic constipation have abdominal distention. The abdomen is usually soft and tympanitic and there may be flaring of the ribs. The degree of distention may vary. In the small child the rectum is an intra–abdominal, rather than a pelvic organ. In anal canal obstruction, the rectum may enlarge to touch the diaphragm, while there may be little colonic dilatation.

Examination of the perineum and rectum should exclude local painful conditions and congenital abnormalities. A long anal canal may suggest short-segment Hirschsprung's disease. A neurological examination to exclude meningomyelocele, other forms of spinal dysraphism and sacral agenesis should also be made. The use of special investigations such as radiology and anorectal physiology studies has already been described.

Treatment

If an underlying cause has been found, it should be treated but the initial management is often symptomatic. The aim of this is to ensure the daily passage of a bulky soft stool. At first, an enema or manual evacuation may be necessary. There appears to be an advantage in combining a bulk laxative such as methylcellulose or sterculia and a stimulant purgative such as senna. The bulk given to the stool will help to dilate the anus, while the stimulant will result in more proximal propulsion. Liquid paraffin should be avoided. Anal dilatation under general anaesthesia may help.

HIRSCHSPRUNG'S DISEASE

Hirschsprung's disease occurs in about 1 per 5000 live births; males are five times more commonly affected. It is associated with an absence of ganglion cells in the myenteric plexus; the extent varies from a short segment of distal rectum to involvement of the entire bowel.

Pathology

There is gross dilatation of the proximal bowel (proximal segment) and a normal appearance in the distal bowel (distal segment) with a tapering zone (transitional segment) between them (Fig. 10.1). The transitional segment appears cone-shaped when it occurs in the distal large bowel. In the neonate the distal segment is usually of smaller calibre than normal and the proximal bowel shows little or no hypertrophy. However, as the condition becomes more long-standing, marked hypertrophy occurs.

Megacolon in children has been recognised for nearly 300 years. Hirschsprung described the disease in 1886 but it was not for 60 years that its essential nature was recognised. A disorder of the proximal segment was thought by many to be the primary disturbance until Ehrenpreis (1946), in a classic study, confirmed that the disorder lay in the distal segment. Shortly after, Zuelzer and Wilson (1948) showed an absence of ganglion cells in the intermuscular plexuses of the undilated segments and this was soon confirmed by others (Bodian, Stephens and Ward, 1949). In addition, hypertrophied unmyelinated nerve trunks in the intermuscular plexuses were identified and found to have intense anticholinesterase activity. Increased numbers of adrenergic and cholinergic nerve fibres have been demonstrated in the aganglionic and transitional segment and reduced numbers of nerve cells are found in the transitional zone; a functional obstruction to the bowel occurs at this level.

Aetiology

The aetiology is unknown. There is an increased familial incidence suggesting that genetic factors are involved. Two per cent of patients have a chromosomal abnormality, mostly trisomy 21 (Down's syndrome). It seems likely that the disorder occurs between the fifth and twelfth week of intra-uterine life. During this time, the myenteric plexuses are formed by the migration of neuroblasts from the caudal cephalic end of the gut tube. Hold-up or retardation of this process might lead to aganglionosis. If environmental factors play a part they would be expected to act during this period.

Clinical features

The distribution of the extent of the disease is shown in Fig. 10.5. In over 70% the transition zone occurs in the sigmoid

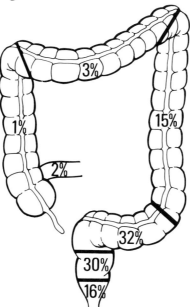

Fig. 10.5 The incidence of the extent of the distal (affected) segment in Hirschsprung's disease. 1% have total aganglionosis.

colon or rectum. Involvement of an ultrashort segment of distal rectum is not uncommon and is the cause in about 10% of children presenting with chronic constipation. There is an association between Hirschsprung's disease and other congenital anomalies.

The clinical presentation varies in time and severity according to the length of aganglionic segment. During the first month of life there may be unremitting intestinal obstruction or intermittent obstructive episodes, relieved either spontaneously or by rectal washouts. In infancy and early childhood symptoms may be traced back to birth but they often develop months later. Episodes of intermittent distension occur with diarrhoea and soiling. Failure to thrive is common. The abdomen is distended (Fig. 10.6) and rectal examination, where there is short-segment disease, may show the characteristic tensely distended rectum above an apparently long anal canal. Anal tone is usually normal.

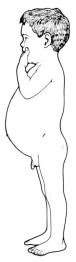

Fig. 10.6

Symptoms can appear for the first time in later childhood or even adult life. Constipation is then the cardinal symptom, there being difficulty in passing even a soft stool. The patient may have a long history of poor general health and poor performance at school. Again, abdominal distension is constantly found and the narrow distal segment can be identified.

Severe enterocolitis can occur in Hirschsprung's disease and is the commonest cause of death. The child presents gravely ill, with diarrhoea, septicaemia and profound water, electrolyte and plasma protein disturbance. There are thought to be two pathological forms; ischemic enterocolitis, with free gas in the bowel wall and patchy gangrene, and superficial enterocolitis which is considered to be an acute sensitivity reaction.

Investigations

Radiology

Plain abdominal x-ray will make the diagnosis of obstruction and to localise the cone a barium enema examination on an unprepared bowel should be performed.

Anorectal physiology studies

The recording of pressure waves from the rectum and a pressure profile of the anal canal is a reliable diagnostic test. There is enhancement of the normal rhythmical waves in the anal canal and of the slow wave component in the rectum. Distension of a balloon in the distal segment causes pain but no simple stimulated pressure wave, whereas if the balloon lies above the segment the rectal pressure wave shows a marked increase. Occasional mass contractions of the segment occur. There is no fall in anal canal pressure in response to rectal distension.

315

Rectal biopsy

The routine diagnosis of Hirschsprung's disease depends on the demonstration of the absence of ganglion cells and the presence of hypertrophied and tortuous nerve trunks. Where specialist facilities are available, stains for acetylcholinesterase and techniques to identify adrenergic fibres should be used.

Treatment

Intestinal obstruction due to Hirschsprung's disease in neonates requires emergency treatment after replacement of fluid and electrolyte losses. A laparotomy is carried out and a relieving colostomy, usually a defunctioning loop colostomy or a double-barrelled colostomy, is made. Biopsies from the abnormal bowel may be taken at the same time. In an older patient with a grossly distended bowel, it may also be advisable to perform a preliminary colostomy some weeks before undertaking curative surgery.

Several operations have been described; the more important are mentioned below.

Swenson's operation

The cone is identified and its level confirmed by biopsy. 10–20 cm of hypertrophied proximal bowel are resected, the ends being oversewn. The distal stump is then evaginated through the anal canal and the proximal bowel pulled through the resulting tube. The anal canal is transected obliquely, effectively carrying out an upper partial sphincterotomy. The proximal bowel is anastomosed to the anal canal outside the anus (Swenson, 1948).

Duhamel's operation

The distal bowel is mobilised as far as the peritoneal reflection. Dissection is continued down in the retrorectal space as far as the attachment of the pelvic floor to the anal canal. A transverse incision is made in the posterior wall of the upper anal canal, just above the zone of stratified cuboidal epithelium. The bowel is divided 10–20 cm proximal to the cone and pulled via the retrorectal space through the incision in the posterior wall of the anal canal. The redundant bowel is excised and an anastomosis between normal bowel and the anal canal is performed (Duhamel, 1960).

The open end of the rectal stump is over-sewn and crushing clamps are applied to the septum between the rectum in front and the colon behind. These separate 5–7 days postoperatively. Alternatively the cut end of the rectum can be anastomosed to the pulled-through colon and the septum can be divided at the time of the operation using a stapling device.

Soave's operation avoids dissection through the pelvic floor structures. The bowel is divided above the peritoneal reflection and the mucosa in the distal stump is excised from the muscle layers to within 1 cm of the anal canal. The proximal bowel is then pulled through the muscle tube and sutured to the peri-anal skin. Approximately three weeks later the excess bowel is trimmed (Soave, 1964).

Soave's operation

A short, ultrashort or residual segment can be adequately treated by extended internal sphincterotomy. The circular smooth muscle is divided under direct vision. It is most useful to know the length of the segment from previous anorectal physiology studies.

Extended internal sphincterotomy (sphincterectomy)

REFERENCES AND FURTHER READING

Bodian M, Stephens FD and Ward BLH. Hirschsprung's disease and idiopathic megacolon. *Lancet* 1949; **1:** 6–11.

Duhamel B. A new operation for treatment of Hirschsprung's disease. *Archives of Diseases in Childhood* 1960; **35:** 38–9.

Ehrenpreis T. Megacolon in the newborn. *Acta Chirurgica Scandinavica* 1946; **94:** supplement 112.

Nixon H and O'Donnell B. *The essentials of paediatric surgery*. London: Heinemann, 1976.

Soave F. Hirschsprung's disease: a new surgical technique. *Archives of Diseases in Childhood* 1964; **39:** 116–24.

Swenson O and Bill AH. Resection of rectum and rectosigmoid with preservation of the sphincter for benign spastic lesions producing megacolon: an experimental study. *Surgery* 1948; **24:** 212–20.

Zuelzer WW and Wilson JL. Functional intestinal obstruction on cogenital neurogenic basis in infancy. *American Journal of Diseases of Children* 1948; **75:** 40–64.

11. Anal and Peri-anal Disorders

ANATOMY

The anal canal runs from the level of the levator ani to the anal margin. It is 4 cm long in the adult and surrounded by muscular sphincters. The arrangement of these muscles, the character of the epithelial lining and the nature of the subepithelial tissues are all relevant to anal and peri-anal disorders.

ANAL SPHINCTERS

All but the most distal part of the anal canal is surrounded by a double sleeve of muscle. The outer layer is striated and comprises the external sphincter and the puborectalis part of the levator ani. The inner layer is made up of circularly-arranged smooth muscle fibres. The layers are separated by a tissue space containing longitudinally-arranged muscle fibres continuous with the longitudinal muscle layer of the rectum. This inter-sphincteric space is important because it often contains the anal glands, structures which are thought to be implicated in the pathogenesis of anal abscess and fistula. There are eight to twelve of these glands and their ducts pass through the internal sphincter and drain into the anal canal at the bases of the anal crypts. The intersphincteric space is important surgically for it provides a plane for excision of the rectum and anal canal in inflammatory bowel disease.

It is usual to divide the external sphincter into subcutaneous, superficial and deep parts. There is, however, little distinction between the three parts and from the surgeon's viewpoint the external sphincter, together with the levator ani, forms a continuous muscle sheet (Oh and Kark, 1972). The deep part of the external sphincter and the puborectalis, together with the proximal part of the internal sphincter, form the palpable anorectal ring.

The longitudinal muscle that lies between the two sphincters ends by fanning out into numerous fascicles which traverse the subcutaneous part of the external sphincter and attach to the overlying epithelium. It is generally agreed that they provide pathways for the spread of peri-anal infections and that the intense pain of peri-anal lesions is due to the way they divide the subepithelial tissue into tight compartments.

In addition to the structures already described are two fat-filled spaces which are important in relation to the anatomy of abscess and fistula. The ischiorectal fossa lies between the fascia over obturator internus, levator ani, the external sphincter and the peri-anal skin. The supralevator space lies between the rectum and the levator muscles and is, therefore, a pelvic structure. These features are depicted in Figure 11.1.

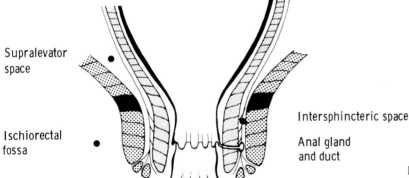

Supralevator space

Ischiorectal fossa

Intersphincteric space

Anal gland and duct

Fig. 11.1 Coronal section of anal canal.

SUBEPITHELIAL TISSUES

The tributaries of the superior and inferior haemorrhoidal veins lie in separate but poorly defined spaces in the subepithelial tissue. Their boundaries, and the nature and attachment of the smooth muscle which they contain, are disputed. Clinical observation suggests that there is some tethering of the epithelial lining of the canal; Parks (1956) suggests that this occurs at the level of the valves, the epithelium being held in place by strands of fibrous tissue which he calls the 'mucosal suspensory ligament'. He considers this to be the site of the watershed between the two systems of venous drainage, and gives the name 'submucous' to the space above the valves, and 'marginal' to the space below (Fig. 11.2).

Whatever the details of its distribution there is undoubtedly more connective tissue underlying the epithelium which covers the distal part of the internal sphincter than that covering the

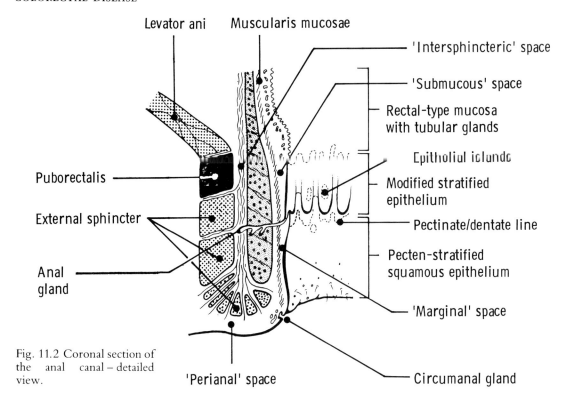

Fig. 11.2 Coronal section of the anal canal – detailed view.

proximal end. According to some, the smooth muscle in this region is merely the inferior extension of the muscularis mucosae of the rectum, while others consider it to consist of separate muscles; the 'corrugator cutis ani' at the anal margin, and the 'muscularis submucosae ani' within the distal part of the canal.

EPITHELIUM AND GLANDS

Between the anal margin and the lower border of the internal sphincter, the anal canal is lined with skin containing hairs, sebaceous and sweat glands and large apocrine glands, the so-called circumanal glands of Gay. The next 10–15 mm of the canal, originally called the 'pecten', is lined by stratified squamous epithelium. This is largely devoid of hairs and glands, but has a thin horny layer. At or below the anal valves the epithelium becomes stratified columnar or thinner stratified squamous epithelium with surface cells more cuboidal than in the pecten. The boundary between epithelial types is very ragged and longitudinal sections of the same anal canal can show differing epithelial relationships (Walls, 1958). It is not unusual to find islands of columnar epithelium amid stratified squamous epithelium. These occur more commonly between

320

anal columns, while the columns themselves are usually covered with stratified squamous, or cuboidal epithelium.

The zone of stratified squamous, cuboidal or columnar epithelium extends proximally from the anal valves for a variable distance of 5–10 mm, to its sinuous, but fairly abrupt, junction with rectal-type mucosa. Rectal-type mucosa, with tubular intestinal glands, lines the canal up to its proximal termination at the level of the levator ani. Although the anal valves and columns are not always obvious, they provide the only unambiguous macroscopic landmark. Because of the possibilities of confusion, terms such as 'anocutaneous' or 'mucocutaneous' are best avoided in descriptions of operative procedures.

REFERENCES AND FURTHER READING

Goligher JC, Leacock AG and Brossy J-J. The surgical anatomy of anal canal. *British Journal of Surgery* 1955; **43:** 51–61.

Lawson JON. Pelvic anatomy. II. Anal canal and associated sphincters *Annals of the Royal College of Surgeons of England* 1974; **54:** 288–300.

McColl I. The comparative anatomy and pathology of anal glands. *Annals of the Royal College of Surgeons of England* 1967; **40:** 36–67.

Oh C and Kark AE. Anatomy of the external anal sphincter. *British Journal of Surgery* 1972; **59:** 717–23.

Parks AG. The surgical treatment of haemorrhoids. *British Journal of Surgery* **43:** 337–51.

Walls EW. Observations on the microscopic anatomy of the human anal canal *British Journal of Surgery* 1958; **45:** 504–12.

Walls EW. Anorectal anatomy. *Scientific Basis of Medicine Annual Reviews*. London: Athlone Press, 1963: 113–24.

ABSCESS AND FISTULA

The usual definition of a fistula is an abnormal communication between any two epithelial surfaces. This must be qualified in the case of anal fistula for reasons which will become apparent. There are several causes of anal fistula and an understanding of pathogenesis is essential to successful treatment. Adequate management also demands an accurate knowledge of the anatomy of the region and the manner in which fistula tracks can ramify within it.

PATHOGENESIS

Most anal fistulae have their origin in the intersphincteric space at the level of the dentate line. Most are due to disease of the anal glands which become chronically infected (Hill, Shryock and Rebell, 1943; Lilius, 1968). Some fistulae, however, are probably related to the lymphoid tissue found around the anal glands, as for instance in tuberculosis and Crohn's disease. Whatever the cause, it is essential that the primacy of infection in the intersphincteric space at this site is understood. Without it, neither the rationale of spread of fistula tracks, nor the essential steps in treatment can be comprehended.

From this primary site in the anal canal infection can spread downwards or upwards in the intersphincteric space; it can also pass outwards through the somatic muscles into the ischiorectal fossa.

Confusion may exist about the relationship between anorectal abscess and fistula. They are, almost certainly, two phases of one and the same disease, originating in the same organ. The abscess may be acute, discharge completely and the infection be totally eliminated, in which case no further trouble arises. If the infection is not totally eliminated, then recurrent abscesses occur, or a chronically discharging sinus and a classical fistula is formed. Abscess, therefore, is the acute phase of the disease, fistula is the chronic phase. This does not imply similarity of treatment, for in the acute phase it is usually wise to make a simple drainage procedure only.

The anatomy of the spread of infection

Longitudinal spread

Infection spreads upwards or downwards in the intersphincteric space. The commonest route is downwards to the anal margin, resulting in a peri-anal abscess. Occasionally pus extends upwards (proximally) and depending upon its relationship to the longitudinal muscle layer, will cause either an abscess within the gut wall (intermuscular abscess), or outside it (supralevator abscess) – Fig. 11.3 (Hanley, 1979).

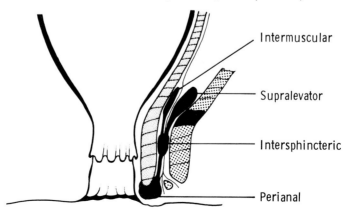

Fig. 11.3 Abscesses – vertical spread of infection.

Infection may spread across the external sphincter at any level into the ischiorectal fossa. Once at this site it may extend downwards towards the skin or upwards to the apex of the fossa and may even extend through the levator ani muscle into the supralevator space. This is therefore another route by which infection may spread to produce a supralevator abscess (Fig. 11.4). Infection may also drain across the internal sphincter to the anal canal.

Horizontal spread

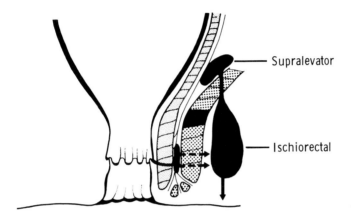

Fig. 11.4 Abscesses – horizontal spread of infection.

Circumferential spread of infection, which is rarely complete, may occur in the intersphincteric space, from one ischiorectal fossa to the other, or between the two supralevator spaces (Fig. 11.5). This is commonly known as 'horseshoeing' and is thought to indicate increased difficulty of treatment. This is not usually the case. The difficulty in dealing with a fistula depends on the level at which it penetrates the external sphincter mass.

Circumferential spread

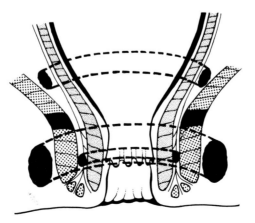

Fig. 11.5 Abscesses – circumferential spread of infection.

323

Differential diagnosis

In a small proportion of cases an anal fistula has an unusual cause such as Crohn's disease, tuberculosis, perforation of the rectum or anal canal by a foreign body, external trauma, carcinoma or postrectal dermoid cysts.

A sinus in the perineum may arise from intrapelvic disease, such as, for example, appendicitis, Crohn's disease of the terminal ileum or diverticular disease of the sigmoid colon. Pus may spread downwards either via the intersphincteric space or by crossing the levator ani muscles to enter the ischiorectal fossa. It is in this group particularly that radiology can be of great help.

Other septic processes may involve the peri-anal area and need to be distinguished from anal fistulae and abscesses. These include pilonidal infection, hidradenitis suppurativa, epidermoid cysts, and simple staphylococcal skin infection. Hidradenitis is not uncommonly associated with an anal fistula.

ABSCESS

An anal abscess usually presents with severe, unremitting, throbbing anal pain, together with pyrexia. It can occur in any of the five main sites. Diagnosis of a high abscess in the rectal wall may be delayed because of the absence of external physical signs. However, unless an obvious cause for the perineal and anal pain is detected, the patient should be examined under an anaesthetic to detect an intermuscular or supralevator abscess. Occasionally a small abscess in the intersphincteric space at the middle of the anal canal causes pain very similar to that of fissure and the diagnosis may be delayed because few physical signs are present (Parks and Thomson, 1973). However, on examination a tender nodule is usually discovered. This is an abscess which has remained localised to the primary site in the anal canal and has not spread.

Management

Abscesses should be drained by the shortest route with minimal muscle section. However, the incision should be adequate to allow the cavity to heal from its highest point without pocketing. There is a good deal of disagreement as to whether a co-existing track entering the anal canal should be laid open at the same time. It is the authors' view that distortion of the anatomy by the acute suppurative processes is so great that severe damage to the muscles can be done by such a manoeuvre.

A primary intersphincteric abscess in the wall of the anal canal should be drained by dividing the internal sphincter medial to it. Abscesses higher in the rectal wall usually burst into the rectum, or should be drained surgically by that route.

However, it is vital to establish that they have an intersphincteric origin and do not arise by extension from the ischiorectal fossa (Fig. 11.6).

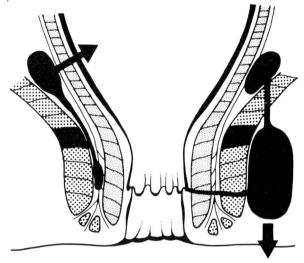

Fig. 11.6 A supralevator abscess is drained directly into the rectum if it originates from upward extension of an intersphincteric abscess (left). If it originates in upward extension from the ischiorectal fossa it should be drained to the exterior (right).

FISTULA

In order to treat fistula successfully it is necessary to know firstly the pathogenesis and secondly the anatomical type. The relationship of the primary track of a fistula to the external anal sphincters is the most important single fact that one needs to know in order to manage such a case, and it is the position of this primary track that forms the basis of the following classification (Steltzner, 1959; Parks, Gordon and Hardcastle, 1976).

Classification

A superficial fistula occurs in association with a chronic anal fissure and runs subcutaneously under a sentinal tag.

Superficial fistula

The primary track lies between the sphincters and from here it may spread upwards or downwards. Extension downwards to the anal margin gives rise to the commonest of all fistulae (Fig. 11.7). An upward extension can give rise to a blind track in the rectal wall; however, this may break backwards into the rectum forming what is often erroneously called a submucous fistula. This is not a strict definition as the track passes deep to the circular muscle on the upper anal canal and lower rectum (Fig. 11.8).

Intersphincteric fistula

325

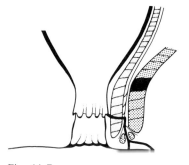

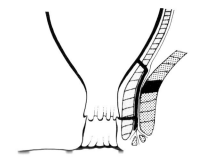

Fig. 11.7   Fig. 11.8

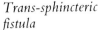

*Trans-sphincteric
fistula*

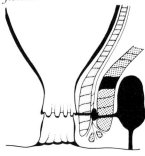

Fig. 11.9

The primary track of a trans-sphincteric fistula crosses the external sphincter from the intersphincteric space to the ischiorectal fossa (Fig. 11.9). It may do this at any level below the puborectalis muscle. Once it is in the ischiorectal fossa it can descend directly to the skin but occasionally sends a secondary track upwards to the top of the fossa or even through the levator plate into the supralevator space. It is this high secondary extension which is the cause of diagnostic difficulty and considerable anxiety from the point of view of treatment.

*Suprasphincteric
fistula*

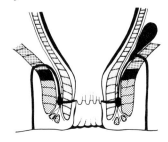

Fig. 11.10

A suprasphincteric fistula is fortunately rare. The track passes from the primary source of the fistula in the intersphincteric space upwards over the puborectalis muscle and then downwards again through the ischiorectal fossa to the skin. It therefore passes over all the muscles of continence. It is often associated with a chronic horseshoe abscess in the supralevator space (Fig. 11.10).

*Extrasphincteric
fistula*

This type passes from the intestinal tract above the anorectal ring to the skin of the perineum entirely outside the external sphincter mass and the puborectalis. In its simplest form this may be an extension of a trans-sphincteric fistula where the supralevator extension has broken back into the rectum (Fig. 11.11). Other causes include pelvic trauma, iatrogenic injury, perforation of the rectum by a foreign body and intrapelvic sepsis (Fig. 11.11).

326

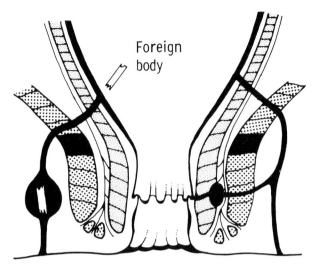

Foreign body

Fig. 11.11 Extrasphincteric fistula (right).
Perforation with abscess due to foreign body (left).

The relative frequency of the different types of fistulae classified in this way seen during a six-year period at St. Mark's Hospital is shown in Table 11a.

Table 11a. *Classification of 769 fistulae (Marks and Ritchie, 1977)*

Superficial	126	16.4%
Intersphincteric	430	55.9%
Trans-sphincteric	164	21.3%
Suprasphincteric	26	3.4%
Extrasphincteric	23	3.0%

The three essential steps in the management of a patient with an anal fistula are as follows:

The precise definition of the anatomy of the fistula.

The operation to excise the primary cause of the fistula and to give adequate drainage to secondary tracts and abscesses.

The postoperative care of the wound created by the operation.

Management

The sites of the external and internal openings of a fistula are usually apparent. The track of a low fistula can usually be palpated under the perineal skin, but if there is no induration then it is likely that the track passes at a higher level. The internal opening in the anal canal can usually be detected by finger palpation as there is a pit at the site with induration underneath it. It is usually tender. A probe can often be passed

Definition of the anatomy

into the anal opening using a suitable proctoscope. It is not always possible to determine completely the pathological anatomy in a conscious patient, especially in the difficult case, and examination under anaesthesia allows the use of anal retractors and probes and will give further information. The final anatomy of a fistula will often not be completely discovered until the operation is almost completed.

The operation

There are three main facets of the operation for fistula:

Unroofing of the intersphincteric abscess of origin in the anal canal.

Laying open of the primary track provided that this does not involve the division of over-much external sphincter.

The drainage of the secondary tracks and the creation of a large pyramidal shape wound which will allow dressings to be inserted to ensure that healing occurs from the apex.

Intersphincteric fistula

An intersphincteric fistula with a low track usually opens into the anal canal at the level of the anal valves and is readily laid open by incising the internal sphincter to the level of the internal opening. It is important to remove all the tissues at the primary site with a curette so that infected glandular lymphoid tissue is completely extirpated.

An intersphincteric fistula with a high extension is again readily treated by dividing the circular muscle as high as is necessary. Fibrosis around the track prevents separation of the divided muscle and as the entire external sphincter mass remains intact there is minimal impairment of anal function.

Trans-sphincteric fistula

The track of a trans-sphincteric fistula usually passes from the primary site in the intersphincteric space across the external sphincter in the region of the mid-anal canal, but it may open at any level, higher or lower than the internal opening. The first step is the opening of the intersphincteric space to expose the abscess of origin. Once this is done the relationship of the primary track to the puborectalis can be determined. Provided the track does not reach this muscle the lower part of the external sphincter may be divided, but it is essential to preserve the maximum amount of muscle. This is particularly true in women and in the elderly.

High tracks which can pass up to the apex of the ischiorectal fossa, or even higher still to the levators although a cause for anxiety, are purely secondary. Provided they are given adequate drainage and form the apex of the fistula wound they will heal satisfactorily.

In this case the track passes over all the muscles of continence, division of which would result in serious anorectal dysfunction. The treatment consists essentially in identifying and excising the primary source of the disease in the anal canal, giving adequate drainage to the ischiorectal and supralevator tracks and preserving at least half of the external sphincter mass. A silicone seton is usually passed around this conserved bar of muscle which may be partially divided if necessary at a later date. A fistula of this type may well take six months before healing is complete (Parks and Stitz, 1976).

Suprasphincteric fistula

In this type of fistula high rectal pressure driving mucus and stool into the track is a second cause for persistance of the condition. Generally speaking therefore a temporary colostomy is required before a cure can be established. Before treatment of this type can be planned, however, the exact cause must be determined. Those which complicate a trans-sphincteric fistula will need the standard treatment of that fistula, together with a formal closure of the opening in the rectal wall with sutures of fine stainless steel wire. If the fistula is traumatic in origin, healing may take place spontaneously after a colostomy alone.

Extrasphincteric fistula

In those cases where an extrasphincteric fistula is due to pelvic disease all that is necessary is the eradication of the site of origin; no operative intervention in the perineum is required. It is therefore imperative to make an exact diagnosis in this type of case.

There are two main functions of a seton. The principal one is to mark a fistula track which has been determined under anaesthesia. Once the patient is conscious the amount of functioning muscle enclosed by the seton can be estimated and further division carried out if necessary at a later date. The second, and perhaps more important, is as a drain to allow a high track to heal from above downwards without premature closure at the external site. It should not be used as a muscle cutting device by tying it tightly around a fistula track.

The use of a seton

At the end of an operation the surfaces of a fistula wound are kept apart by a light gauze dressing soaked in hypochlorite or some other suitable solution. Oily dressings are best avoided as occasionally a chronic inflammatory reaction occurs (an

Dressing the wound

oleogranuloma) which impairs and greatly delays healing. The postoperative care of the wound is of the greatest importance. The patient has a bath twice daily, the wound is irrigated with weak hypochlorite solution (Fig. 11.12) and a light dressing

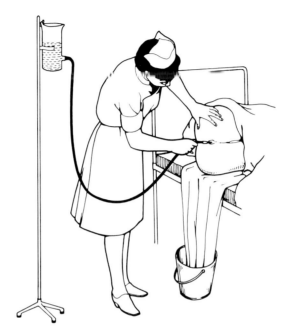

Fig. 11.12

replaced on each occasion. The aim of such treatment is to keep the wound clean with its surfaces gently apart; it is not to pack the cavity in any way. The wound will heal from the apex downwards and pocketing of pus will be avoided.

Postoperative function of the anal sphincters

Anal function will depend not only on how much muscle has been divided, but on how effective muscle function was before the operation. Many women have poorly functioning anal sphincters and even minimal division will cause serious impairment of function. It is therefore important to divide as little as possible and it is here that the seton is of such value. When in doubt it is far better to divide only the lower part of the external sphincter. If necessary more can be divided at a later operation when it has been established that residual sphincter function is adequate.

The principle behind the management of this type of case is to keep operative intervention to a minimum. It will be necessary to drain abscesses, but the Crohn's disease process will often prevent total healing and radical operations are generally contra-indicated. The use of drugs, such as salazo-pyrin, metronidazole, steroids and azathioprin may be helpful, but the treatment is often governed by the other manifestations of the disease. Nevertheless the behaviour of Crohn's lesions in the perineum is capricious and occasionally complete healing occurs quite unexpectedly, after relatively minor drainage procedures. The disease may, on the other hand, become more extensive, resulting in destruction of the sphincters and incontinence; it may then be necessary to excise the rectum completely.

REFERENCES AND FURTHER READING

Hill MR, Shryock EH and Rebell FG. The role of the anal glands in the pathogenesis of anorectal disease. *Journal of the American Medical Association* 1943; **121:** 742–6.

Lilius HG. Fistula-in-ano. *Acta Chirurgica Scandinavica* 1968; Supplement **383.**

Hanley PH. Anorectal supralevator abscess–fistula in ano. *Surgery, Gynecology and Obstetrics* 1979; **148:** 899–904.

Parks AG and Thomson JPS. Intersphincteric abscess. *British Medical Journal* 1973; **2:** 537–9.

Steltzner F. *Die anorectalen fisteln.* Berlin: Springer, 1959.

Parks AG, Gordon PH and Hardcastle JD. A classification of fistula-in-ano. *British Journal of Surgery* **63:** 1–12.

Marks CG and Ritchie JK. Anal fistulae at St. Mark's Hospital. *British Journal of Surgery* 1977; **64:** 84–91.

Parks AG and Stitz RW. The treatment of high fistula-in-ano. *Diseases of the Colon and Rectum* 1976; **19:** 487–99.

HAEMORRHOIDS

THE NATURE OF HAEMORRHOIDS

Few aspects of colorectal surgery are more confusing in nomenclature than haemorrhoids. The obvious pathological anatomical entity associated with most anal symptoms is the swollen submucosal vascular structure we call a haemorrhoid. From the times of John Hunter and Morgagni it was thought that haemorrhoids were varicose veins in the submucosal space of the anal canal and a variety of explanations were proposed. The erect posture of man, obstruction of the haemorrhoidal veins by sphincter spasm or faecal impaction or even a local weakness in the vein walls resulting from trauma or infection were all blamed. However, what these varicose vein theories did not explain adequately is the apparent return to complete normality of an anal canal that once contained huge prolapsing haemorrhoids, either spontaneously or after such simple procedures as manual dilatation.

Some have likened haemorrhoids to erectile tissue with prominent arterio-venous connections; citing as evidence the fact that bleeding is usually profuse and bright red and therefore cannot come from veins. A third theory is that haemorrhoids result from laxity of the muscular connective tissue in the upper part of the anal canal allowing the mucosa to prolapse during defaecation. However, it can be observed that haemorrhoids are much more frequently associated with a tight rather than a lax anus, and that patients with rectal prolapse do not have haemorrhoids.

In a detailed anatomical study a logically argued case was made by WHF Thomson (1975). Discounting the varicose vein and vascular hyperplasia (erectile tissue) hypotheses, he proposed that the cause was a sliding of the anal lining, composed of vascular and muscular tissue (anal cushions), leading to congestion by a tight anal sphincter. He found that three anal cushions were the normal configuration even in embryo and that they formed an integral part of a distensible yet completely watertight sphincter mechanism.

The anal cushions are normal structures analogous to the lips of the proximal end of the alimentary tract. A simple experiment of holding a tight rubber band around ones own pouted lips soon shows how congested the anal cushions might become if gripped by a tight anal sphincter. It is easy to imagine how readily hypertrophy could occur as the result of congestion. If the muscle fibres that normally hold the vascular cushion in its anatomical site become stretched or even disrupted by continuous prolapse, it is easy to imagine how irreducible prolapse could occur.

The analogy of anal cushions to the lips helps to explain the profuse bright red bleeding that can occur and the rapid healing of any surface breach. The principal difference between the anal cushions and the lips is that the cushions are permeated by the longitudinal muscle fibres arising from the outer smooth muscle layer of the bowel. Presumably, these fibres normally help to retract the anal cushions into their correct position after they protrude during defaecation. In permanently prolapsed haemorrhoids the longitudinal muscle fibres may be so stretched that they can no longer fulfil their retractile role. However, the muscle fibres are presumably not irrevocably damaged as manual dilatation or internal sphincterotomy, by relieving the constricting effect of the sphincter, can allow permanently prolapsed haemorrhoids on occasions to return to their normal position, size and, function.

Thomson (1975) has demonstrated by anatomical dissection that there is no basis for the popular belief that the common left lateral, right posterior and right anterior position of haemorrhoids is due to the anatomical position of the principal branches of the superior haemorrhoidal artery. Such branches are variable, whereas the positions of the major anal cushions tend to be quite constant in the right anterior and posterior and left lateral positions. The cause of haemorrhoids or swollen anal cushions is, therefore, either failure of the normal submucous musculature to withdraw the cushions into the anal canal after defaecation or a tight anal sphincter causing congestion and consequently hypertrophy of the anal cushions. The size of haemorrhoids varies from day to day or hour to hour and when prolapsed or congested after defaecation they can, after a period of rest, look quite small on proctoscopy. Patients often state that their haemorrhoids are very large at some times and not at others; they describe 'attacks of piles' lasting for days or weeks. The traditional classification of 1st, 2nd, 3rd, or even 4th degree piles is therefore of limited clinical or scientific value.

SYMPTOMATOLOGY AND DIFFERENTIAL DIAGNOSIS

Symptoms associated with disorders of swelling of the anal cushions are bleeding, anal discomfort after defaecation, perianal swelling, acute anal pain and, as a partially related symptom, itching. As anal cushions are normal structures, it is extremely unwise to ascribe anal symptoms to haemorrhoids just because swellings are visible on protoscopy. The lay public tends to relate all anal symptoms to 'piles' and although the doctor may feel encouraged to make this diagnosis, he must be aware of the possibility of serious anal and rectal disease.

Bleeding

Bleeding from haemorrhoids occurs characteristically after defaecation when the mucosa is prolapsed through and congested by the anal sphincter. Bleeding is often profuse, always bright red and the pan may be spattered with a jet of blood. It is rare for any other disease to give these characteristic symptoms but a prolapsing adenomatous polyp may do so. Haemorrhoids sometimes bleed spontaneously unrelated to defaecation, and occasionally they produce blood mixed with, or streaked on, the stool. A rectal adenoma or carcinoma causes rectal bleeding,

333

usually with blood on the stool and, like the bleeding from haemorrhoids, it is often intermittent.

Apart from haemorrhoids, most lesions in the lower half of the rectum will be felt on digital examination but full sigmoidoscopy is necessary, particularly to detect distal proctitis. Proctoscopy alone is insufficient to differentiate haemorrhoids from proctitis. The symptoms of proctitis are often similar to those of haemorrhoids, although the blood is usually mixed with the stool and accompanied by mucus. Furthermore, the treatment of haemorrhoids by haemorrhoidectomy, rubber band ligation or cryosurgery can cause severe problems in patients with inflammatory bowel disease. To subject all patients with rectal bleeding to full examination by either barium enema or colonoscopy might be the counsel of perfection in a society with unlimited resources, but in a patient with a pattern of rectal bleeding characteristic of haemorrhoids and in whom no abnormality is found on a full sigmoidoscopy to 25 cm it is probably not necessary. However, in patients in whom there is blood on the stool or where blood and mucus are seen on sigmoidoscopy, or in those who are anaemic, a double contrast barium enema or colonoscopy is advisable. This is also reasonable in an aged patient or where there is a family history of bowel cancer.

Discomfort and pain

What is discomfort to one man may be pain to another. Pain and discomfort are subjective but doctors should be able to recognise the difference between the dull discomfort that a patient may describe when haemorrhoids are protruding and the very sharply localised pain of a newly thrombosed external pile. It is difficult to establish objective criteria by which to classify anal pain and it is necessary to rely on the fallible methods of observation and clinical experience. It is possible that discomfort is caused by nerve endings being stretched by tissue distension and pain is associated with anal sphincter spasm. Haemorrhoids may cause discomfort after defaecation when they are 'prolapsed', that is when the anal cushions are congested by the internal sphincter. Discomfort lasts until the swelling subsides or the cushions return within the anal canal above the strangulating effect of the sphincter. Very few other conditions present the same clinical picture. Although a low rectal carcinoma, anal canal carcinoma or acute inflammatory disease of the prostate may give similar symptoms, these should be identified by digital examination.

Acute anal pain is rarely associated with internal piles unless they are complicated by thrombosis, which results in acute swelling and possibly secondary anal spasm. The commonest cause of acute anal pain is fissure-in-ano, which may also cause rectal bleeding, particularly blood on cleansing after defaecation. It is extremely common for a patient with a fissure-in-ano to describe his complaint as 'piles'. A fissure can be readily differentiated from haemorrhoids by anal canal inspection.

In thrombosis of the external haemorrhoidal veins there is intense local swelling and tenderness, rarely associated with bleeding but often diagnosed by the patient as an 'attack of piles'. This condition is not a peri-anal haematoma but a true intravascular thrombosis. It is frequently, but not necessarily, associated with the presence of engorged anal cushions and can be differentiated from haemorrhoids by finger palpation and inspection in a good light.

Prolapse

The appearance of lumps at or around the anal orifice is often misdiagnosed by patient and doctor. Normal anal cushions prolapse to some extent during defaecation. In prolapsed haemorrhoids the anal cushions swell as they prolapse with defaecation and are trapped by a tight sphincter (Fig. 11.13). The congestion and swelling can often be felt by the patient or seen with the aid of a mirror. Once reduced inside the anal sphincter, these lumps return towards normal size as the congestion subsides. Sometimes, as the result of persistent prolonged congestion by a tight sphincter, the skin component of the haemorrhoids undergoes hypertrophy and remains as a swollen skin tag. These tags cannot be returned within the anal canal and are sometimes incorrectly referred to as irreducible haemorrhoids. Fibrous polyps of the anal canal, which are usually due to gross hypertrophy of anal papillae, are sometimes mistaken for prolapsing haemorrhoids, but can be differentiated since they are felt on digital examination, whereas haemorrhoids once they have been returned into the anal canal are usually not palpable. Skin tags are also often misdiagnosed as piles, particularly when they are oedematous and associated with skin maceration in pruritus ani.

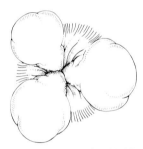

Fig. 11.13

Itching

Pruritus ani is a complex condition due to a combination of factors that include skin sensitivity, skin maceration and local bacterial or fungal infection. The condition does not appear in the differential diagnosis of haemorrhoids but when the haemorrhoids do not return completely into the anal canal and mucous membrane remains permanently exposed, the leakage of mucus gives rise to maceration of the skin causing pruritus. Pruritus is sometimes the only indication for treating haemorrhoids.

TREATMENT

General considerations

As anal symptoms associated with haemorrhoids are so common it is obvious that most patients go untreated or treat themselves with local applications. The efficacy of local applications has rarely been assessed critically but anecdotal evidence suggests that they do produce some symptomatic relief. Most of the preparations used contain several ingredients including topical anaesthetics, steroids and antiseptics. There seems to be no indication to give an antiseptic or an antibiotic. Although topical anaesthetics may give temporary relief they can provoke hypersensitivity. There is no evidence that topical steroid therapy is any better than a local anaesthetic alone in relieving symptoms nor that any of these preparations are better than a simple soft paraffin application. Soft paraffin is frequently used by sufferers as self-medication and probably works by lubricating swollen haemorrhoids or skin tags so that they do not rub together during walking or movement. Astringent or hygroscopic agents are often used, aimed presumably to reduce tissue oedema.

In contrast to the traditional topical medicaments, some orally or parenterally administered drugs have been used. Some have advocated hydroxyethylrutosides, which are vaso-active drugs with an anti-inflammatory action. They appear to be more widely prescribed on the continent of Europe than in Great Britain but there are few critical assessments of their value.

Straining at stool is one of the commonest causative, or at least aggravating, factors in the genesis of haemorrhoids. Measures to prevent straining are usually helpful. Counselling may help, the patient being advised to defaecate only when there is a positive desire to do so and to spend not more than one and a half minutes in the act of defaecation. Bulk forming aperients usually help.

It is important to realise that schemes and methods of treatment have not evolved logically but empirically. Accounts of the available methods of treating haemorrhoids written in the last century show that many of the so-called new developments are nothing more than a rediscovery or resurgent popularity of methods known and used a hundred years ago.

For convenience the principles of surgical treatment of haemorrhoids can be classified under three headings – those designed to prevent mucosal prolapse through the anus, to correct anal outlet obstruction or spasm and to remove redundant tissues.

Prevention of mucosal prolapse

Mucosal prolapse alone does not cause the symptoms normally associated with haemorrhoids, unless congestion of the prolapsed mucosa also occurs. However, symptoms cannot occur without prolapse of the mucosa and submucosal vessels.

Injection treatment, apparently first used in Dublin about 100 years ago, was not widely adopted by the medical profession until the beginning of this century. Originally the active liquid was injected into the substance of the haemorrhoid but now the technique is to inject into the submucosal space above the haemorrhoid. A special syringe and a locking needle, with a guarded end to prevent too deep penetration, is used to inject through a wide bore proctoscope (Fig. 11.14). Two to five ml

*Injection
sclerotherapy*

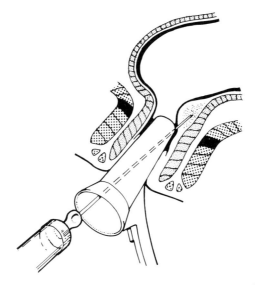

Fig. 11.14 Injection sclerotherapy.

of 5% phenol in arachis oil are placed into the submucous space. Rather than causing haemorrhoidal veins to thrombose as some believe, the injection works by producing submucosal fibrosis. If thrombosis does occur, fortunately a relatively rare complication, a painful surgical emergency may be created. It was suggested that the improvement after injection treatment might be due to the carrier oil rather than the phenol. However, Clarke, Giles and Goligher (1967), in a controlled trial, showed that phenol in oil was significantly more effective than oil alone.

Most descriptions of the technique emphasize that the injection should be placed high in the anal canal at the base of each haemorrhoid. However, if the principle is not to cause thrombosis but fibrosis then the exact site of the injection in relation to the haemorrhoid is immaterial. Some authors suggest that the injection may be repeated at intervals of three or four days but it has proved equally effective to inject circumferentially at the first treatment session and leave one or two months between sessions. If injections fail on the first occasion they are only rarely successful subsequently.

The injection technique, judged in clinical comparative trials, appears to give satisfactory short-term results particularly in patients whose only complaint is bleeding. If correctly sited it produces little pain and does not cause the reported complications, such as submucous abscess or oleogranuloma.

Freezing

Rapid freezing of tissue results in its destruction. The subsequent ulceration of the mucosa heals by granulation leading to fibrosis and fixation of the mucosa to the muscle wall. The most effective equipment uses liquid nitrogen, which rapidly lowers the temperature of the probe to $-196°C$. A tissue 'ice-ball' is produced at the tip of the cryoprobe, the visible edge of which sharply defines the area of destroyed tissue while adjacent tissue remains unaffected. At these very low temperatures nerve endings are destroyed and so cryosurgery can be employed without anaesthesia. However, if the cryodestruction involves the mucosa at the anorectal junction or the anal skin, the patient usually experiences severe pain as thawing occurs. For this reason cryosurgery is used almost exclusively to produce destruction of the mucosa within the anal above the area with somatic sensory innervation. As liquid nitrogen is expensive the cheaper nitrous oxide cryoprobe which produces temperatures of only $-60°$ to $-80°$ is more commonly used. The nerve endings are not so rapidly destroyed and several minutes are required to produce a satisfactory 'ice-ball'.

One of the principal disadvantages of this technique is the profuse watery discharge that tends to occur from the anal region, particularly if tissue is frozen distal to the dentate line.

Treatment of external skin tags by cryosurgery is more painful than excision under local anaesthesia and the watery discharge following cryosurgery is inconvenient and uncomfortable for the patient. Preliminary results of a prospective comparative trial of cryosurgery and rubber band ligation show no advantage for cryosurgery. It takes longer to perform and the equipment is more expensive than that for rubber band ligation.

Ligation

Ligation of an entire prolapsed haemorrhoid, including the skin covered portion, was the standard treatment in the middle ages. As this ligature included the sensitive part of the anal canal it must have been a painful procedure, and this prevented its widespread use. Ligation without excision fell into disuse until it was re-introduced with ligation of the mucosa above the level of cutaneous innervation. The method gained popularity after Barron (1963) developed a more sophisticated instrument employing a strong rubber ring or band. The band gripped the mucosa sufficiently to cut off its blood supply and cause localised necrosis and ulceration. Initial experience of the rubber band ligation technique following Barron's description of ligating the haemorrhoid itself, invariably caused pain that was often severe. By placing the rubber band more than 1 cm above the line of the anal valves, the pain was much less and the ligation was equally effective. No evidence of congested veins can be seen at this level and it is not possible to recognise the sites of the primary haemorrhoids. Rubber band ligation removes excess tissue and produces an ulcer which leads to mucosal fixation after it has healed. It does not work by producing thrombosis (Fig. 11.15).

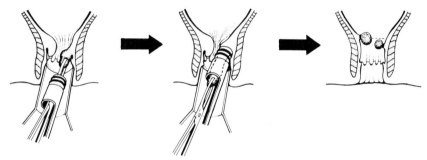

Fig. 11.15 Rubber band ligation.

Secondary haemorrhage may occur between the 7th and 14th day when the necrotic tissue sloughs and separates. The incidence is the same whether the slough is created by ligation, freezing or suture, and there seems to be no way of preventing it. Patients should be warned of this possibility and are advised not to go on safari or solo yacht races for fourteen days after ligation.

It is difficult to repeat rubber band ligation within a few weeks of the original ligation as the mucosa is not sufficiently lax. Patients are advised to return in two months and if the symptoms are not completely controlled, two further ligations are performed laterally at 90° to the original ligation. About 70% of patients have their symptoms controlled by the first ligation and a further 15% by the second. It has not been found necessary to employ freezing or topical anaesthesia, either before or after ligation. Patients can be provided with a mild oral analgesic but with high placement of the bands these are now rarely necessary. They can leave the clinic directly and, if they wish to, return to work immediately. They are advised to attempt to suppress the desire to defaecate for the remainder of the day. If there is a tendency to constipation, a lubricating or bulk forming aperient should be prescribed. Little time is lost from work as a result of rubber band ligation.

As with any treatment of haemorrhoids, the longer the follow-up period the greater will be the number of recurrences. Panda, Laughton, Elder and Gillespie (1974) have reported a recurrence rate of 11%, a rate that corresponds closely with that of 14% in a long term survey of the results of rubber band ligation conducted by Steinberg, Liegois and Alexander-Williams (1975). However, many recurrences can be treated by repeated ligation. Although the rate of cured or satisfied patients is very high (over 90%), it should be realised that they are not necessarily all permanently asymptomatic.

Infra-red coagulation

The newest tool in the proctological armamentarium is the infra-red coagulator. This is a simple device employing a quartz halogen lamp, a reflector and light-conducting handle. A one-second pulse of infra-red radiation produces accurately defined necrosis 3 mm deep and 3 mm in diameter. The probe can be used *via* a proctoscope at exactly the same site as one does rubber band ligation, cryosurgery or injection. The procedure is quick and precise, the equipment much less expensive and the apparatus probably safer than that used for cryosurgery. The results of planned clinical trials are awaited with interest.

Correction of anal outlet obstruction

Dilatation

It is difficult to see how forceful dilatation of the anus could have been conceived as a logical therapy for patients with haemorrhoids. It has, however, been known as a method of treatment for some time; the ancient Greeks practised it. Lord (1975) recounts that his first experience with manual dilatation of the anus happened by chance when he was attempting to make the anus larger in order to reduce acutely prolapsed congested haemorrhoids that otherwise could not be reduced. He then discovered that, on the following day, the haemorrhoids appeared to be 'cured' and did not recur. Lord describes circular constricting bands around the anal canal at more than one level and considers that these must be thoroughly stretched before the symptoms of haemorrhoids are relieved. Biopsies of these bands have shown them to consist of normal muscle fibres. Manual dilatation of the anus has proved to be effective in the management of haemorrhoids and this technique has been adopted in many centres throughout the world. Its success has also led to a reconsideration of the aetiology of haemorrhoids and many surgeons question the necessity of excising enlarged anal canal tissues. It is a frequent observation that enormously enlarged haemorrhoids can disappear and the anal canal eventually becomes completely normal on proctoscopy.

Where the symptoms are predominantly those of prolapse and the patient is elderly with a low resting anal pressure, manual dilatation is less effective. It is in this group that incontinence may be caused.

In trials comparing manual dilatation with rubber band ligation and lateral subcutaneous sphincterotomy, there was little difference between the three methods. Manual dilatation is easy to perform, requires little training and few special instruments. It is, however, comparatively costly requiring general anaesthesia and a short hospital stay.

Internal sphincterotomy

Partial division of the internal anal sphincter is an established method of treating chronic anal fissure. Many surgeons have adopted this procedure, first for fissure and, more recently, for haemorrhoids. Lateral sphincterotomy is preferable to posterior sphincterotomy since healing is quicker and soiling less common. The operation can be performed under general or local anaesthesia and a description of the technique is given by Allgöwer (1975).

Removal of redundant tissue

Haemorrhoidectomy

Excision of prolapsed haemorrhoidal tissue has been practised since ancient times. However, it was well known that simple excision or ligation or cautery were associated with considerable pain and the risk of haemorrhage. In Great Britain it was Salmon in the 19th Century who was responsible for the greatest advance in the surgical treatment of haemorrhoids when he showed that the principal vessels feeding prolapsing haemorrhoids could be dissected free from sensitive mucosa and ligated at their base. The operation most commonly used in Britain today is that described by Milligan and his colleagues in 1937 (Fig. 11.16). They carried their incision to the upper anal canal but an area of sensitive mucous membrane can become incorporated in the ligated pedicle and may be the reason for the postoperative discomfort so often experienced. Parks (1956) has described a method of submucosal dissection by which it is possible to dissect out the haemorrhoid without having to

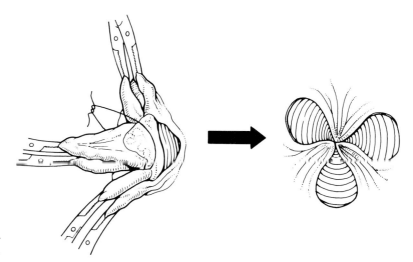

Fig. 11.16 Ligature and excision haemorrhoidectomy.

sacrifice much of the epithelium of the anal canal. It is claimed that the method produces less pain than the classical low-ligation haemorrhoidectomy. A similar technique of so-called 'closed haemorrhoidectomy' has been described by Ferguson and his colleagues (1971) (Fig. 11.17). The technique of sub-

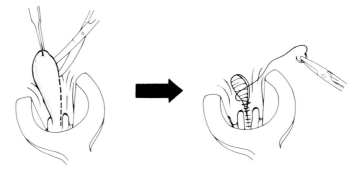

Fig. 11.17
Closed haemorrhoidectomy.

mucosal dissection, with or without primary suture of the epithelium, has not become popular. Part of the reason for this is that it is more difficult to learn the mucosal dissection technique than the simple excision haemorrhoidectomy. This is particularly true in patients who have previously had injection therapy, rubber band ligation or cryosurgery. Many surgeons have furthermore been influenced by the results of trials which indicate that pain was not significantly different after excision with low ligation, excision with clamp and cautery or sub-mucosal excision. It appears that the individual patient's reaction to pain after haemorrhoidectomy is probably more important than the type of operation used. On average only 5% of all patients with haemorrhoids require a haemorrhoidectomy and almost all of these have had some form of previous conservative treatment.

Haemorrhoidectomy can be complicated by reactionary haemorrhage which is due to poor haemostatic technique and should be preventable. Secondary haemorrhage, which occurs in 2% of cases, is due to the late separation of necrotic infected tissue at the site of ligation of the haemorrhoidal pedicle. Thrombosis of peri-anal venous plexuses can occur. Anal stenosis is a late complication which occurs less often after submucosal haemorrhoidectomy than after ligation and excision.

COMPLICATION OF HAEMORRHOIDS

An acute intravascular thrombosis in the veins beneath the peri-anal skin will produce a painful tender swelling. The episode may last seven to ten days before the swelling subsides as the thrombosis organises.

Thrombosed external haemorrhoids

When this condition involves the whole anal margin it is best treated by bed rest, the application of ice packs or an evaporating lead lotion, analgesics and a lubricant laxative. If it involves only a part of the circumference a discrete swelling occurs. This is sometimes called a *peri-anal haematoma* and may have a different pathology. Whilst it may be treated in the way described above it can, after infiltration with local anaesthetic, be evacuated with instant relief of pain.

Acute irreducible haemorrhoids associated with gross oedema, often with venous thrombosis and invariably with severe pain, are often referred to as being strangulated. They may be treated as described above but the symptoms may persist for several days and residual symptoms are almost always the rule (Grace and Creed, 1975). Manual dilatation may relieve the congestion and oedema and relieve the pain. Internal sphincterotomy may have a similar effect. Haemorrhoidectomy also has a place especially if the haemorrhoidal masses are hard. Whilst this is straightforward for a single prolapse thrombosed haemorrhoid, it may not be so easy to perform when the problem is circumferential; there is a danger of removing too much skin and mucosa which may be followed by anal stenosis.

Thrombosed, prolapsed haemorrhoids (strangulated piles)

PLANNING TREATMENT

Patients may be relieved of symptoms simply by avoiding straining. When symptoms persist there is available a graduated armamentarium of therapy, the choice depending on the nature and severity of the principal symptoms. In the young patient presenting with bleeding, good results may be expected from any of the methods of mucosal fixation; injection, freezing, or rubber band ligation. In the young patient with high anal tone and, in particular, in those patients in whom pain or discomfort are prominent features, it is usually best to rely on measures that relieve the congesting effect of the internal sphincter. If facilities for general anaesthesia are available, manual dilatation of the anus is the simplest technique that reliably relieves most patients of their symptoms. Once the technique of lateral subcutaneous sphincterotomy has been perfected it is a reliable alternative and can be used under local anaesthesia.

In patients over the age of 60, those with a lax anus and women who have had parturition perineal injury, dilatation or sphincterotomy should be avoided and mucosal fixation is preferred. Whilst skin tags do not usually give rise to symptoms they are occasionally the principal indication for advocating haemorrhoidectomy. Haemorrhoidectomy may be carried out for other reasons such as resistance to other forms of treatment, patient preference or thrombosis.

REFERENCES AND FURTHER READING

Allgöwer M. Conservative management of haemorrhoids. 3 – Partial internal sphincterotomy. *Clinics in Gastroenterology* 1975; **4**: 608–18.

Barron J. Office ligation for internal haemorrhoids. *American Journal of Surgery* 1963; **105**: 563–70.

Clarke CG, Giles GR and Goligher JC. Results of conservative management of internal haemorrhoids. *British Medical Journal* 1967; **2**: 12–4.

Ferguson JA, Mazier WP, Ganchrow MI and Friend WG. The closed technique of haemorrhoidectomy. *Surgery* 1971; **70**: 480–4.

Grace RH and Creed A. Prolapsing thrombosed haemorrhoids: outcome of conservative management. *British Medical Journal* 1975; **2**: 354.

Lord PH. Conservative management of haemorrhoids: 2 – Dilatation treatment. *Clinics in Gastroenterology* 1975; **4**: 601–8.

Milligan ETC, Morgan CN, Jones LE and Officer R. Surgical anatomy of the anal canal, and the operative treatment of haemorrhoids. *Lancet* 1937; **2**: 1119–24.

Panda AP, Laughton JM, Elder JB and Gillespie IE. Treatment of haemorrhoids by rubber band ligation. *Digestion* 1975; **12**: 85–91.

Parks AG. Surgical treatment of haemorrhoids. *British Journal of Surgery* 1956; **43**: 337–51.

Steinberg DM, Liegois H and Alexander-Williams J. Long term review of the results of rubber band ligation of haemorrhoids. *British Journal of Surgery* 1975; **62**: 144–6.

Thomson WHF. The nature of haemorrhoids. *British Journal of Surgery* 1975; **62**: 542–52.

FISSURE

Fissure-in-ano is a common and minor disorder but merits careful attention because it is painful and treatment is simple and effective. A fissure is a longitudinal ulcer situated in the anal canal, it usually lies posteriorly in the midline and may be up to 1.5 cm in length.

AETIOLOGY

It is often suggested that an episode of constipation causes a fissure, a hard stool being forced against the posterior margin of the anus. Posteriorly the internal sphincter is poorly supported by the external sphincter which firmly embraces it laterally. The unsupported posterior anal mucosa is easily damaged. Frequently there are larger anal crypts in the midline posteriorly and these too are liable to be traumatized by the stool.

Measurements of intra-anal pressure using a sensitive pressure probe have shown that patients with a fissure have an abnormally high anal pressure and slower waves of contraction of the internal sphincter (Hancock, 1977). These contraction waves may account for the pain but they also raise the possibility that there is an underlying abnormality of the internal anal sphincter.

PATHOLOGY

The fissure commences as a linear ulcer in the base of which the fibres of the longitudinal muscle are clearly visible. The ulcer may then develop certain features associated with *chronicity* becoming deeper and exposing the pale transverse fibres of the internal sphincter. Granulation tissue forms around the edges of the ulcer and undermining between the edge and the internal sphincter allows a small abscess to develop just superficial to the internal sphincter. Because of the spasm of this sphincter, the abscess is unable to drain. The chronic inflammatory tissue may become heaped up at the proximal part of the fissure to form a fibrous anal polyp at the level of the dentate line (present in 16% of patients) (Fig. 11.18). An external anal skin tag (sentinel pile) may be found in 40% of patients, being more common in women than men. Distally this external skin tag may itself become undermined, forming a bridged fissure (superficial fistula). Fissures frequently occur adjacent to the right posterior haemorrhoid as a result of traction upon the haemorrhoid at the time of defaecation.

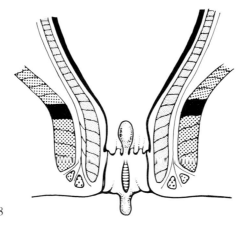

Fig. 11.18

CLINICAL FEATURES

Fissures have classically been divided into acute and chronic but the length of history bears no relationship to the type of fissure found. A patient with a long history of intermittent fissure may have recurrent simple tears whereas a patient with a single episode, sometimes as short as one week's duration, may already have developed a florid undermined lesion. It is, therefore, most informative to consider fissures as either simple or complex rather than acute or chronic.

History

The length of history may vary from several years to a few hours. There is usually more than one symptom of which the commonest is pain (90%), followed by bleeding (80%), pruritus (45%), complaint of an anal lump (30%) or of an anal discharge (5%). In the simple type of fissure, the patient complains of acute pain in the anal area upon defaecation whereas in the more complex fissure the pain is usually a dull ache coming on after defaecation and lasting up to two hours. Bleeding usually occurs as a few spots of blood noted on the lavatory paper. Complaints of an anal lump or discharge are not usually related to the presence of an external anal skin tag or to a discharging fistula.

Occasionally the patient will give a history of an episode of diarrhoea or constipation antedating the onset of anal symptoms and it should be remembered that such symptoms may be the result of inflammatory intestinal disease. Constipation is more usually secondary to the pain associated with defaecation in the presence of the fissure. Ten per cent of mothers have a fissure at some time during the puerperium, the incidence being greater following a difficult delivery; some of these fissures persist.

With the patient in the left lateral position, it is usually possible to examine the peri-anal area and lower anal canal by gently parting the buttocks (Fig. 1.5). It should be emphasised that the condition can be extremely painful and even at this stage the patient may complain of severe discomfort unless the examination is undertaken with the utmost care. Peri-anal excoriation, a skin tag or a related haemorrhoid may be seen. Digital rectal examination will probably cause severe pain and further examination is probably best carried out using a pediatric sigmoidoscope of the Lloyd-Davies pattern – diameter 10 mm (Fig. 1.11). This small-bore instrument allows the distal rectal mucosa to be examined to exclude the possibility of inflammatory disease, as well as the anal canal. It must be emphasised that if sigmoidoscopy is not performed at this stage, it must be done at some point during the early management of the patient, since other pathology may be present.

Sixty per cent of anal fissures occur in men and this male predominance is present in all decades except in those under 20 when fissures are more than twice as common in women as in men. Seventy-five per cent of fissures occur posteriorly, only 15% are anterior and a further 8% of patients have both posterior and anterior fissures. Lateral fissures are uncommon (2%) as primary pathology but may occur in combination with posterior and/or anterior fissures. There is a sex difference between the position of fissures; in women 20% of fissures are anterior, whereas in men only 10% are anterior.

Special investigations are rarely required. If a barium enema is requested in order to exclude other pathology, it may be too painful to perform until after the fissure has been cured. In addition to co-existing pathology in the rectum or abdomen, the differential diagnosis of a primary anal fissure includes Crohn's disease in which case there are usually other manifestations of the disorder such as violaceous skin discoloration and oedematous tags. Tuberculosis, primary chancre, leukoplakia, leukaemic infiltration, reticulosis, squamous cell carcinoma, Bowen's disease and Paget's disease of the anus have also presented as fissures, but less than 1% of all cases are due to these. Foreign bodies passing through the anal canal in either direction may also traumatize it.

TREATMENT

Nonoperative

A large number of patients with anal fissures are never seen in hospital. The episode may be so trivial that the patient does not seek treatment or the condition may be treated by the general practitioner with a wide variety of proprietary creams and pastes. It is not known how successful treatment with these applications is, but from first principles it seems unlikely that they are efficacious. On presentation in the clinic, careful assessment of the fissure is essential to determine the precise method of treatment indicated. Only simple fissures are suitable for conservative treatment and the more complex varieties require early operation.

It has long been recognised that simple fissures can be cured conservatively. Methods recommended in the past included a non-constipating diet, laxatives and attention to personal hygiene. Topical treatment arose historically by the application of ointments containing opiate to relieve pain, belladonna to alleviate sphincter spasm and silver nitrate or pure ichthyol to promote healing, the ingredients being mixed in a bland base to protect the fissure from further trauma. The mixture was introduced on the finger or a short rectal bougie to ensure its application to the proximal part of the fissure. The modern practice is to insert an anal dilator (Fig. 11.19) well lubricated with lignocaine gel both to act as a lubricant and as a local anaesthetic. This should be done two to three times a day for about five minutes at a time. It is recommended that the instrument is passed before the passage of stool to prevent exacerbation of symptoms during defaecation.

Complications of this treatment include pruritus due to sensitisation of the skin to the local anaesthetic and loss of the dilator in the rectum. Patients should be seen frequently until the fissure has healed. If healing has not taken place within two weeks, the patient should undergo operative treatment without delay, since persistence with this treatment is uncomfortable. Other forms of conservative management are practised elsewhere but have not found favour. They include the application of phenol to the fissure or the injection of lignocaine into its base, the complication most feared being the production of an intersphincteric abscess.

In children, in whom it is frequently difficult to visualise the fissure, treatment should be by oral stool softening agents. The majority of fissures will respond to this conservative therapy but it must be remembered that a child may rarely, secondarily to the pain of the fissure, retain stool in the rectum and develop secondary overflow incontinence.

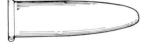

Fig. 11.19

Operative

Operation is indicated following a failed course of conservative treatment. It is also indicated for a fissure complicated by fibrous anal polyp at the level of the dentate line, by an external anal skin tag, haemorrhoids or infection in the base of the fissure including the presence of a bridged fissure (superficial fistula). It has been shown (Lock and Thomson, 1977) that fissures complicated by any of these factors will not heal spontaneously and will not respond to conservative treatment.

The rationale of operative treatment is to destroy the spastic contraction of the internal sphincter and thus to alleviate the pain of the fissure, allowing it to heal.

Reduction of the internal sphincter tone may be performed either by stretching (Watts, Bennett and Goligher, 1964) or by partial sphincterotomy. Sphincterotomy is usually performed in the left or right lateral position either in an open or closed procedure (Notaras, 1977). A dorsal sphincterotomy still has a place when there is associated sepsis. Lateral sphincterotomy (Fig. 11.20) is preferred by many since the operation is more

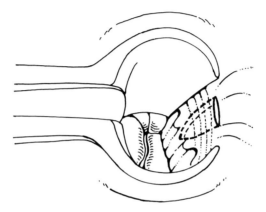

Fig. 11.20 Lateral (partial internal) sphincterotomy.

precise than stretching the whole anal canal and does not carry the disadvantage of possible damage to the entire anal musculature which may, especially in the elderly, cause temporary or permanent anal incontinence. In addition, an anal polyp, associated haemorrhoid or sentinel tag should also be excised.

Results of operation

Dividing the sphincter in the base of the fissure (posterior or dorsal sphincterotomy) was widely practised until recently. It has now been shown (Hawley, 1969) that whereas lateral sphincterotomy provides an almost 100% cure rate, the posterior operation only achieved cure in 90%, and carries a much higher risk of minor soiling due to the formation of a 'key-hole' deformity at the site of operation. At the present time lateral sphincterotomy is the treatment of choice.

REFERENCES AND FURTHER READING

Hancock BD. The internal sphincter and anal fissure. *British Journal of Surgery* 1977; **64:** 92–5.

Hawley PR. The treatment of chronic fissure-in-ano. *British Journal of Surgery* 1969; **56:** 915–18.

Lock MR and Thomson JPS. Fissure-in-ano: the initial management and prognosis. *British Journal of Surgery* 1977; **64:** 355–8.

Notaras MJ. Fissure-in-ano. Lateral subcutaneous internal anal sphincterotomy. Todd IP, ed. *Colon, rectum and anus*. (3rd ed. Operative surgery.) London and Boston: Butterworths, 1977: 354–60.

Watts J McK, Bennett RC and Goligher JC. Stretching of anal sphincters in treatment of fissure-in-ano. *British Medical Journal* 1964; **2:** 342–3.

PRURITUS ANI

More than 90% of patients referred to a dermatologist from the proctological clinic complain of pruritus ani. It is a symptom only and steps must always be taken to establish an underlying cause.

Pruritus may accompany anal disorders such as haemorrhoids and fissure or it may be due to minor physical disturbances, such as excess sweating, lack of cleanliness or obesity. Hirsute fat patients have to be more particular about washing than the lean and hairless. Persistent pruritus may not only be due to physical causes, but also to emotional factors, but it should not be assumed that an anxious patient itches because of his anxiety, since any patient with persistent pruritus may become emotionally upset. Not only is itching socially embarrassing, it may also interfere with sleep. Other commoner causes of pruritus ani include skin infections and infestations, allergies, steroid local effects and primary dermatological problems.

ASSESSMENT

Clinical

A full history is taken with special reference to skin disease elsewhere: has the patient had any diseases requiring broad spectrum antibiotics recently? Has he ever had psoriasis or atopic eczema? Has he a family history of these? A full examination is carried out including an assessment of peri-anal hygiene and detection of anorectal disease by sigmoidoscopy and proctoscopy. The simplest way to diagnose threadworms is to see them on the rectal mucosa during sigmoidoscopy, or on 'sellotape-swabs'.

Investigation

Urine testing – glycosuria should always be excluded as patients with diabetes mellitus are prone to skin infections.

Ultra-violet light – The peri-anal skin should be examined under ultra-violet light. Infection with *Corynebacterium minutissimum* (erythrasma) results in a salmon-pink fluorescence.

Skin scrapings – The taking of skin scrapings is essential, especially when no other cause has been found and where there is scaling. This is done with a scalpel blade and the scrapings examined on a microscope slide for the presence of hyphae. To prepare the slide the scrapings are macerated in a 10% solution of potassium hydroxide. A separate sample is sent to the laboratory for mycological culture on Sabouraud's medium.

High vaginal swab – In female patients pruritus ani may occur with pruritus vulvae. This may result from a primary vaginal infection such as candidiasis.

Patch testing – Patch testing may be needed to confirm the diagnosis of allergic contact dermatitis and identify the allergen. It is usually carried out using a large range of allergens so that unsuspected positives may be found. It is also wise to patch test with any cream the patient may have been applying.

The tests are performed very simply on the patient's back. A drop of the test substance is placed on a small piece of filter paper heat-sealed on to aluminium foil. It is then fastened to the back with zinc oxide plaster for 48 hours. The patches are then removed and the skin inspected. Any vesiculation or redness is looked for immediately on removal of the plaster, 15 minutes later, and again 48 hours later – i.e. 96 hours after application.

Biopsy – The morphological characteristics of any skin condition are modified by local factors. This is particularly true of the peri-anal region which tends to be warm and moist. Lesions that would normally scale become reddened and exuberant, and secondary inflammation frequently occurs. Despite this, the peri-anal appearances of many of the common dermatoses are characteristic to the trained eye. Histological examination may, however, be necessary, especially if malignancy is suspected, or in making a differential diagnosis in bullous diseases. Either a conventional biopsy or a 3 mm punch biopsy may be taken.

INFECTIONS

Infections of the peri-anal skin which produce itching may be bacterial, viral, fungal or parasitic.

Bacterial infections

Erythrasma is a well-defined browny-red condition of the peri-anal skin and genitocrural folds due to infection with *Corynebacterium minutissimum*. The diagnosis can be confirmed by examination under ultraviolet light, as well as on microscopic examination of a scraping. The treatment is erythromycin 250 mg six-hourly for ten days.

351

Viral infections

Viral infections, such as molluscum contagiosum and condylomata acuminata are discussed elsewhere (Chapter 12).

Fungal infections

Candidiasis – Infection with *Candida albicans* is characterised by scattered peripheral reddened papules, some of the lesions having white edges. A scraping will show the organisms, and frequently also hyphae. The organism has two growth phases – yeast cells and hyphae; the yeast cells alone may be commensals, but when there is a predominance of hyphae there is infection. Candidiasis is common when cellular immunity is reduced and in patients with diabetes.

Epidermophyton and trichophyton infections – *Tinea cruris* and other fungal infections may affect the peri-anal skin. A lesion is characteristically circinate and scaly. It may be associated with lesions elsewhere especially in the groin and feet. The treatment of choice is topical clotrimazole, miconazole or econazole.

Intertrigo of the peri-anal region is common, and usually extends into the groin and natal cleft. Inflammation in the body folds occurs more frequently in the obese and sweaty, and those wearing occlusive clothing or dressings. Secondary infection with Candida is common, but it is often difficult to determine whether this is primary or secondary. There may be similar lesions elsewhere on the body. The main complaint is soreness and on examination an ill-defined reddened area, which may be fissured and oozing, is seen. An antibiotic or antiseptic combined with a local steroid preparation may be used for a short period initially. If Candida is present, nystatin should be used as well.

Parasitic infections (infestations)

Threadworms are effectively eliminated using piperazine hydrate as a single oral dose (adults 2 g, children 120 mg/kg body weight) repeated after two weeks. All members of a family should be treated simultaneously.

Lice are treated using malathion 0.5% lotion and scabies by γ-benzene hexachloride 1.0% lotion. Again, other contacts should be examined and treated if necessary.

REACTIONS TO MEDICINES

Contact dermatitis

In *allergic contact dermatitis* the peri-anal region is reddened and oedematous. It most commonly follows the application of medicaments, common 'offenders' being lanoline, local anaesthetics, neomycin, and soframycin, topical antihistamines and parabens (a preservative added to many creams and ointments). Perfumed sprays, nylon clothes and rubber contraceptives have also been incriminated. If a contact sensitivity is suspected, there may also be a dermatitis of the tips of the fingers. Discrete eczematous patches may be seen peri-anally in patients with nail varnish dermatitis and are due to digital contact.

Primary irritant dermatitis may follow the use of wart remedies or disinfectants, either on first exposure or after repeated applications. It subsides quickly on withdrawing the irritant. Calamine cream or a dilute corticosteroid cream should be applied for a short period. Saline or potassium permanganate baths (1/10 000) are soothing in the acute stages of both primary irritant and contact dermatitis.

Steroid effects

Local reactions to steroids are well described on the face, and also occur in the peri-anal region although they are not so often recognised. Prolonged use of the more potent steroids produces atrophy of the skin and erythema. There is usually soreness and burning which is initially relieved by further applications of the offending substance. The treatment is to remove the cause.

Broad spectrum antibiotics

Oral administration of some antibiotics may be followed by pruritus as a result of a disturbance in the bacterial flora of the gut.

PRIMARY DERMATOLOGICAL PROBLEMS

Eczema

Eczema of any type, if widespread, may involve the peri-anal area, although this is relatively rare even in quite severe and extensive atopic eczema.

Lichen simplex (neurodermatitis) of the peri-anal area may be found to alternate with other patches of lichen simplex on the nape of the neck or anywhere – but it tends to be even more itchy in the peri-anal area than elsewhere and it is only very rarely scaly. The lichenification may be severe and give rise to a 'warty' raised appearance.

Seborrhoeic eczema is found quite frequently in the peri-anal area and in the groins. Unlike intertrigo there is a well marked edge to the erythema. Histology shows characteristic appearances of eczema, but frequently features of psoriasis may also be seen. Local antiseptic and antibiotic combinations are helpful, but should only be used for short periods to avoid secondary sensitisation (contact dermatitis).

Psoriasis

Psoriasis often involves the peri-anal area. In this site it appears somewhat atypical having a sharp outline and a bright red glazed appearance. As it spreads away from the anus the

353

edges may have the characteristic scaly appearance. Patches of psoriasis on the elbows, knees and scalp, or nails are usually found.

Histological examination even of atypical areas shows typical features of psoriasis.

Corticosteroids may be used in the treatment, but the stronger preparations should only be used for limited periods since they may produce striae, atrophy and soreness. Mild preparations, such as oils, and zinc and castor oil cream, may be found to help.

Bullous dermatoses

Epidermolysis, familial benign chronic pemphigus, pemphigus vulgaris, pemphigus vegetans and erythema multiforme may all affect the peri-anal region. Lesions are always found at other sites.

Atrophic dermatoses

Lichen sclerosis et atrophicus and lichen planus are atrophic dermatoses which may involve the peri-anal area.

The treatment is the removal of irritants and application of bland soothing creams. One percent hydrocortisone cream may be prescribed, but stronger local steroids should be avoided as they may cause further atrophy.

Atrophic lesions may become malignant, and a close watch must therefore be kept for the development of leukoplakia. Patches of *thickened* and whitish skin which are not influenced by treatment should be biopsied, as should ulcers which do not heal.

SYSTEMIC DISORDERS

Systemic diseases may become manifest as pruritus of the peri-anal region. These include diabetes mellitus, obstructive jaundice, Hodgkin's disease and polycythaemia.

Peri-anal lesions in Crohn's disease are present in approximately half the patients and may be the presenting feature. Oedema and violaceous peri-anal tags are common, as are indolent ulceration and abscesses. Unfortunately excision of the affected bowel does not always lead to clearing of the skin and scarring is frequent even if these lesion heal.

Other rare causes of anal skin disorders include acanthosis nigricans, Darier's disease and neurofibromatosis.

REFERENCE AND FURTHER READING

Alexander S. Dermatological aspects of anorectal disease. *Clinics in Gastroenterology* 1975; **4**: 651–7.

PILONIDAL SINUS

It is surprising that such a well-known benign condition as pilonidal sinus should still excite controversy. There still remains uncertainty as to its true aetiology and pathogenesis or, indeed, as to whether there is a single cause. Its reputation for recurrence after treatment has provoked surgical ingenuity to devise numerous operations with multiple modifications varying from simple measures to radical excision.

GENERAL DESCRIPTION

A typical sinus consists of one or more pits lined by squamous epithelium in the crease of the natal cleft leading to a subcutaneous cavity lined by granulation tissue and containing a mass of loose hair. The midline or primary pits appear to be the route of entry of foreign material and hairs; when viewed under magnification they look like the orifices of sweat glands or sebaceous follicles. From the main underlying cavity hair may track subcutaneously, giving rise to secondary cavities and openings on to the skin. Tracking most frequently occurs in a cephalad direction either in the midline or laterally into the buttocks; in less than 10% the tracking is towards and to one side of the anus. It is rare to find more than one or two tracks with such secondary openings.

Histology

The midline primary pits are lined by squamous epithelium but hair follicles are not present. The underlying cavity is lined by a vascular granulation tissue in which some foreign body giant cell systems may be seen as well as hair and hair fragments. There is no histological evidence of any cyst wall or even a wall partly destroyed by infection, so the term pilonidal cyst should probably be abandoned. Secondary tracks and skin openings are all lined by granulation tissue.

AETIOLOGY

Postanal pilonidal sinus occurs most commonly in young adults between the ages of 18 and 30 with a male predominance of 70%. Hirsutism, chronic irritation, intertrigo and sepsis are precipitating factors. The war-time term 'Jeep-seat' suggested a traumatic origin but civilian practice suggests that this is not so, although the sitting posture may be a contributory factor. Over 90% of affected male patients have been noted to have an excessive growth of hair in the glabella region.

The epithelial-lined skin pits in the natal crease appear to be the site of entry of hair and other foreign material which form the subcutaneous cavity but the origin of these pits has caused controversy.

A congenital origin of pilonidal sinuses was postulated but evidence has now accumulated to support the suggestion that the condition is acquired. The congenital theory invoked imperfect midline skin union, associations with spina bifida and neural canal vestiges, vestiges related to the preen gland in birds, vestigial sex glands and traction dermoids in the sacro-coccygeal region. These theories are untenable when they are related to the factors of age and sex distribution, the rarity of associated congenital defects, recurrences after wide excision and the histological appearances with the absence of hair follicles and epithelial lining to the main underlying cavities.

Although the condition is now generally accepted as being acquired the disagreement over the origin of the primary midline pits continues. They may be produced as a result of direct puncture by loose hairs or by hairs growing on the side of the natal cleft. Alternatively, the pits may be sweat or pilo-sebaceous follicles into which foreign material and other hairs can be drawn because of their situation. Support for the hair puncture theory is suggested as similar sinuses can be seen in the webs of the fingers and other sites in barbers. Barbers' sinuses, however, have cut hairs which have chisel-like ends capable of penetrating the skin and it is less likely that normal loose hairs or local hairs bending into the natal cleft could puncture the skin unless it was softened by intertrigo.

It has been postulated that squamous epithelium proliferates down the puncture wound to form a primary pit into which loose hair and debris can penetrate, setting up a granulomatous and septic tissue response to form the underlying cavity. Loose hair can be rolled together into a bundle or 'drill' by buttock movements, which might puncture the skin or enter the already formed sinus. Lateral traction on the buttocks in the sitting posture may produce a suction effect aiding the entry of loose hair. Furthermore, the arrangement of the scales on a hair will tend to propel it in the direction of its root, explaining how the tip of a hair can project from a pilonidal sinus although it has not, in fact, grown inside the sinus and how it can track in the subcutaneous tissues.

The origin of the primary pits may, however, not be that of direct hair puncture and in almost half the cases hair cannot be demonstrated in the underlying cavities. It has been suggested that the sinuses originate in pilosebaceous follicles activated after puberty, susceptible to infection and enlarged by the lateral tractions of the buttocks.

Most sinuses will progress through a long history of suppuration and discharge and following incision or natural discharge of an abscess there may be intervals of apparent healing. Smaller sinuses can undergo spontaneous cure if the contents of this cavity are completely discharged, but this is less likely if extensive tracking has occurred.

DIAGNOSIS

A pilonidal sinus has one or more external openings in the midline about 6 cm posterior to the anus and hairs may be seen projecting from them. It is distinguished from an anal fistula by the absence of any internal opening in the anal canal or any palpable indurated track extending towards the anus. A congenital skin dimple may be associated with a spina bifida but lies over the sacral hiatus and has shelving margins unlike the usual pits of a pilonidal sinus; it can be the site of suppuration but does not have an extensive underlying subcutaneous granulomatous cavity.

Simple boils and epidermoid cysts have typical appearances and are situated on the buttocks and around the anus rather than the natal cleft. They have no indurated track felt connecting with the midline.

Hidradenitis suppurativa produces extensive subcutaneous tracking but involves not only the natal cleft and adjacent buttocks but the perineum and groins and the axillae, back of the neck and mammary regions are involved in 90% of cases. The sinuses are multiple but the immediate peri-anal skin is usually clear.

Following a blow on the buttock traumatic fat necrosis may occur and cause a sinus. The openings of high sinuses due to pelvic inflammatory disease lie in the ischiorectal fossae. Sacro-coccygeal cysts lie between the rectum and the sacrum; infection with abcess formation can form a sinus close to the posterior border of the anus.

The rare complication of squamous carcinoma has been described in longstanding cases of pilonidal sinus so that the routine histological examination of chronic lesions is advisable.

Pilonidal disease in other sites

Granulomatous cavities and tracks containing hair have been reported in sites other than the natal cleft. Pits containing hair are sometimes seen in the corrugated skin around the anus and hair-containing tracks may occur in the perineum and scrotum. There are reports of similar conditions in the umbilicus, axilla, pubis, prepuce, front of chest and in the midthigh amputation stump. The accumulation of sharp ended hairs in the interdigital clefts of barbers' hands has been mentioned and hair splinters

357

can also penetrate the skin of the feet. The stiff udder hairs of cows can penetrate the hands of milkers and animal hair splinters are described in wool shearers. The cause of sinuses in these abnormal sites is either the existence of a pre-existing hole or cavity into which debris and hair can accumulate, or the special circumstances of cut or especially stiff hairs.

TREATMENT

Simple measures

It is apparent that spontaneous cure after discharge of the contents of some of the smaller sinuses can occur. Thus in the absence of acute suppuration, large cavities and tracking the simple measures of removal of the hairs from the sinus followed by meticulous local hygiene and shaving of the surrounding skin gives results comparable to or better than surgery. Presumably these measures prevent recrudescence and allow natural healing of the sinus. Epilatory creams and abrasives keep the hair short until the scar is sound; irradiation for effective epilation is unjustifiable.

Operative methods

Wide excision with closure of the defect

The whole of the sinus cavity and its track are excised through healthy fat down to the glistening fascia overlying the sacrum. If the defect is not too large a primary suture can be performed, employing deep sutures to include the sacral fascia and tied in such a way as to hold the dressing in place. Larger defects may be closed by using relieving incisions, rotation flaps from the buttocks, Z-plasty or immediate skin grafting.

Wide excision with healing by granulation

Large wounds following wide excision will heal satisfactorily by granulation. Although convalescence may be prolonged the results are comparable with those of other major procedures. A silicone foam sponge has been advocated to facilitate healing but there is doubt as to whether this influences the long-term results.

Incision and laying open

These procedures involve incision with local excision of the midline pits, extending into the central cavity and laying open lateral tracks. All the hair and foreign material is removed and early bridging of the skin edges is prevented during frequent follow-up examinations. Various modifications have been advocated to prevent early closure of the skin over the cavity and to avoid long wounds extending into the lateral tracks.

Marsupialization involves suturing down the skin margins to the edge of the granulomatous cavity.

Alternatively, the midline pits may be locally excised to lay open the main cavity which is thoroughly cleaned, the lateral tracks being brushed or curetted and secondary openings excised by a circular incision to provide full drainage (Millar, 1977).

Small quiescent sinuses have been injected with pure phenol under general anaesthesia with a cure rate of 80% and an inpatient stay of only 36 hours. This method is not suitable for tracking extensive or infected sinuses.

Injection of phenol

Cryosurgical techniques have been applied in the treatment of pilonidal disease but final evaluation of the long-term results is awaited.

Cryosurgery

Treatment of the acute pilonidal abscess by simple incision over the pointing abscess results in a very high recurrence rate and for this reason has been largely regarded as a temporary expedient before definitive surgery. If, however, the sinus pits are excised and the whole cavity laid open and thoroughly cleaned, a high percentage of cures result. Marsupialisation and unroofing of the central cavity by a cruciate incision have also been successfully used.

Pilonidal abscess

Treatment of recurrent sinuses is either by total re-excision and closure by suture or skin-flaps or by laying open the sinus which is as effective and simpler.

There is a wide choice of treatment for pilonidal disease but all methods have in common an obligatory careful period of follow-up until there is firm healing. For the small, simple and uncomplicated sinus, simple measures should be tried in the first instance before resorting to surgery. It seems that extensive surgical procedures give no better results than simple ones. Excision and primary suture, if reserved for small, uncomplicated sinuses, gives quick results with periods of hospitalisation of about a fortnight. Extensive, infected and recurrent sinuses should be treated by an open method but wide total excision gives no better results than laying open and *débridement*. The methods of marsupialisation and laying open are suitable for outpatient use for the smaller sinuses and although complete healing may take a month the patient loses little time off work.

Results of treatment

Most 'recurrences' occur within six months and are largely avoidable by the correct choice of method. They denote failure of the treatment rather than true recurrence and account for the wide variation in the reports of the results. 'Recurrences' occurring a year or more after surgery may be new sinuses and should be treated as such.

It is significant that simple measures are as effective in the treatment of small sinuses as any of the current surgical procedures.

If primary suture after excision is reserved for small uninfected sinuses a low recurrence rate is to be expected. The attempted suture of large defects, however, and factors which may impede primary healing such as the presence of infection and the use of drains, will result in early recurrence in nearly 40% of cases. The completeness of the excision, as indicated by the injection of dyes, is not significantly associated with reduction in the recurrence rate.

Excisional defects may be closed by Z-plasty or rotation flaps but whilst these procedures give anatomical results superior to primary suture they must be regarded as significantly major procedures with no better cure rates than the simpler treatments.

Firm healing in the natal cleft is essential to prevent early recurrence. Soft scars and intertrigo permit hair to penetrate the skin and a true sinus or a granulomatous ulcer can result.

Meticulous shaving or the use of epilatory creams or abrasives, prevents this until the healing is sound, and the patient should not be discharged from follow-up until this is obtained.

For infected and extensive sinuses the best consistent results are obtained by methods which leave the wound open to granulate. There is no evidence to suggest that total excision of the lesion has any advantage over simple laying open or marsupialisation, provided that all the foreign material is removed from the tracks. These methods still require postoperative follow-up. If the above principles of treatment are followed the early recurrence rate due to delayed healing or failure of primary healing can be in the region of 10%. Late recurrences after a year are less common. There is evidence to suggest that these are new sinuses and are not related to the previous treatment.

REFERENCE AND FURTHER READING

Millar DM. Procedures for pilonidal sinus. In: Todd IP, ed. *Colon, rectum and anus.* (3rd ed. Operative surgery.) London and Boston: Butterworths, 1977: 379–81.

12. Sexually Transmitted Diseases

The failure to control the incidence of sexually transmitted diseases is one of the least satisfactory developments in medicine during the past 25 years. The sexually transmitted diseases are now the commonest notifiable communicable diseases in most industrial countries and in the United States of America the prevalence of gonorrhoea has reached 410 per hundred thousand of the population. In Britain there was a rise from 95.6 per hundred thousand in 1968 to 104.2 in 1976. The World Health Organization has recently suggested that each year more than 250 million people are infected with gonorrhoea and between 40 and 50 million people with syphilis.

Not only have the sexually transmitted diseases become increasingly common in most communities but the older classical venereal diseases such as syphilis, gonorrhoea and chancroid account for only a minority of the infected patients and a new generation of sexually transmitted diseases are being recognised with increasing frequency. These include infections with *Chlamydia trachomatis, Mycoplasma hominis, Trichomonas vaginalis, Candida albicans,* Herpes virus hominis, the wart virus, *Sarcoptes scabiei, Phthirius pubis,* the virus of molluscum contagiosum and more recently infection with the virus of hepatitis B, the cytomegalo virus and probably the virus responsible for Marburg disease. Despite great improvements in diagnostic techniques a significant proportion of patients with sexually transmitted diseases have diseases which cannot be classified and which are therefore called non-specific genital infections.

Because of the broadening of the scope of the specialty the older term 'venereal disease' is slowly being replaced by 'sexually transmitted disease'. There is also a tendency to change the name of the physician who is responsible for dealing with patients with these conditions. The older term 'venereologist' is being replaced by 'genito-urinary physician' and the specialty is referred to as 'genito-urinary medicine'. It

361

must be appreciated that sexually transmitted diseases are not limited to the genito-urinary tract but involve many other parts of the body and quite frequently the two extremes of the alimentary tract, namely the mouth and throat and the anus and rectum.

The great increase in the prevalence in the majority of sexually transmitted diseases is one of the paradoxes of modern medicine. The reasons for this trend are complex and include medical, social and economic factors. Some of the more important factors that may be responsible include the recent liberalisation and change of sexual attitudes and behaviour, the appearance of organisms that are less sensitive or even totally insensitive to antibiotics, the asymptomatic carrier state in many infected patients, the availability and ease of modern travel and greater opportunities for casual sexual encounter, the very high incidence of infection among homosexual men and ignorance among doctors and members of the public.

Sexually transmitted diseases of the anorectal region have frequently been underdiagnosed in the past and indeed many surgeons and physicians do not have the necessary experience in the diagnosis of these diseases to enable them to recognise the presence of such infections in their patients. Recent developments and changes in public attitudes to sexual matters and the great changes in sexual practices which have occurred make it increasingly important that all doctors should be aware of the common manifestations of the sexually transmitted diseases particularly in the anorectal area.

SYPHILIS

In the modern world syphilis is most frequently contracted by homosexual activity among men. In the majority of large cities, including London, as many as 70% of patients diagnosed as having infectious syphilis are homosexual men. The majority of patients presenting with lesions in the anorectal area have either primary or secondary syphilis and it is easy to miss the diagnosis of the disease as the physical signs may be minimal.

Primary syphilis

The incubation period of primary syphilis is usually from 4–6 weeks but may be from 9–90 days. A primary chancre usually develops 4–6 weeks after infection and may be situated either at the anal margin or in the anal canal. Anorectal primary chancres may be symptomless but in some cases there will be discomfort, pain on defaecation, soreness, irritation and discharge.

On physical examination there is usually ulceration or erosion of the anal canal. Because the primary lesion in the anorectum may appear trivial the diagnosis is often missed. In the majority of instances the inguinal lymph nodes will be painlessly enlarged and on palpation they will be found to be rubbery, discrete, indolent and non-tender.

The earliest and most satisfactory way of diagnosing primary syphilis is to demonstrate *Treponema pallidum* in serum from the chancre by dark ground examination. The investigation requires experience and skill in taking the specimens and identifying the organism. Serological tests for syphilis do not become positive until the primary chancre has been present for many days or a week or two. Several conditions have to be distinguished from anorectal primary syphilis and include anal fissures, haemorrhoids, herpes simplex, ulcerative colitis, Crohn's disease, basal or squamous cell carcinoma and the erosions occurring in secondary syphilis. If there is any doubt about the diagnosis repeated dark ground examination of serum from the anorectal lesions and weekly serological tests for syphilis are advised.

In the secondary stage the treponemes are widely diffused throughout the body and produce a multitude of symptoms and a wide variety of physical signs. The characteristic lesions in the peri-anal area are condylomata lata which are usually found in association with a maculo-papular skin rash of the trunk, limbs, palms and soles, generalised lymphadenopathy and erosions of the palate and pharynx. Condylomata lata consist of multiple, flat, oval or rounded papules which may become hypertrophic and dusky pink or greyish in colour. They are highly infectious and are teeming with treponemes. In addition there may be erosions of the mucous membrane of the anal canal and rectum forming circular patches of whitish-grey colour, surrounded by a reddish areola.

Secondary syphilis

In the secondary stage the diagnosis is confirmed by demonstrating *Treponema pallidum* under the dark ground microscope in material obtained from lesions. The serological tests for syphilis will be positive in almost all cases and usually the titre will be high. It is advisable to suspect the diagnosis of syphilis in all cases with unexplained ulceration or erosion around the anal canal. The suspicion should be enhanced by the discovery of enlargement of the lymphatic nodes. The patients will usually be unmarried men who will confide in the doctor that they are homosexual or bisexual.

Tertiary lesions of the anorectum usually take the form of gummata of the rectum and of the peri-anal tissues and are extremely rare at the present time.

Tertiary syphilis

363

Treatment

The diagnosis should be confirmed and the patients informed of the nature of the disease and the full implications of the infection. They should be told that they are infectious to sexual partners and should not have sexual contact until tests have indicated that they are free from infection. The necessity of tracing all the sexual contacts should be stressed and the patients' co-operation requested. All sexual contacts for at least the past 3 months should be examined and treated when the patient has primary syphilis and all the contacts for the past year should be seen in cases of secondary syphilis.

Penicillin is the treatment of choice and the usual regime is to give procaine penicillin 600 000 units daily intramuscularly for 10 days for both primary and secondary syphilis. For those who are sensitive to penicillin, erythromycin 500 mg orally every 6 hours for 15 days is also effective, as is tetracycline at the same dosage. Long-acting penicillins such as benzathine penicillin should not be used at the present time as it is probable they do not get into the cerebro-spinal fluid in adequate concentrations.

The possibility of a Herxheimer reaction should be explained to the patient and arrangements should be made for careful follow-up and repeated examinations. Quantitative serological tests should be carried out at each outpatient visit and for a total period of two years. If the patient is seronegative and there are no signs at the end of that period he can be discharged as cured and fully reassured that the disease has been eliminated.

GONORRHOEA

Gonorrhoea is one of the commonest acute infections in the world today and attacks susceptible mucous membrane surfaces such as the urethra, the cervix, the rectum and the oropharnyx. The diagnosis is made by demonstrating the causative organism, *Neisseria gonorrhoeae*, on Gram stained specimens of discharge from the various mucous membrane surfaces. The gonococcus appears as a pink, kidney-shaped organism occurring in clumps and in pairs in the intracellular position. Culture techniques are essential for complete identification and for sensitivity studies to antibiotics. Owing to the emergence of strains of β-lactamase producing organisms which are totally resistant to penicillin, sensitivity tests have become increasingly important.

In men infection of the rectum usually occurs from anorectal intercourse. In women, on the other hand, the condition is frequently spread to the rectum from the genital tract but may also result from anorectal sex. The lower part of the anal canal is not involved because of its stratified squamous epithelial lining, but the upper part of the anal canal, the lower end of the rectum and the ducts and crypts of Morgagni may be infected. Upward extension of infection as far as the sigmoid colon is rare. The gonococcus provokes an inflammatory reaction which may be acute but is more commonly subacute and results in the production of varying quantities of mucopus.

In the vast majority of men and women infection of the anorectum is symptomless and is diagnosed when bacteriological tests are taken during proctoscopic examination. This most commonly occurs when a patient is seen as a passive partner of a homosexual man known to have gonococcal urethritis. It can also be the only manifestation of gonorrhoea of a woman who is the wife or regular sexual partner of a man with urethral gonorrhoea. Symptoms, if they occur, are usually mild and include soreness of the anus, burning, discomfort and pain on defaecation. There is sometimes a feeling of fullness in the anorectum and staining of the underwear by discharge.

Frequently there may be no signs of gonococcal proctitis. In a few cases there may be peri-anal excoriation together with a purulent discharge. Proctoscopy reveals a rectal mucosa that may be injected, oedematous and friable. The surface may be covered with thick, creamy tenacious pus or there may only be a few strands of mucopus adherent to the rectal wall. Ulceration is very uncommon.

Complications of gonococcal proctitis are relatively uncommon and they may take the form of septicaemia; this usually presents as a febrile illness with malaise, fleeting joint pains and a scanty pustular and petechial skin rash usually found at the distal end of the limbs. The rectal infection is often quite symptomless but microbiological tests will reveal the presence of gonococci in the rectal secretions. The condition is usually subacute but it may be acute and cause serious complications such as pericarditis, endocarditis, meningitis and perihepatitis which can threaten the patient's life. Gonococcal arthritis may also be a complication of gonococcal proctitis.

Diagnosis

The diagnosis of gonococcal proctitis is a microbiological procedure. Slides of specimens from the rectal mucosa are stained with Gram's stain and must be examined for Gram negative intracellular diplococci. Confirmation by growing the organism on cultures is extremely important. A selective medium, such as the modified Thayer-Martin medium, should be inoculated with material from the rectal wall and sent immediately to the laboratory to be put in the incubator in the presence of carbon dioxide. If such facilities are not available Stuart's transport medium is also satisfactory. There is unfortunately no suitable serological test for the diagnosis of gonorrhoea.

365

Treatment

Despite the prevalence of partially insensitive strains of gonococci and the recent appearance of β-lactamase producing strains which are totally resistant, penicillin remains the antibiotic of choice in the majority of instances. In uncomplicated patients a single intramuscular injection of 4.8 million units of aqueous procaine penicillin will produce a high cure rate. Some physicians prefer to obtain a higher serum level by giving 1 g of probenecid orally to block the renal excretion of penicillin and 10–15 min later a single injection of 5 million units of benzyl penicillin G dissolved in 5 ml of a half per cent solution of lignocaine. This treatment gives a high cure rate but treatment failures are not infrequent and tests of cure are essential. Patients sensitive to penicillin may be treated with either 2 gm of kanamycin intramuscularly or with cotrimoxazole orally at a dose of 3 tablets twice daily for 3–5 days. These preparations are useful as they are not treponemacidal and therefore do not mask the manifestations of syphilis. Many other antibiotics are available for the treatment of gonorrhoea but they have no special advantages and pencillin, cotrimoxazole and kanamycin will usually provide adequate treatment for the majority of patients with the disease.

Tests of cure should be performed at regular intervals and include proctoscopy. As syphilis is common in homosexual men, serological tests for syphilis should be carried out 3 months after the treatment has been completed and all the sexual contacts should be traced, examined and treated if they are found to be infected.

HERPES

Herpes simplex is a commonly recognised condition of the genitalia and occurs in the anorectal area, especially in passive homosexual men. It is caused by herpes virus hominis, type 2, and is usually spread by sexual activity. Lesions develop 5–25 days after intercourse and the condition has a strong tendency to relapse. The symptoms may consist of itching and soreness in or around the anus some hours before the development of severe anal and rectal pain. The pain is usually severe, leading to complete and absolute constipation and a great reluctance on the part of the patient to permit any form of examination. There may be generalised malaise and difficulty in walking because of pain. There is often retention of urine with painful distention of the bladder and some patients may notice difficulty in emptying the bladder with a poor urinary stream.

Examination of the peri-anal area reveals some red erythematous areas with either small groups of vesicles or multiple superficial ulceration with small ulcers surrounded by a red areola. If the ulcers become secondarily infected they may coalesce to form larger ulcers. The inguinal lymph nodes may be slightly enlarged and tender.

The ulcers start to heal after a few days and frequently become crusted. They disappear in 10–14 days leaving no residual scarring. It is now known that herpes virus invades the nerve sheath and the posterior root ganglion of the area concerned. When relapses occur they are thought to be due to the migration of the herpes virus from the posterior root ganglion down the nerve sheath to the skin where the virus provokes a new attack of the condition. The diagnosis may be confirmed by growing the virus on tissue culture. A sample of material from the lesions is taken on a cotton wool swab and placed in a virus transport medium. The virologist will usually be able to grow the virus and demonstrate a typical characteristic cytopathic effect within 24–48 hours. Antibodies appear in the blood but are not helpful in diagnosis of the acute case.

Treatment

Unfortunately there is no effective treatment or cure for herpes. The majority of substances that have been used to try to shorten attacks and prevent recurrence prove disappointing. Examples of these are idoxuridine, cytosine arebonoside, sulphonamides and steroids. The best procedure is for the lesions to be kept clean with repeated applications of normal saline and by frequent warm baths. Suitable analgesics should be given to relieve the pain which may be very severe. If secondary infection occurs it should be treated with a sulphonamide such as cotrimoxazole which will usually control it.

It should be explained to the patient that he or she is infectious sexually while there are open, active lesions of herpes. As herpes quite frequently occurs together with syphilis in the same patient, care should be taken to exclude the possibility of syphilis by carrying out serological tests for syphilis and repeating them in 3 months time.

WARTS

Warts are also known as condylomata acuminata and are caused by a papilloma virus. In the anorectal area they are usually sexually transmitted and are frequently found in homosexual men. The incubation period is considered to be from 1–6 months or longer. Warts are frequently found in association with gonococcal proctitis. They appear as minute pink swellings and grow rapidly into grouped, pedunculated, filiform lesions. They may completely surround the anus and form large cauliflower swellings. They may extend up the anal canal as far as the anorectal line and are found occasionally on the rectal mucosa. They are usually not difficult to diagnose from their appearance but they must be distinguished from condylomata lata of secondary syphilis, from skin tags and in some cases, from haemorrhoids. In occasional instances it will be necessary to carry out biopsy to exclude carcinoma.

Treatment

Any other associated sexually transmitted disease should be dealt with but if the warts are not extensive they are best treated with local applications of a solution of 25% podophyllin in spirit which is applied carefully twice or three times a week until the warts have disappeared. The patient should be instructed to wash the painted area 6–8 hours after the application of podophyllin to prevent damage to the surrounding skin and burns. If the warts are very extensive then they should be removed surgically by the scissor excision technique (Thomson and Grace, 1978). The use of electrocautery or diathermy usually leaves a series of burnt erosions with painful edges which heal slowly. The scissor excision technique under general anaesthesia is more satisfactory and healing occurs rapidly and almost painlessly.

All the sexual contacts should be examined and treated if necessary. There is a strong tendency for warts to recur and therefore follow-up should be thorough and newly-formed lesions should be treated immediately.

MOLLUSCUM CONTAGIOSUM

Molluscum contagiosum is a virus infection spread by close body contact and usually by sexual contact. The virus is one of the largest of the pox group and has an incubation period of 3–6 weeks. Typical lesions of Molluscum contagiosum are small, white or pink in colour, dome-shaped, waxy in appearance and with a characteristic central depression. They are filled with a soft plug of semi-solid white material which can be expressed by squeezing them. The lesions are usually symptomless but they may become secondarily infected. They occur most frequently on the abdomen, thighs, perineum and buttocks of both sexes, the penis and scrotum in men, the vulva in women and the peri-anal and anal area in homosexual men.

Molluscum contagiosum should be regarded as a marker that the patient may have another form of sexually transmitted disease.

Treatment

The aim of treatment is to destroy each individual lesion and this is best done by applying neat phenol on the tip of a sharpened orange stick to the centre of each individual lesion. The papule will become white in colour and will heal in about

2–3 days. New lesions frequently occur after apparently successful treatment and these should be dealt with quickly. All the sexual contacts should be examined.

NON-SPECIFIC GENITAL INFECTION

Proctitis

Non-specific genital infection is the commonest form of sexually transmitted disease, producing urethritis in men and cervicitis, vaginitis and urethritis in women and proctitis in both sexes. Recently evidence has accumulated to suggest that the agent *Chlamydia trachomatis* may be responsible for about half the cases of non-specific infection.

Chlamydial proctitis will be found most frequently in homosexual men following anorectal intercourse. It may also occur in women either as a result of anorectal sex or from the penis coming into contact with the peri-anal tissues during sexual intercourse. Symptoms are of soreness, irritation and a mild anal discharge which may stain the underwear. On proctoscopy there may be slight inflammation of the wall of the rectum and some adherent mucopus. Gram stained slides will show an excess of polymorphonuclear leucocytes and on Giemsa staining inclusion bodies will be found. *Chlamydia trachomatis* can be grown from the secretions from the rectum and in the majority of instances the disease will be found in passive homosexual men whose active partners have non-specific urethritis or chlamydial urethritis. Occasionally there are ocular or skeletal complications of the disease and these include conjunctivitis, punctate keratitis, uveitis, Reiter's disease and a form of sacro-iliitis resembling ankylosing spondylitis.

Treatment

The best treatment for chlamydial and non-specific proctitis is to give tetracycline or oxytetracycline at a dose of 250 mg 6 hourly for 7–15 days depending upon the severity of the condition. Erythromycin may also be used at a similar dosage and tests of cure should be carried out as relapses are frequent. All the sexual partners should be examined.

LYMPHOGRANULOMA VENEREUM

Lymphogranuloma venereum is uncommon in industrial countries and is caused by a member of the chlamydial group of agents. There is usually an incubation period of 7–28 days before a small vesicular lesion appears at the site of inoculation. This disappears rapidly within 24–48 hours but the inguinal lymphatic nodes then become enlarged and tend to mat together forming tender, large, fluctuant masses. The overlying

369

skin is frequently red. There may be constitutional symptoms including malaise, fever, headaches, joint pains and anorexia. If the initial lesion is in the area of the cervix or upper vagina the perirectal and pelvic lymph nodes become enlarged and may produce pelvic pain. The rectal wall may become ulcerated producing a type of proctitis with a purulent, blood-stained rectal discharge. Similar rectal changes may occur in passive homosexual men.

Chronic inflammation leads to damage to the lymphatic channels resulting in oedema, ulceration and the formation of fistulae. Rectal strictures may develop in women but are usually situated distally within the reach of the examining finger and can be relatively easily dilated.

The diagnosis of lymphogranuloma venereum can be confirmed by complement fixation tests. In patients with recent lesions, a rising titre of antibody should be regarded as diagnostic and in more chronic cases a titre of more than 1 in 32 is usually regarded as significant. An intradermal test called the Frei test used to be performed but the antigen is difficult or impossible to obtain.

Treatment usually consists of one of the tetracycline antibiotics at a dose of 500 mg 6 hourly for 10–14 days. Fluctuant bubos should be aspirated and not incised and rectal strictures can usually be dilated, but abscesses, fistulae and elephantiasis require careful surgical treatment. All the sex partners should be examined and followed up to exclude infection.

CHANCROID AND GRANULOMA INGUINALE

Both of these diseases are very rare in developed industrial countries. Chancroid, caused by *Haemophilus ducreyi*, produces painful multiple ulcers associated with painful lymphadenopathy and fluctuant abscesses. Sometimes the ulcers of chancroid are found in the anorectal area. The condition is easily confused with herpes and the diagnosis is based on clinical observation confirmed by culture of the organism on solid culture medium containing defibrinated rabbits' blood or alternatively a liquid medium containing the patient's own serum. The best treatment is with the sulphonamides at full doses or with the tetracyclines for 10–14 days.

Granuloma inguinale is usually only seen in South-east Asia but occurs sporadically elsewhere. It is a chronic granulomatous condition caused by the Gram negative rod-shaped bacillus, *Donovania granulomatis (Calymmatobacterium granulomatis)*. It produces beefy red, shiny, granulomatous masses on the genitalia and around the anus which extend slowly resulting in scarring of the tissues and occasionally in anal stenosis. The diagnosis is confirmed by biopsy and the treatment is with either streptomycin or tetracycline in high doses. The incubation period is long and contact tracing should go back over several months.

OTHER SEXUALLY TRANSMITTED DISEASES

Lesions in the anorectal region may result from other sexually transmitted diseases such as scabies, pediculosis pubis, candidiasis and other fungal infections. Homosexual men may transmit enteric diseases to each other by oro-anal sexual contact. Minor epidemics of amoebiasis, giardiasis or shigeliosis have occurred in several non-tropical areas of the world and those treating diseases of the colon, rectum and anus should be aware of this method of transmission and of the importance of tracing sexual contacts and treating them if they are infected. It is now well established that the virus causing hepatitis B is commonly sexually transmitted, particularly by homosexual contact, and a possible route of spread of the virus is via the anorectum. Other conditions that are not sexually transmitted may appear around the anus following sexual intercourse and may be thought by the patient to have been acquired sexually and lead to considerable anxiety.

The sexually transmitted diseases are now extremely common in every section of society in every country in the world. Proctologists will meet them in their practices and it is particularly important that they bear them in mind in diagnosis if they are not to be missed and further spread of infection encouraged. Anorectal lesions are particularly common amongst homosexual men but their manifestations may be subtle and difficult to detect unless the observer is knowledgeable and experienced in this growing field of medicine.

REFERENCES AND FURTHER READING

Catterall RD. *A short textbook of venereology*. London: English Universities Press, 1974.

King A and Nicol C. *Venereal diseases*. London: Baillière Tindall and Cassell, 1969.

Morton RS. *Gonorrhoea*. London: W.B. Saunders, 1977.

Nahmias AJ, Dowdle WR, Naib ZM, Josey WE, Malone D and Domescik G. Genital infection with type 2 herpes virus hominis – a commonly occurring venereal disease. *British Journal of Venereal Diseases* 1969; **45:** 294–9.

Thomson JPS and Grace R. Peri-anal and anal condylomata acuminata – a new operative technique. *Journal of the Royal Society of Medicine* 1978; **71:** 180–5.

Index

carcinoma (*cont.*)
   surgery 269–81
   treatment 269–86
   undifferentiated 254
castor oil 62, 128
cathartic colon 92
cauda equina syndrome 122
Celevac *see* methyl cellulose
Chagas' disease *see* trypanosomiasis, South
   American
chancroid 370–1
chemotherapy
   antibacterial 129–32
   cytotoxic 284–6
cholestyramine 59
cholinergic agents 53
   antagonists 62–3
chlamydial proctitis 370
codeine
   diarrhoea 57
   irritable bowel 73
colectomy, subtotal 140, 169
colitis
   acute 223–5
   aetiology 208–10
   amoebic 29
   chronic 225–6
   classification 185–6
   Crohn's 202–3, 227–30
   diagnosis 16, 210–14
   drug therapy 216–18
   epidemiology 204–8
   fulmination 203–4
   granulomatous, *see* Crohn's disease
   infective 187–99
   ischaemic 28, 71, 297–301
   mucous *see* irritable bowel syndrome
   pseudomembranous 29, 186
   surgery 218–20
   ulcerative *see* ulcerative colitis
Colofac *see* mebeverine
colon
   absorptive function 42–3
   anatomy 134–5
   bacteriology 44–5
   benign tumours 236–46
   blood supply 136–7
   carcinoma 231–5, 246–54, 269–72
   cathartic 92
   drug effects 53–4
   electrical activity 49–50
   fluid handling 42–4

   function 41
   gangrene 293–6
   haustration 47–8
   hypertrophic 99
   inflammation *see* inflammatory bowel disease
   injuries 175–6
   intraluminal pressure 48
   ischaemia 290–3
   lymphatic drainage 137–8
   malignant tumours 246–55
   mass movements 48
   motility 47–52, 64–5
   mucosa 41–2
   nerve supply 52–3, 138
   obstruction 161–5
   paper-thin 98
   perforation 165–9
   pressure waves 48–9
   resection 84–5
   segmentation 48–9
   spastic *see* irritable bowel syndrome
   transit 45–6
   polyps *see* polyps
colonic ileus 161
colonoscopic polypectomy 37, 264–5
colonoscopy 31–8
   complications 37–8
   limited *see* fibre-sigmoidoscopy
   medication 33
   preparation for 32–3
   technique 34–6
colostomy
   barium enema 19–20
   defunctioning 127
   double-barrelled 147
   divided 147
   loop 146–7
   rectal excision with 220
   temporary 277–8
   terminal 146
   transverse 163
colovesical fistula 169–70
computerised tomography 30
condylomata acuminata *see* warts
connective tissue defects 99
constipation 59–60, 87–93
   classification 88–9
   chronic paediatric 311–13
   colonic motility in 49
   diagnosis 88
   drug-induced 89
   drug treatment 60–2

paediatric assessment 302–6
  disorders 306–17
Parks' colo-anal anastomosis 142
Paul-Mickulicz operation 168
pelvic floor
  anatomy 102–4
  muscle function 103
  muscle ring repair 124–5
  nerve supply 104, 138
  neurological disorders 122–4
  postanal repair 118–20, 123–4
peppermint oil 63
peptides, colon regulation 55
peranal, anastomosis 274–5
  local excision of carcinoma 278
  polypectomy 264–6
perianal, benign tumours 255–6
  dermatological problems 353–4
  examination 4–5
  infections 351–2
  intertrigo 352
  irritation 2, 350
  malignant tumours 256–7, 278–9
  warts 367–8
perineum, Crohn's lesions 330
  descending 108–11
  paroxysmal pain 126
  postanal repair 118–19, 123–4
  wound management 150–1
peritonitis
  anastomotic breakdown 172
  colonic perforation 167
  diverticular disease 83–5
pethidine 33, 82
Peutz–Jeghers polyps 237–9, 263
phenolphthalein 60
phthalylsulphathiazole 192
physiology
  anorectal 39–40, 104–8
  colon 41–55
pneumatosis coli 71
  diagnosis 16
pilonidal abscess 359
  sinus 355–60
polypectomy, colonoscopic 37, 264–5
  surgical techniques 265–6
polyposis, familial adenomatous 266–8
  inflammatory 25–6
polyps 6, 21–4
  adenomatous 240–6
  diagnosis 258–60
  familial adenomatous polyposis 266–8

hamartomatous 237–40
heterotopic 237
inflammatory 236–7
metaplastic 237, 263
non-adenomatous 263–4
pathology 235–46
removal 260–1, 264–6
postanal repair
  in incontinence 123–4
  in rectal prolapse 118–19
Potassium, colonic absorption 42–3
Probanthine see propantheline
proctalgia fugax 126
proctitis see inflammatory bowel disease
  chlamydial 369
  gonococcal 365
  non-specific 369
  radiation 199–200
  traumatic 183
proctocolectomy with ileostomy 219–20
proctoscopy 6–7
prolapse
  anal 2, 336
  mucosal 114
  rectal 113–120
propantheline, irritable bowel effects 73
  shigellosis treatment 191–2
  spasmolytic effect 63
prostaglandins
  colonic effects 54
  synthesis inhibitors 58–9
Prostigmine, colonic effects 53
protozoal infections 12
pruritus ani 2
  causes 351–4
  in haemorrhoids 335
  investigation 350–1
pseudomembranous colitis 29, 186, 198
pseudopolyps see inflammatory polyps
psoriasis, perianal 353–4
psychological factors
  in constipation 88
  in irritable bowel syndrome 66–7, 75
  in paediatric soiling 312

radiation enterocolitis 199–200
radiology 13–31
radiotelemetry capsules 47
radiotherapy 281–3
Rae's mixture 98, 100
rectopexy 118